ART-POUNDING SOUL-BARING EYE-

TH-WATERING TONGUE-TWISTING

THIGH-SLAPPING BREAST-BEATING

URNING NOSTRIL-FLARING HAIR-

NG LIP-SMACKING FINGER-POPPING

FOOT-STOMPING ARM-WRESTLING

THE Body Shop BOOK

THE Body Shop BOOK

SKIN, HAIR AND BODY CARE

Introduction by Anita Roddick

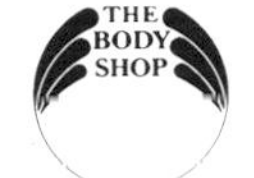

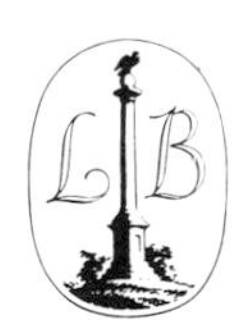

Little, Brown and Company

BOSTON • NEW YORK • TORONTO • LONDON

credits & acknowledgements

A Little, Brown Book

First published in Great Britain in 1994 by Little, Brown and Company
First reprint March 1995

A CIP catalogue record for this book is available from the British Library

ISBN 0-316-91031-7

10 9 8 7 6 5 4 3 2

Written, Designed and Researched by The Body Shop Team
Thanks to: Tim Blanks (Editor); Sharon Leece (Assistant Editor)
Jason Brooks and Peter Sutton (Illustrators)
Marion Hume, Susan Irvine and Juliet Warkentin (Writers)
Mark Johnston and Stephen Milton (Researchers)
Photographers:
A. Abbas - Magnum p.18; Bruno Barbey - Magnum p.168; Carol Beckwith - Robert Estall pp.9, 156;
Claude Coireault p.184; Angela Fisher - Robert Estall p.80;
Melanie Friend - Hutchison Library p.118; Hutchison Library p.134; Peter Jordan - Network p.40;
Thomas L. Kelly p.13; Daniel Lainé - Actuel p.60; National Windpower p.12;
Louie Psihoyos - Matrix/Contact Press Images/Colorific! p.102; Antonio Vizcaino p.13; Michael Zinn p.8.

Printed in Italy

Little, Brown and Company (UK) Ltd
Brettenham House, Lancaster Place, London WC2E 7EN

This book is printed on paper made from 100% chlorine-free bleached pulp
from a source certified as sustainable by the manufacturer.

The Body Shop thrives on the energy,

enthusiasm and commitment of all the people who

work in our shops around the world.

That is why we are dedicating this book to them.

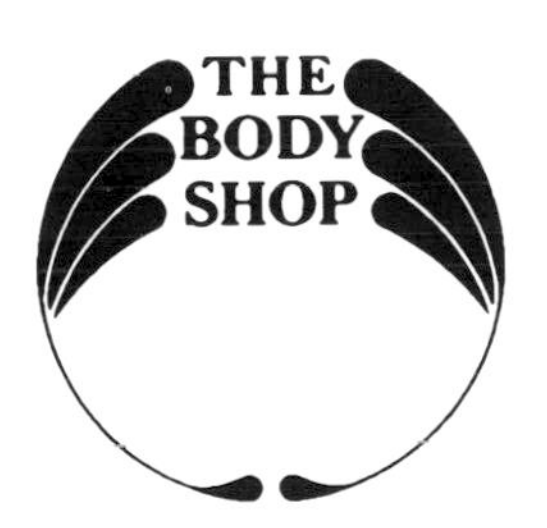

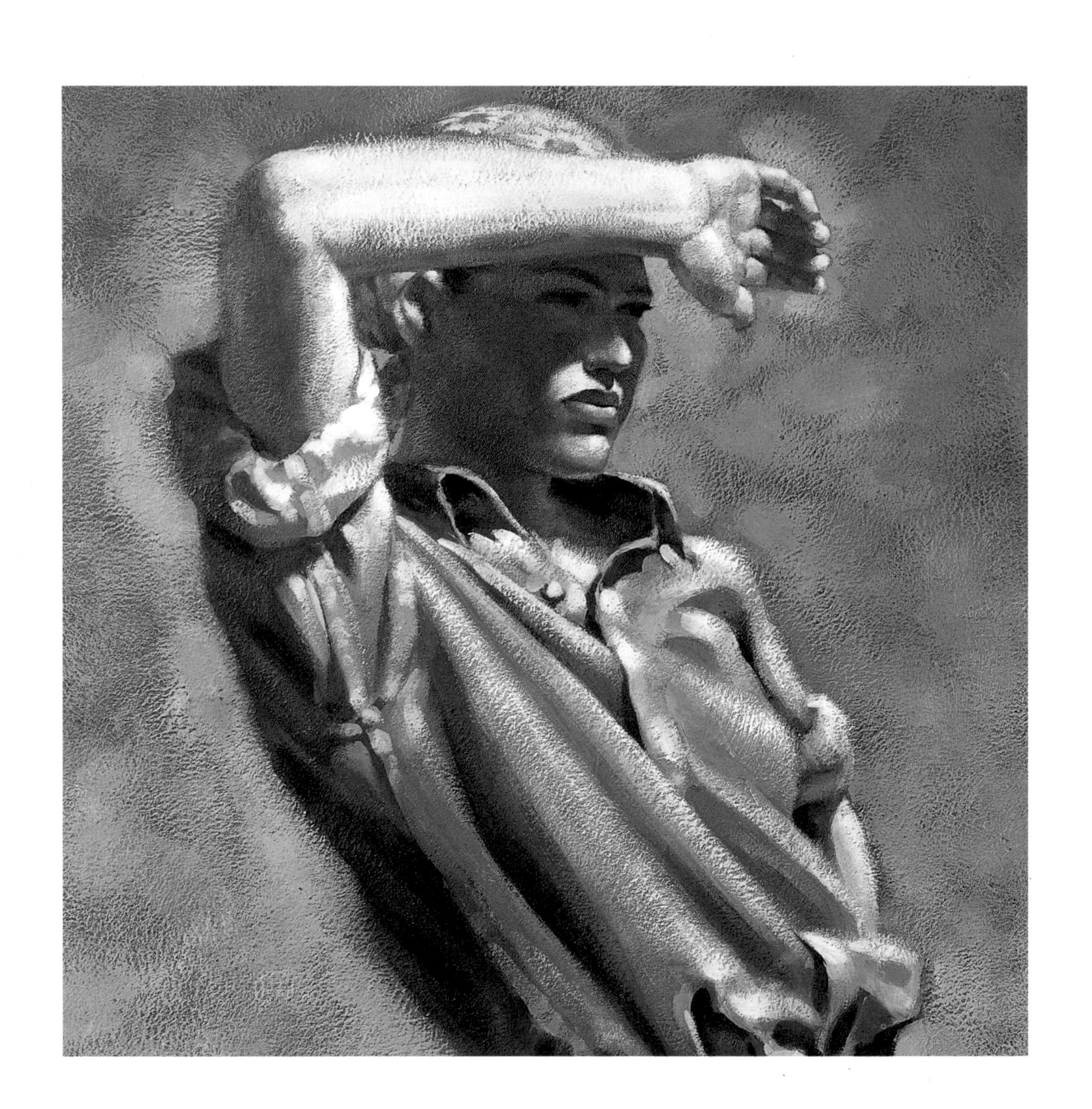

contents

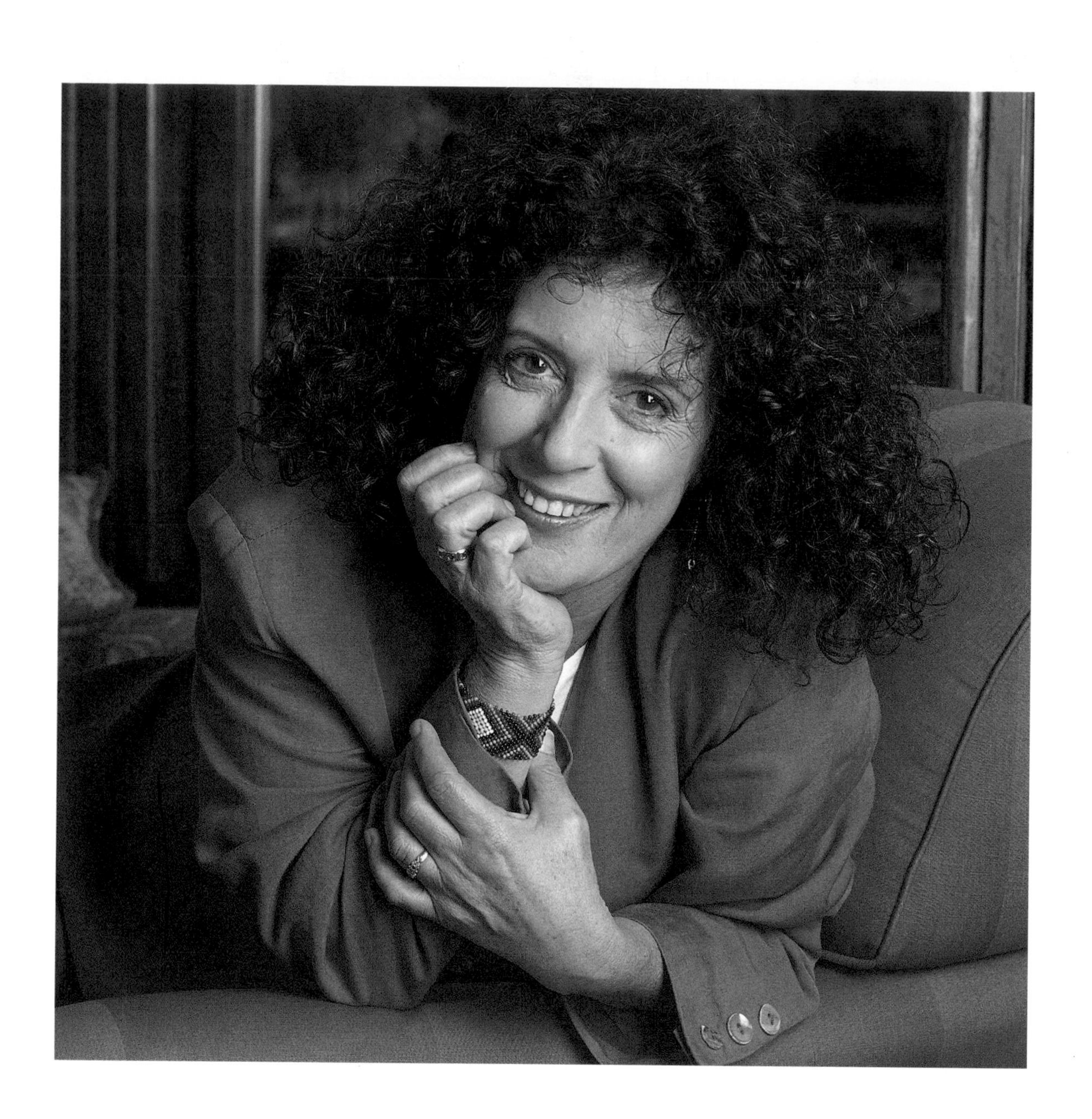

introduction

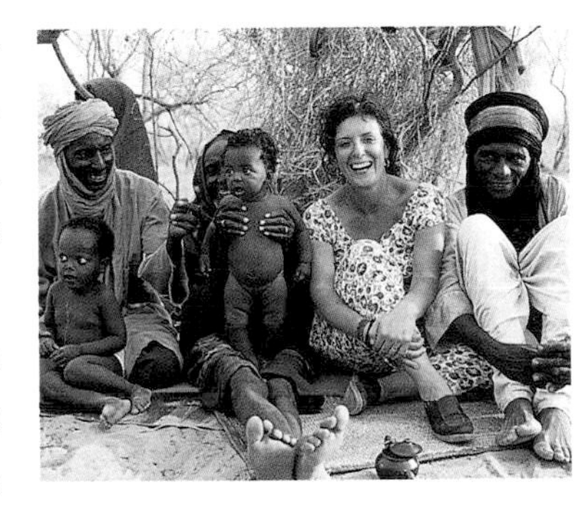

Simply stated, beauty means vitality, imagination, energy - personality traits that have more to do with an individual's character than his or her age or some idealised arrangement of physical features. There is nothing more attractive than love of life or the curiosity of a child.

These are the ideas that have inspired The Body Shop's approach to skin, hair and body care. They've got nothing to do with the "hope in a jar" sold by the cosmetics giants of the past and present, but I believe they've helped The Body Shop become expert at another much more human level. From the beginning, we have developed products to be easily understood, practical and interesting. Before I opened the first shop in 1976, I'd been around the world and seen how women in other cultures cared for themselves. The skin of Tahitian women looked pretty good for all their regular cocoa butter massages. And fresh pineapple seemed to get skin clean and clear in Sri Lanka. Why not use the successful traditions of other peoples to develop new products back home in England? I found something very reassuring about ingredients that had been used safely by human beings for hundreds, even thousands of years. And they certainly made good stories to pass along to customers.

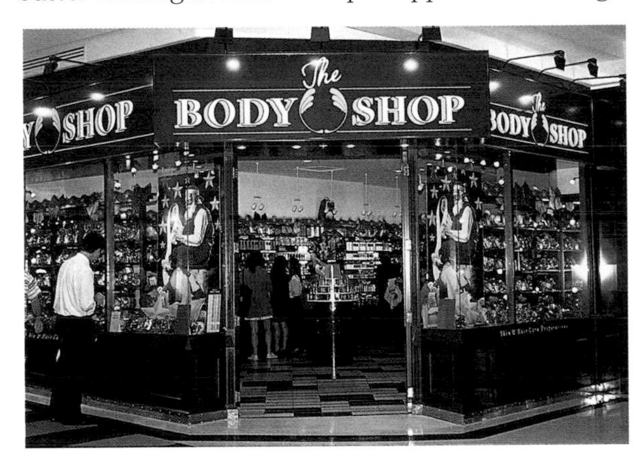

I can't make enough of that last point. From the beginning, The Body Shop was about communication between shops and customer. In the early days, it was a case of "Tell me what you want and we'll try and get it". That eagerness led to some of our greatest successes - Peppermint Foot Lotion, for example, was inspired by the need of marathon runners for something that would soothe hot, sore feet. Now the dialogue is somewhat different of course. There are over a thousand shops around the world so we give out a lot more information on our products and on the issues we care about. And we get a lot more information back. We're always learning. But we've never really had one vehicle that collected in one place all the knowledge we've acquired in the last 18 years. That is why I feel this book is as valuable for the Company as it is for our customers. And for anyone who doesn't know what The Body Shop is all about, here's a brief resumé.

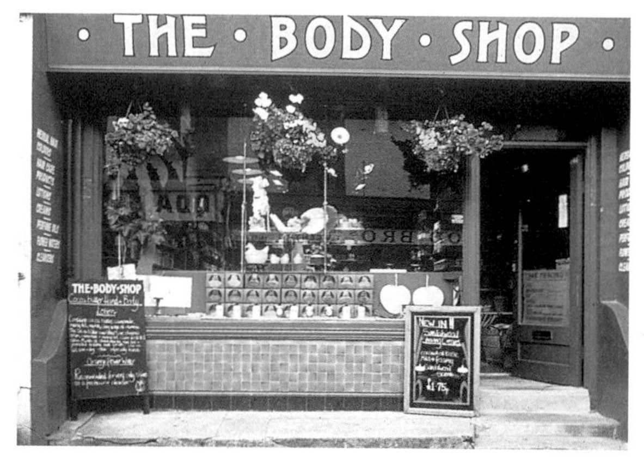

As I said, the first shop opened in 1976 in Brighton on England's south coast. At the time, you could have written everything I knew about the cosmetics industry on the head of a pin, but I trusted my instincts. I knew hype and unrealistic promises weren't doing women any favours. And I knew that fancy packaging not only jacked up the price of a product but also created a hell of a lot of unnecessary waste. I reasoned that there were a lot of people as fed up as I was with having to buy more of this lotion or that shampoo than they needed or could afford. Common sense really. Why shouldn't I sell skin- and hair-care products the way the greengrocer sold his goods, so customers could buy as much or as little as they wanted?

We were environmental activists without even knowing it. Green became the company colour because that's what covered the damp patches on the walls best. We used plastic bottles in five sizes so customers could buy as much or as little as they wanted. And we had to offer a refill service - I couldn't afford to buy more bottles so I needed customers to bring theirs back.

We reused everything we could find, from boxes and decorations to gift baskets and paper. My mother once said I ran my shop the way she ran her household during the Second World War. Then, she wasn't being environmental. She was simply a good housekeeper. I was doing the same. And it worked. Common sense usually does.

Later, when we discovered that common sense had a positive impact on the planet as well as on our purses, we consciously became activists and shared our lesson with others. Our activism was the best kind - it sprang from our own experiences. And we could personalise and humanise an issue that might otherwise be hard for customers to grasp.

Looking back, it all seems so logical. At the time, we just did what felt right. That is how our success came to be a vehicle for our values. The interweaving of profit and principle is, I believe, the major point of difference between The Body Shop and other cosmetics companies. It's the guiding light of every aspect of our business, from the way we find our ingredients to the volunteer work done by our staff in their communities all around the world. I'm not fool enough to believe you can change the world with a new face cream, but you *can* do something with the money that accrues from the sale of that face cream.

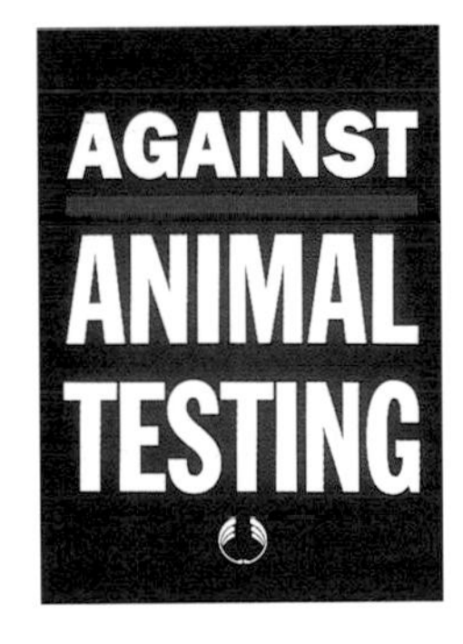

The best place to see our values at work is in what we make - and the way we make it.

We don't test our products or ingredients on animals. Nor do we commission others to do so. But we're realistic enough to acknowledge that no cosmetics company can claim that its manufactured ingredients have never been tested on animals by somebody, at some stage, for someone else. So we believe the best we can do is:

• refuse to test or commission others to do so.

• help fund research into and use alternative testing methods.

• use our purchasing power to persuade ingredient suppliers to stop animal testing.

• educate the public so that they will demand a ban on animal tests.

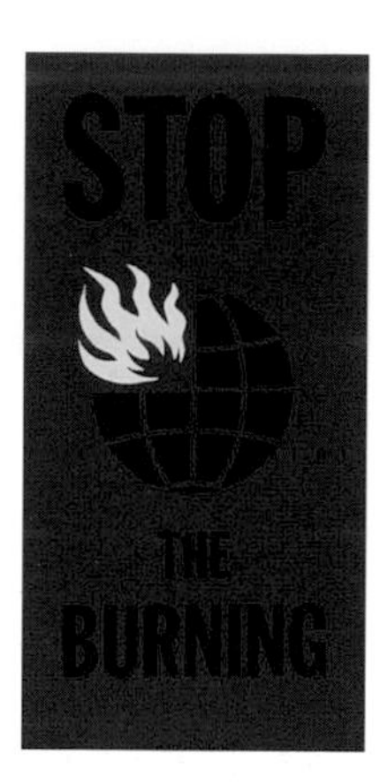

We take care in the manufacture and merchandising of our products to minimise damage to the environment. We don't think it's possible for any business to be truly environmentally friendly, because all business involves some environmental damage. The best we can do is take responsibility for the waste we create, and clean up our own mess.

• We try to avoid excessive packaging, and make the packaging we do use as reusable or recyclable as possible.

• We try to ensure that our raw materials come from renewable sources.

• The refill policy that was so necessary in The Body Shop's earliest days now offers customers the opportunity to bring back their empty, clean containers and have them refilled with the same product at a discount.

• We also have dump bins in shops for customers to drop off any containers they don't want refilled. These are then recycled by us.

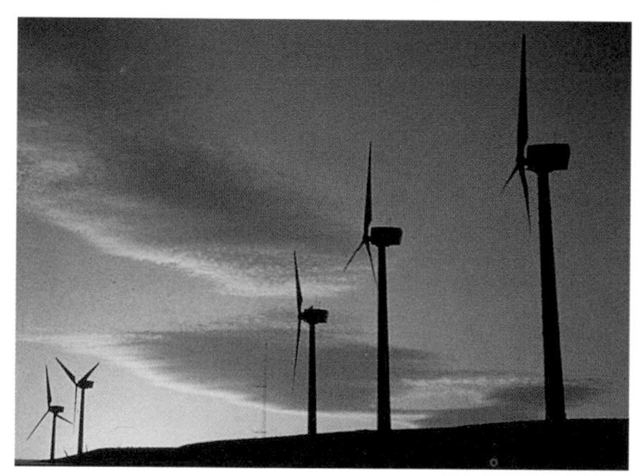

All of this conserves resources, reduces waste and saves everyone money, which is why we're always looking for creative new ways to reduce our impact on the environment. One of the most exciting is the wind farm we're building in Wales. That should match all our UK energy needs.

Increasingly, we are attempting to buy our ingredients from communities in need, mostly in the majority or developing world, who can use our business to help build a future for themselves.

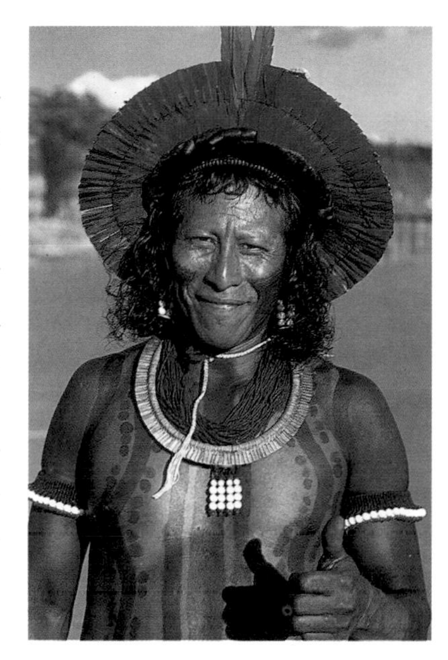

Although direct sourcing from such communities is currently just a small percentage of our trade, it is a direction we strive to work towards. Hand-outs don't always work - it's much better to provide people with the tools and resources they need to help themselves. And because The Body Shop is a huge company with a great need for raw materials, it's easy to see how useful it would be if we could satisfy that need by building trading relationships with groups who would otherwise have no secure livelihood. Take the Kayapo Indians in the Amazonian rain forest. They are selling logging rights to their lands, which poses a threat to their traditional way of life. Now they have another source of income: nuts harvested and processed by them are the basis of our Brazil Nut Conditioner.

As I said before, we like to have stories to tell our customers. Fair trading is the stuff of fair exchange: let consumers know that neither places nor people have been exploited in getting the products to market and you can help them make informed, responsible choices. Because that's what it's all about: responsibility, both individual and corporate. And if you've ever wondered how a company that makes shampoos and skin creams could really help the world, here's how. By breeding a sense of responsibility and communal obligation in their customers, a cosmetics company - or an ice-cream manufacturer or a T-shirt maker, for that matter - can make a difference. In fact, when I think about it, a cosmetics company, which deals with nothing less than the way people see themselves, has a strong obligation to bring about positive change.

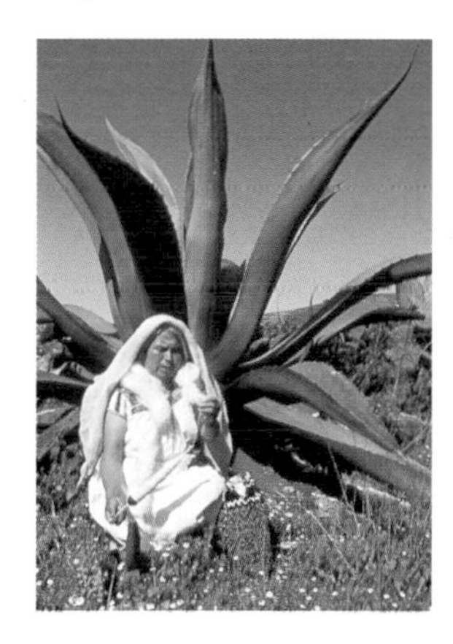

Our goal is simple: to leave the world a better place than we found it. How irresistible that sounds! It undoubtedly helps explain the glamour of the green connection - what business doesn't want to be seen to do good? But it's much more complex than simply bandying around marketing buzzwords like "all-natural" and "environmentally friendly". The Body Shop has been at it long enough to take a sensible long view. Progress towards our goal comes through trial and error. We learn as we go, and pass that learning along.

Here's just one example. When The Body Shop started up, we emphasised the fact that we were making naturally-based skin- and hair-care products, but our evolving relationship with natural ingredients has taught us that "natural" is a loaded word. For one thing, it isn't always best. Look at natural musk, a very popular fragrance ingredient, which is cruelly extracted from the male musk deer. So we developed our own nature-identical synthetic to scent our best-selling White Musk perfume.

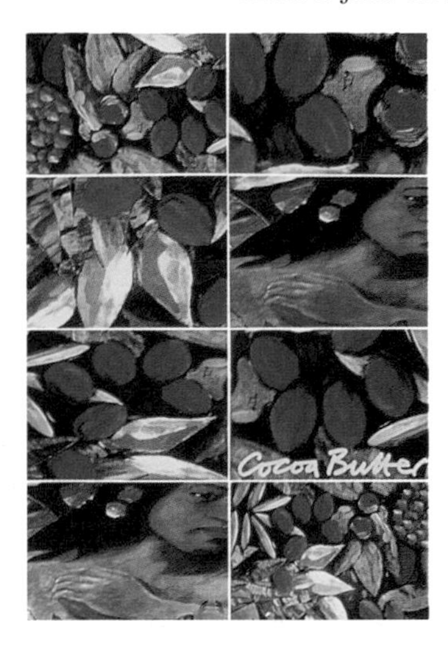

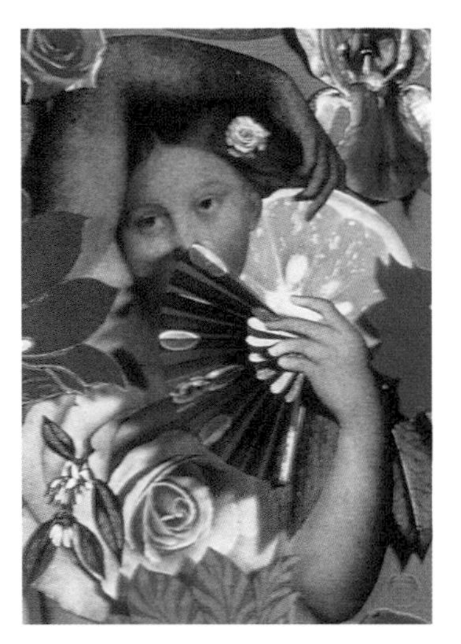

And "more natural" doesn't necessarily mean better. We combine traditional uses of natural ingredients with the benefits of modern science. Our products contain different levels of natural ingredients depending on how much is required to achieve peak product performance. Brazil Nut Conditioner, for example, has 1.5 per cent Brazil nut oil - any more, and it would be too oily, any less, and it wouldn't do what we say it does.

I know that "natural" is a reassuring term in the eco-conscious 1990s, but I'm sure many people would be surprised to learn that synthetics are often necessary. As our products contain natural materials, they may be susceptible to bacterial contamination. Preservatives are used wherever necessary to prevent this. Because some people are concerned about the use of chemical preservatives, we are looking for natural alternatives. We already use natural colorants

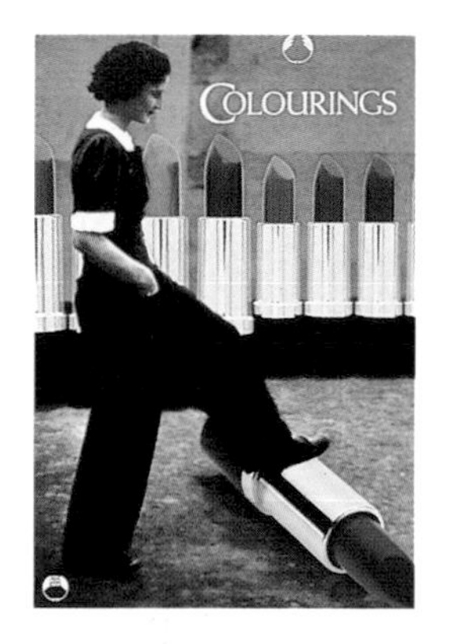

but they have a tendency to be unstable, so we'll continue to use synthetics until suitable natural alternatives are available. And much as we'd love to use only natural fragrances, many are prohibitively expensive (or, like musk, cruelly derived from animals). So nature-identical synthetics are a useful stop-gap.

All the issues I've been talking about - from animal testing to the nature of "natural" - are the forces which will shape the cosmetics industry over the next few years. I think the power structure in the beauty business has shifted a little. I've always believed our customers' expectations are much more realistic than the industry will admit. After all, how many people really think that the antidote to ageing can be found in a face cream? What they're seeking is something that's good to use, that makes them feel like they're looking after themselves, because they know that will make them feel better. Then they're going to look better, regardless of how old they are.

But now that consumers are increasingly well informed, they're going to be asking trickier questions - not just "How does this work?" but "Where does this come from?" So that is a whole new set of needs the cosmetics industry must be prepared to meet.

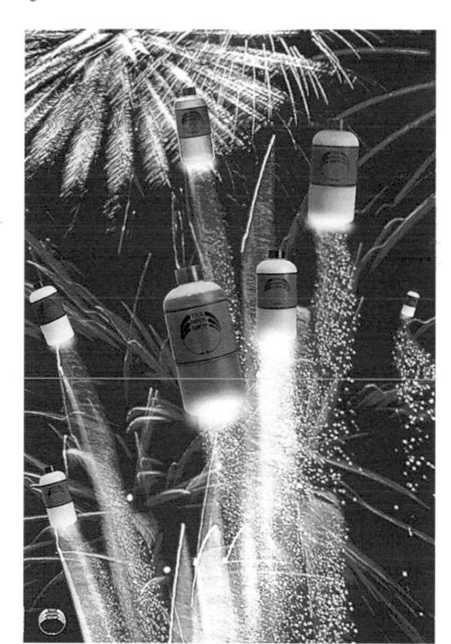

It's an exciting challenge, one that, in a way, this book takes up. I hope *The Body Shop Book* is inspiring. It is designed to entertain while it informs (surely the best way of learning); to make the mysterious simple, and to underline the commonality of human experience by placing the rituals of skin, hair and body care in various contexts - historical, anthropological and cultural. And if that all sounds too grand, just look on it as a favourite cookbook, something you dip into for everything from "hows" and "whys" to "oohs" and "aahs". In other words, a celebration of life.

And every little celebration helps us to a brighter future.

Anita Roddick

BODY

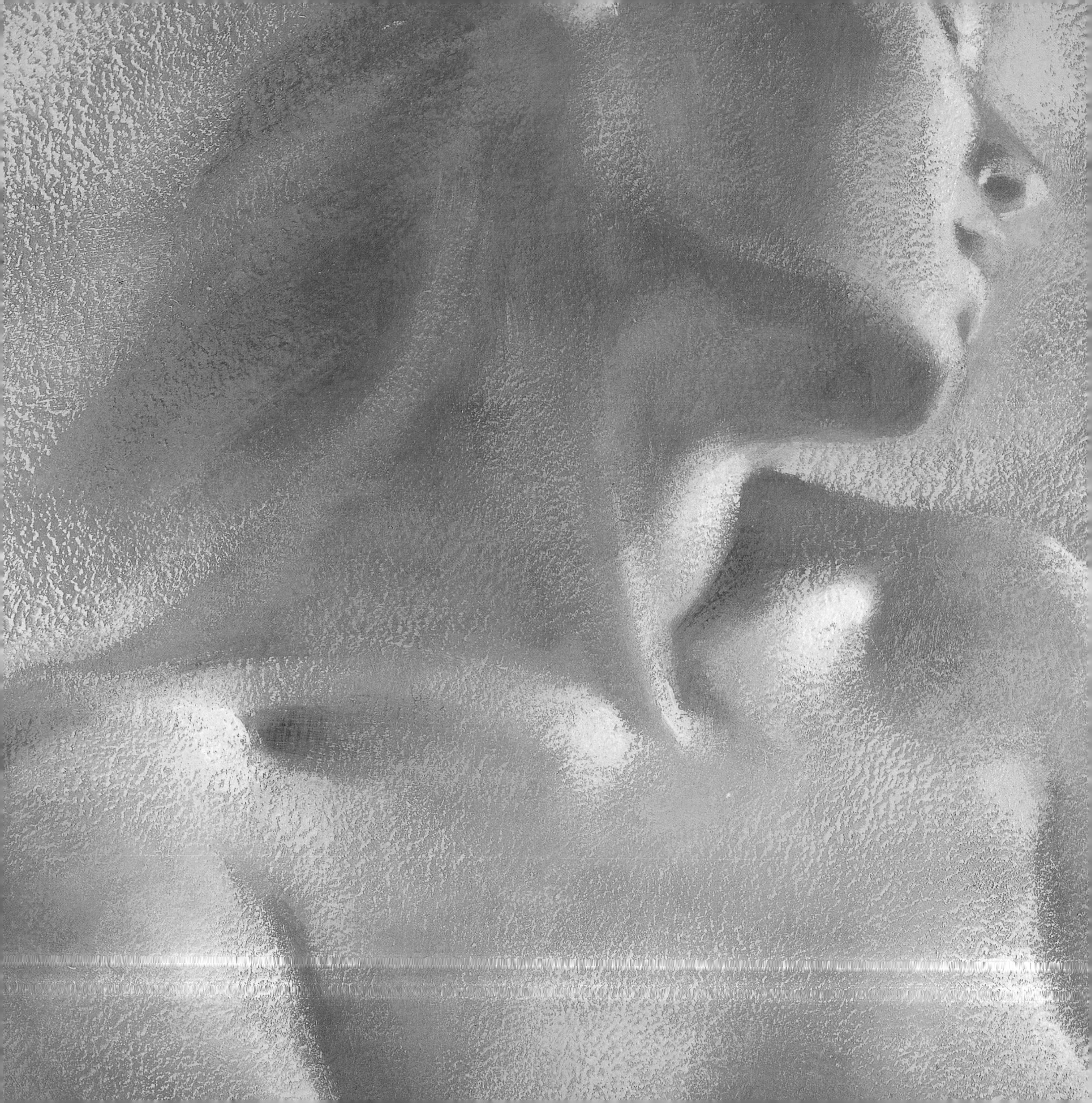

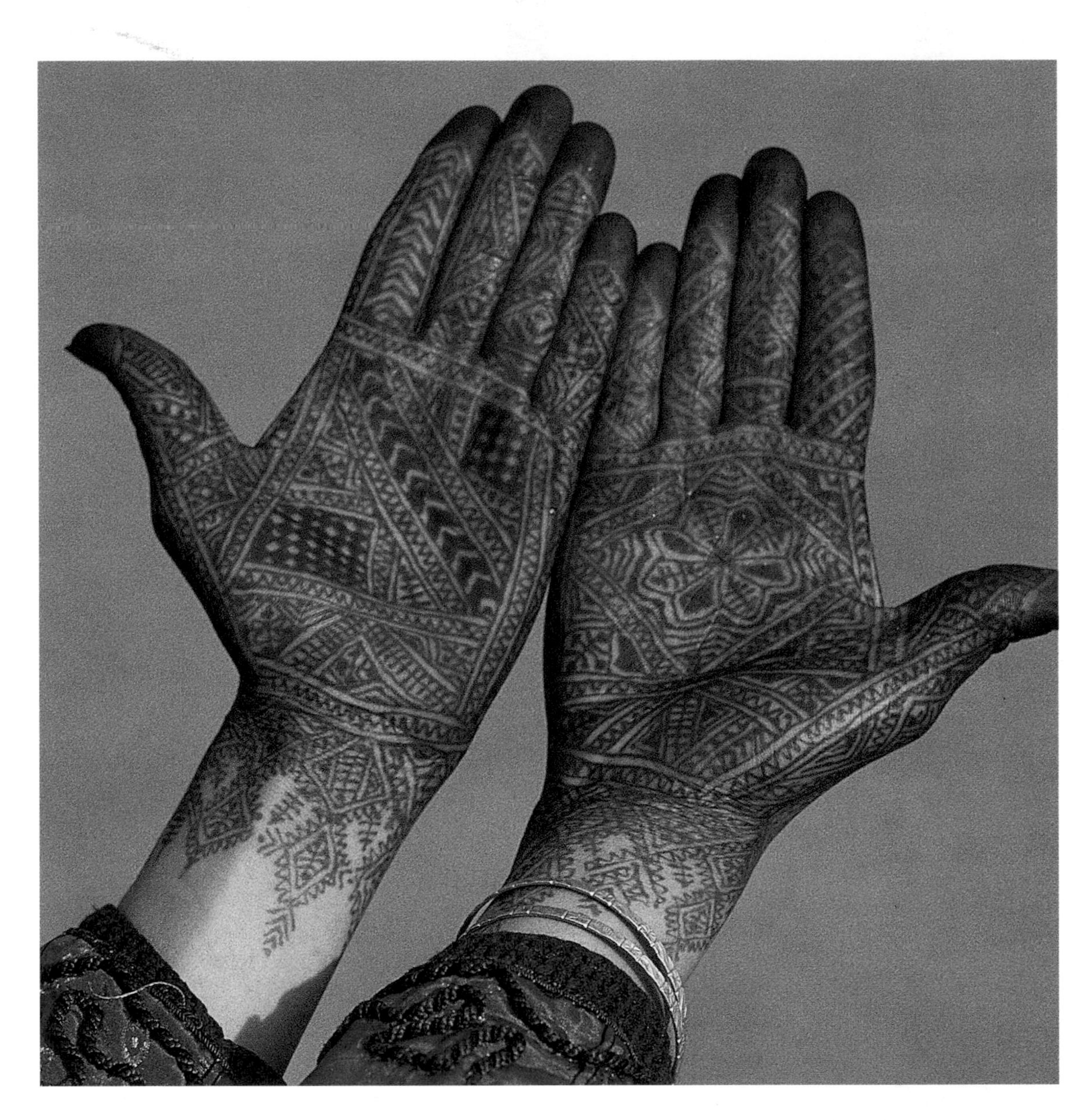

In the Middle East, women have their hands decorated with intricate patterns of red henna for special occasions.

body

Medieval man believed that his body was created in God's image. He was convinced that this god-given substance was directly connected to the soul. Therefore, what was done to the body was done to the inner man too. And so he treated it with enormous respect, however seldom he may have washed it.

In the modern world, we may know all about the benefits of bathing and life-preserving hygienic practices but we could also do ourselves a favour by taking heed of our ancestors' ways and paying more loving attention to what we do to our bodies.

Part of the problem is that we are continually bombarded by the media with visions of an ideal other. This creates dissatisfaction with what we've got. Our culture tells us, repeatedly, that beauty means slim, taut and young. Those who are ample, curved or not young must therefore be found wanting.

But let's not turn the searchlight on the cosmetic giants of the Western world alone - even though they make millions out of breeding anxieties which can lead people to yearn for some unobtainable, illusory optimum beauty. Obsession with the body perfect is not just a Western preoccupation. It can be just as perverse in other cultures.

The body is a miraculous machine, often taken for granted until something goes wrong. We need to wake up, listen to our own rhythms, rediscover our lost instincts. After all, if we don't look after our bodies, where else are we going to live?

To the Tuareg of the Sahara, beauty means obesity. "Ideal" women with rolls of fat hanging from fleshy necks must crawl because their legs can no longer carry their weight. While some Western women deny themselves enough food to keep their bodies healthy, there are women in Africa who are penned up by their tribes and fattened by force-feeding with balls of bread so that they will be thought beautiful.

But in Western culture, obsession with our version of the "perfect body" is perhaps more disturbing than some African ideals because, with a lot of money and a lot of pain, we think we can have what we want. Advances in cosmetic surgery mean you can have the slender body of a teenage girl for life, if that is your heart's desire.

But at least cosmetic surgery - whether one is for or against it - is an adult choice. One by-product of medical research into foetal development means that scientists are almost at the point where they can screen unborn babies for possible health problems so that these may be rectified in the womb or the foetus aborted. Imagine a culture that valued thinness to the point where an unborn child could be aborted on the grounds that it would have a weight problem in later life. Shockingly, this isn't unthinkable - in a poll already conducted among adults in New England, more parents said they would abort a child if it was likely to be fat than if it was likely to develop Alzheimer's disease.

Data like this suggests we are losing sight of our body as a thing of marvels and instead learning to hate it for being the "wrong size". Right now, 5 to 10 per cent of American women are estimated to be anorexic while vast numbers are enduring the weight fluctuations of unhealthy "yo-yo" dieting. In 1991, America spent $33 billion on diets more than the gross national product of Ireland.

OUR BODIES ARE NOT MACHINES

Today we appreciate that a regular change of underwear is vital to cleanliness. But our thinking is diametrically opposed to Victorian beliefs. In order to keep their children from colds and chills, many mothers smeared their infants with goosefat and then sewed them into their underwear for the duration of the winter.

We have declared war on our bodies. We no longer bother to listen to their rhythms or the signals they send out to us. So we push them too hard. We deny our bodies enough sleep and we deprive them of valuable nutrients. To men and women in the Middle Ages - backward though they might seem to us in terms of personal hygiene and medical practices - this would have seemed like lunacy.

We need a reminder. Most of us are born with the requisite number of body components. By taking care of them, we can ensure health and looks and stave off premature signs of advancing years. Feeling good is looking good. It's really very simple.

THE BODY CELEBRATED

For more than two thousand years, artists have portrayed the naked bodies of men and women as the epitome of beauty, power and energy. The body has been eulogised in poetry and painting and celebrated in song. In the Middle East it is the rounded female form, signifying maternal abundance, that is praised. In an anonymous ode to an Indian bride, the lovely woman is of a shape contemporary Americans would deem extraordinary: "Moon-faced, elephant-hipped, serpent-necked, antelope-footed, swan-waisted, lotus-eyed".

Imagine how boring it would be if we all had the same expectations of the body beautiful; if we could all be shaped, pulled, twisted and tweaked into "the ideal". Homogenised so that we were all identikit "perfect", not one of us would be special. As the Mexican writer Octavio Paz wrote, "Life is plurality, death is uniformity".

DECORATING THE BODY

In tribal culture, the body can be a blank canvas for intricate patterning caused by nicking the skin with thorns and other sharp implements to cause welts. The process is called scarification. In Southern Sudan, these scars on a Dinka woman's back are a sign of great beauty, and they are more than decorative. The patterns also relate to the sense of touch, as Dinka lovers can decode their erotic messages written in human braille.

Scarification is strong visual evidence of the key moments in an individual's experience, a map of a life which is patterned with skin souvenirs of significant stages. The scars also relate to one's identity within a group. Other groups can read where someone comes from by the marks on his or her skin. In Scotland, where the climate is less friendly, the same function was filled by the intricate, elaborate knitting patterns of Arran sweaters, which originated so that drowned sailors could be identified by their families.

In the Western world, we try to keep skin as smooth as possible and, though we paint our faces, our bodies are unadorned - except for the increasingly popular tattoo. We can probably thank Tahiti for that. Captain Cook reported seeing tattoos on Tahitian men and women in 1769. The word itself may come from the Tahitian "tatau", meaning to strike.

THE UNAVOIDABLE FACT - WE ARE WHAT WE EAT

What we put in to our bodies determines what we get out of them. We require proteins, vitamins, fibre, fatty acids, starchy carbohydrates and minerals - particularly iron and calcium. Most important are vitamins C and those of the B complex. They are soluble in water and should be replenished daily.

We know what's good and bad for us, but persist in eating junk. That is usually because it is the easy option. But even if we find thinking about what we eat boring in the extreme, we can still help ourselves without turning into bean-eating vegans. Two successful secrets for looking better are right at hand. And neither of them involves the tedium of counting calories or reading through long lists of ingredients. *The secrets are water and fresh air.*

The rise in mass-market popularity of bottled water means that within easy reach is a pick-me-up which is much better for you than a cup of coffee. Water gives our internal organs a work-out. It keeps them healthy, it prods them out of sluggishness and it helps eliminate waste.

Fresh air famously has the same effect. Even if you can't nip out for a hearty hike at lunchtime, sit back, inhale deeply through the nose, hold your breath and breathe out slowly. This helps ease tension and tiredness. Our bodies need oxygen to survive. Breathe it in and let your lungs and heart do the rest. Blood vessels courier the oxygen around the body. But beware: obesity, alcohol, cigarettes and inactivity all work to impede the proper action of the blood vessels and make them far less effective at transporting oxygen-rich blood and essential nutrients.

Chinese women use a scrub of rice husks as a fragrant exfoliator. The Body Shop Rice Bran Scrub has ground rice to exfoliate, and rice bran oil to moisturise.

STARTING WITH YOUR SKIN

There is not a people anywhere on earth that doesn't, traditionally, spend time and effort on trying to look better. In order to care for our bodies, we need to know what the body is and something of what it does for us and why. We need to spend a little time getting to know the marvel of engineering that is a human foot, the intricate tool that is the human hand. But we start our tour of the body with its largest organ, the skin.

THE SKIN'S STRUCTURE

That's right, the skin is the body's largest organ, weighing between four and six pounds. The complexity of its structure and workings make it an admirable model for the whole human organism.

The skin is multifunctional. It acts as a barrier to hold our internal organs in place - a protective envelope keeping vital substances in and harmful ones out. It also regulates temperature, ensuring that the body does not overheat. Thirdly it is a delicate sensory organ that enables us to touch and feel. Touch is usually the sense that serves us longest. The elderly can often touch and feel and thus stay in contact with the world, long after their sight or hearing have deserted them.

The body is covered with two types of skin: hairy and glabrous. Glabrous skin, which is found on the soles of the feet and the palms of the hands, is hairless and smooth, while the rest of the body is covered with hairy skin that varies in texture, thickness and hair density depending on its location.

Structurally, the skin is made up of layers of skin cells, the outer layers being known as the epidermis and the lower layers as the dermis.

THE EPIDERMIS

The epidermis is the part of the skin we see and touch. It is mostly made up of dead or dying cells that are created in the stratum germinativum, the very lowest level of the epidermis, and gradually pushed closer to the surface as new cells form below. This bottom layer is where melanocytes, the cells that produce melanin which protects the skin from the sun, are produced.

By the time the cells have reached the surface layer - the stratum corneum - they have hardened, flattened and compressed, creating a fairly unbreachable barrier which protects the living cells below. By this point the cells are completely dead.

"Desquamation", the process by which skin cells fall naturally off the skin, is constant. The life cycle of the skin is from 21 to 28 days, older skin renewing itself the slowest. It's a complete cycle of birth, maturation and death — all in a space less than one millimetre thick.

THE DERMIS

The thicker, underlying layer, the dermis, performs housekeeping duties for the epidermis, providing the blood capillaries and the lymphatic system necessary for nourishing and clearing waste from the new skin cells. But it also performs other essential functions. The hair follicles and nerve endings found in the dermis make it one of the body's sensory centres. It also houses the sebaceous glands (which are larger on the face, neck and shoulders than elsewhere on the body) as well as two kinds of sweat glands - apocrine and eccrine - which are present in varying numbers on different parts of the body and are used to control the body's temperature.

To aid in the protection of the skin, a mixture of sweat and sebum is produced in the dermal layer and expressed through pores in the skin. This forms a thin film called the acid mantle, which is the skin's first line of chemical defence against harmful bacteria and infection. In addition, the acid mantle helps to moisturise the stratum corneum until it is ready to be sloughed off.

BATH ADDITIVES

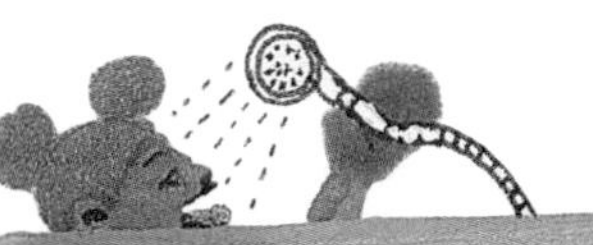

EPSOM SALTS
To relax tired muscles and joints, dissolve Epsom Salts in warm water and massage lightly with a mitt.

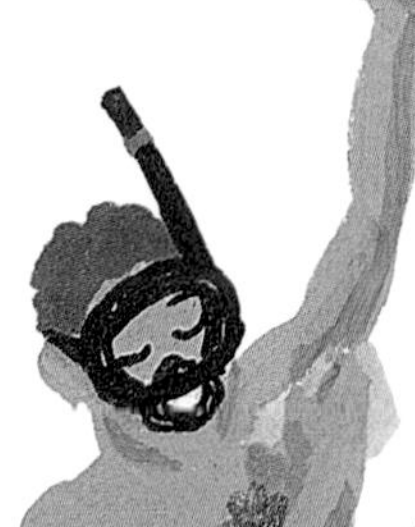
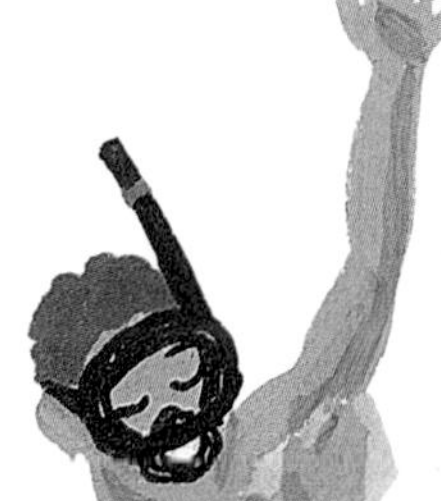

SEA SALT
Rub coarse sea salt all over your body - but not your face! Then wash it off in a warm bath. Alternatively add sea salt directly to your bath for an invigorating and reviving cleansing session.

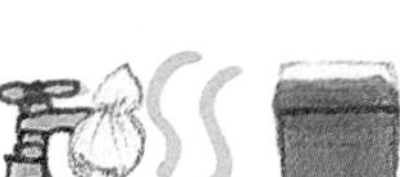
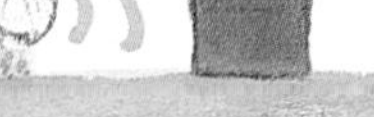

PERFUME
Add a few drops of your favourite perfume to your bath. For super-smooth skin, add some unfragranced baby oil too.

OATMEAL OR BRAN
Tie a cupful of oatmeal or bran in a square of muslin and hang it from the hot tap. Oatmeal and bran both have a cleansing and soothing effect on the skin.

AROMATHERAPY OILS
Add a few drops of the aromatherapy essential oil of your choice to a warm, full bath. Simply choose the oil to match your mood - relaxing, reviving, invigorating or soothing.

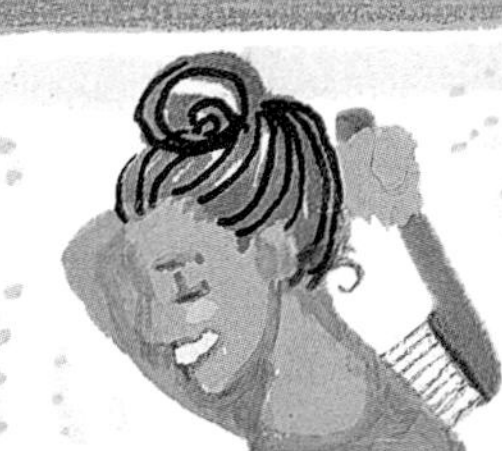

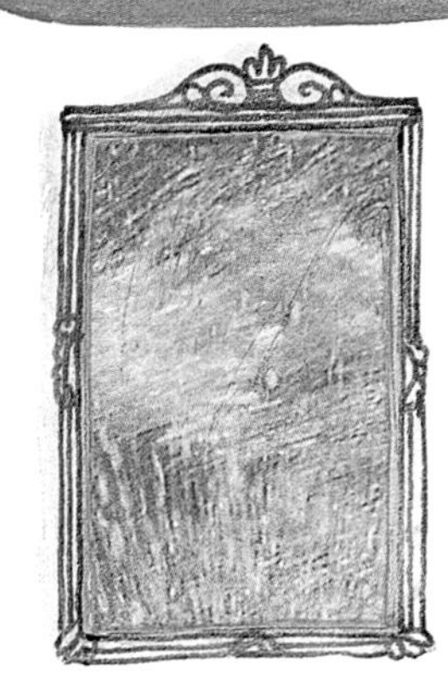

HERBS
For a perfumed herbal bath, steep 2oz of herbs in one pint of boiling water for half an hour, then strain the liquid into your bath. Alternatively fill muslin bags with a selection of herbs, tie them over the hot taps, and let the water run through.

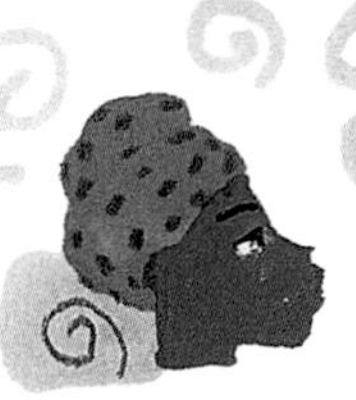
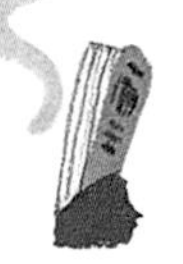

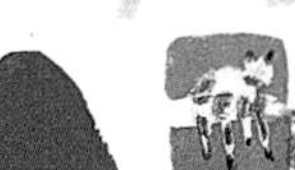
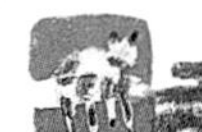

MILK
Make your own moisturising milk bath by adding one cup of powdered skimmed milk to the water. Relax and enjoy!

CIDER OR WINE VINEGAR
Add a cup to your bath to soothe dry skin for a great pick-me-up and relaxer all in one.

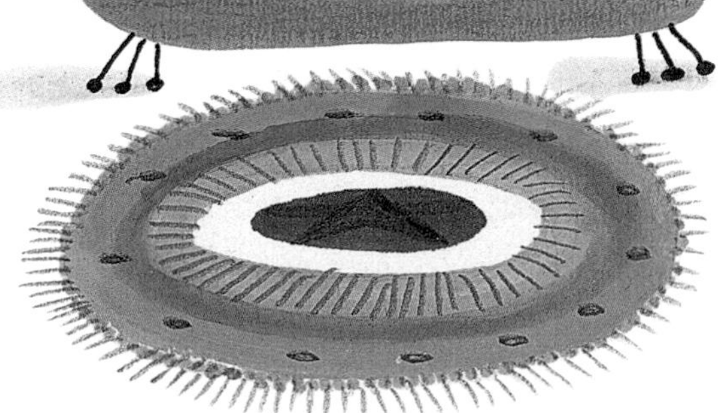
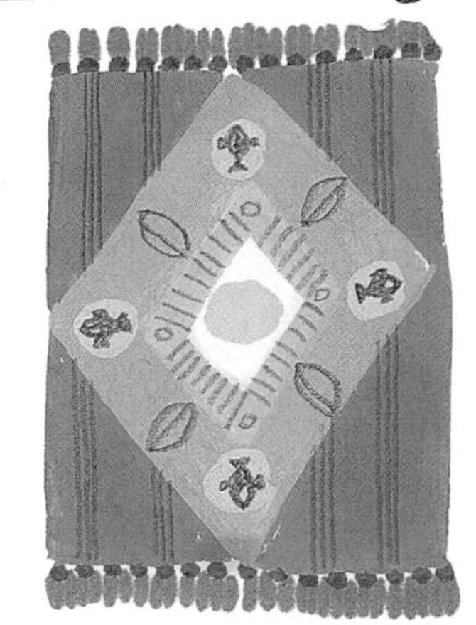

Finally, the dermis also nurses the protein fibres - collagen and elastin - that provide the skin with the elasticity it requires to fit our bodies and the resiliency needed to withstand knocks and bumps. Collagen fibres, by nature tough and resilient, make up 75 per cent of the dermis's weight and are interwoven with elastin fibres which are naturally stretchy and able to expand and contract so the skin fits the body, regardless of shape or size. It is the gradual disintegration of these fibres thanks to environmental stresses and a slower replacement rate as we age that causes wrinkles and sagging, the main signs of ageing in the skin.

The skin is also a habitat, home to hosts of different benign bacteria - 100 million in each armpit alone - which fight off alien germs. This outer defence system can be upset when we take antibiotics, which can disturb the skin's natural flora. Hence the itchy feeling which is occasionally a side effect of taking prescription drugs. You probably won't even make the connection between the drugs and the itch, but everything in the body is connected. The skin is a mirror of the internal condition of the body, and many signs of what is happening within are evident to those who pay it close attention. In the Orient, there exists a remarkably accurate system of diagnosis based solely on the texture, colour and odour of the skin.

SLEEPING BEAUTY

One of the best ways to maintain the lustre of the skin, whether it is decorated or smooth, is to let it rest. Beauty sleep is well named. During sleep, cells are renewed and waste disposal carried out. The skin regenerates because the energy needed for this is not siphoned off elsewhere, as it is during the active day.

The skin smooths out as the body relaxes, easing tiny wrinkles. A bath or shower before bed will aid relaxation.

FOR A GOOD NIGHT'S REST...

- Make sure the bedroom is dark and quiet and the bed is comfortable.
- Unwind in a relaxing aromatherapy bath before bedtime.
- Rest your head on a soothing herbal pillow packed with thyme, mint, lemon verbena, marjoram and spices.
- Light an aroma jar and let the scent of soothing essential oils pervade your bedroom.
- Try a late night banana snack. Bananas are a natural relaxant because they contain the sleep-inducing amino acid, tryptophan. Milk is a good late night drink.

CLEANING THE BODY

Cleanliness is next to the goodliness of a night's healthy rest. Cleansing loosens particles of dirt and flakes of the dead, outer epidermis that are ready to be shed. But washing the body can also be a delightful personal ritual. Far more than just a place to get the body clean, the bath can be a place of relaxation, sweet with the scents of perfumes; a centre for health cures in a tub filled with muds or seaweeds; and of course, a sanctuary. In the bath, sore muscles relax, surface wrinkles are soothed and inner aches and pains can be washed away. Also dirt, sweat and flakes of dead skin are dislodged from the body, which is why the Japanese find the British habit of lying in the bath without having pre-washed so appalling.

THE BEST KIND OF CLEAN

The best kind of cleansing is still the simplest - soap and water.

The Body Shop has a wide range of soaps, all made with 100 per cent vegetable base - a mixture of palm oil and coconut oil. But as soap removes grease, it also removes some of the body's natural oils so:

DO massage in moisturiser while the body is still slightly damp to counter dryness.

DO pay special attention to legs - they tend to be particularly dry because they have fewer sebaceous glands.

DO use superfatted soaps with jojoba oil on dry skins.

DO use milk and honey soaps for sensitive skins, including children's skins.

DO use translucent glycerine soaps for extra mildness. Less alkaline than other soaps, they produce less lather and rinse off easily.

CHECKLIST FOR THE IDEAL BATH

- Warm Bathroom
- Aroma Jar
- Soothing Music
- Warm Towels
- Bubbles/Oil/Salts
- Body Scrub/Loofah
- Back Brush
- Soap
- Sponge
- Flannel
- Face Mask
- Nail Brush
- Pumice Stone
- Body Buddy and Massage Oil
- Champagne, Wine or Herbal Tea
- Body Moisturiser
- Bathrobe
- Lots of time - lock the door!

HISTORY OF THE BATH

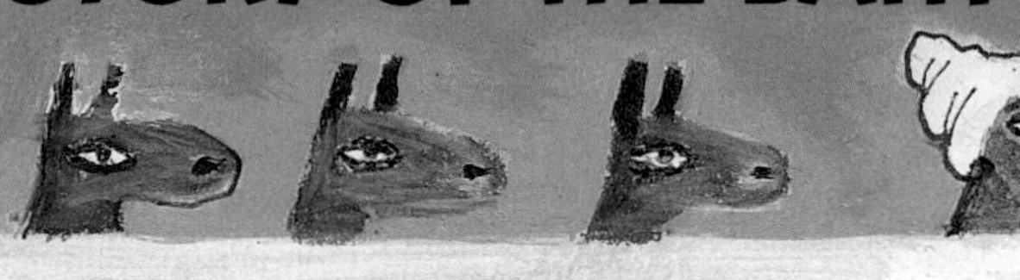

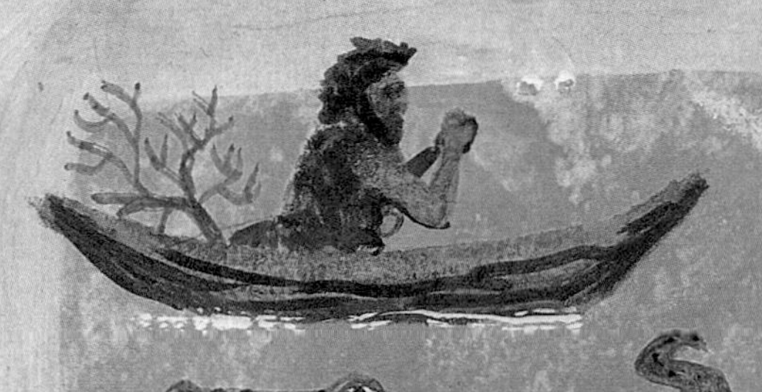

Emperor Nero's queen Poppaea travelled with a train of asses to be milked for her fresh bath. Cleopatra is also said to have enjoyed the skin-cleansing, softening and whitening properties of milk.

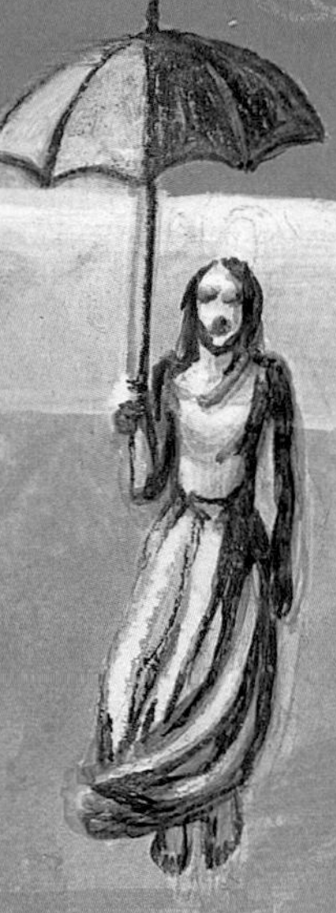

Early man stank in self-defense. It is thought that he smelt bad so that predators would avoid him.

With the rise of Christianity, bathing became associated with the pagan and godless. The early Christians took particular pride in not washing. St Agnes died unwashed at the age of 13.

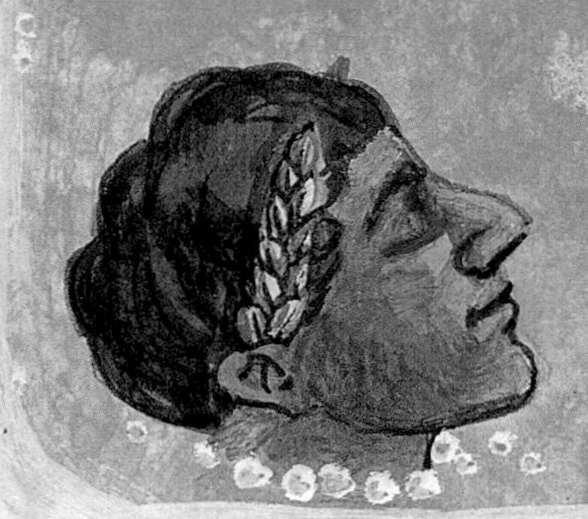

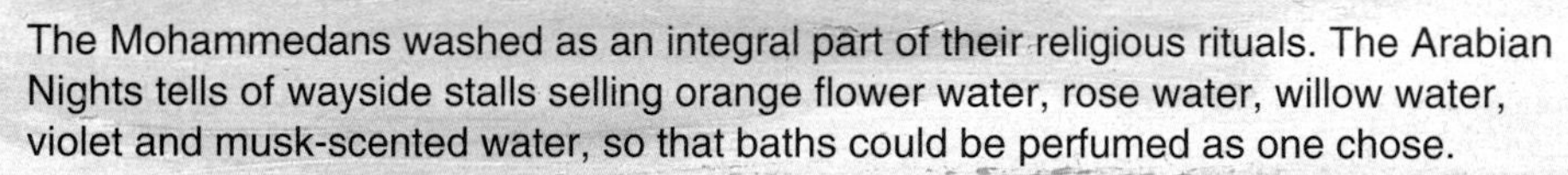

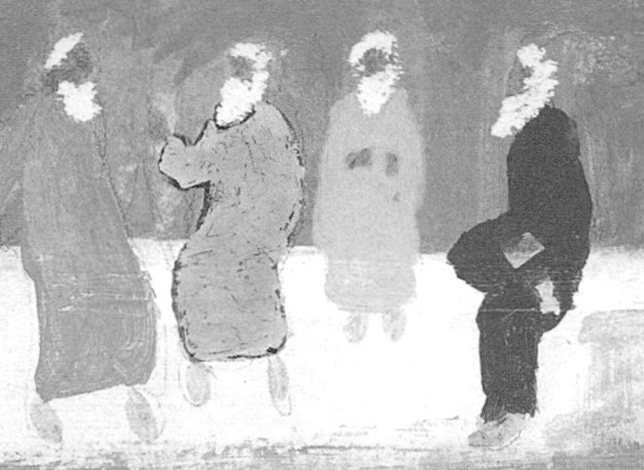

The Mohammedans washed as an integral part of their religious rituals. The Arabian Nights tells of wayside stalls selling orange flower water, rose water, willow water, violet and musk-scented water, so that baths could be perfumed as one chose.

Cleanliness was a high priority for the Romans. They were so horrified by the stench of the races they conquered, they set about building bath houses wherever they set up colonies.

According to medical theories of the Renaissance, the body was composed of four delicately balanced "humours". The body's balance would be thrown if exposed to too much water. So bathing was frowned upon.

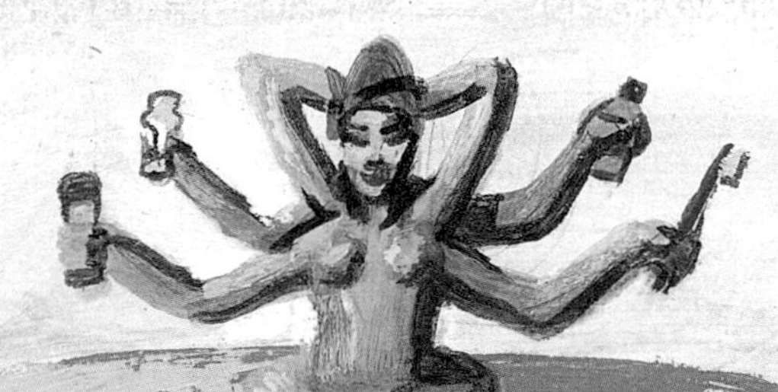

In the folklore of India and the Orient, the scented bath has been used to attract good spirits, new lovers and to obtain and preserve happiness.

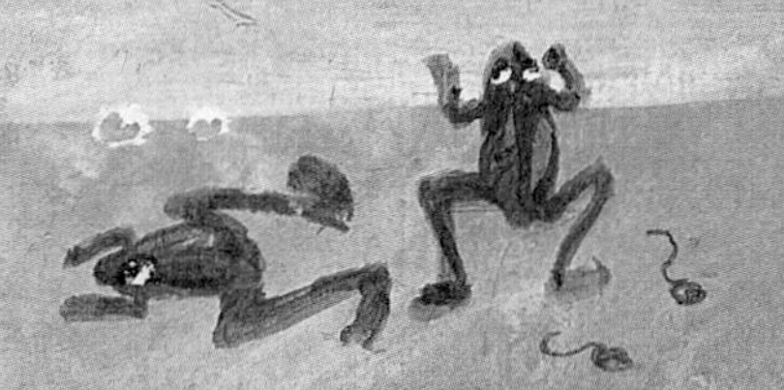

In addition, public bathhouses were little more than brothels. They also had a tendency to be infested with tadpoles and frogs. No wonder Henry VIII ordered all public baths to be closed in 1500. France followed in 1538. They remained closed in England for 200 years.

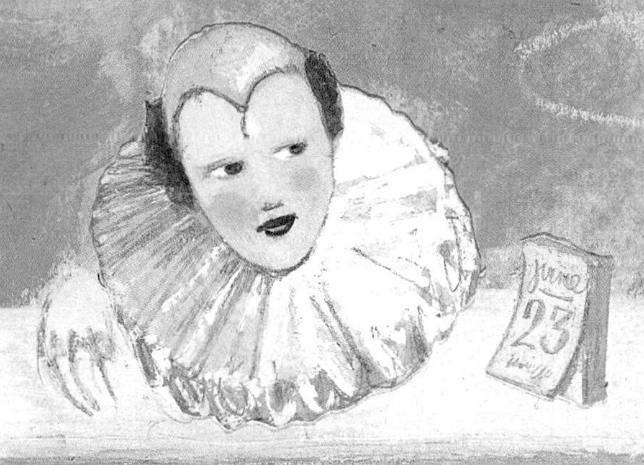

Mary Queen of Scots bathed in wine, which is possibly effective as a disinfectant to kill off the parasites that infested the seldom washed flesh of Tudor times. Her cousin Queen Elizabeth I boasted of bathing “once a month whether she needed it or no”.

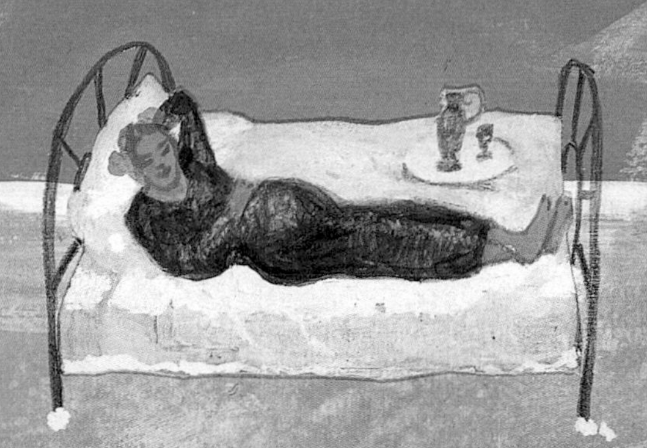

By the 18th century, taking too many baths was thought to be a cause of infertility and a danger to beauty. Pregnant women were warned off them altogether.

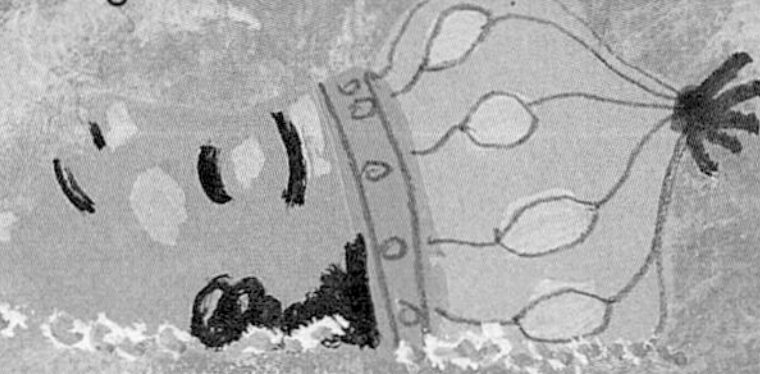

But the craze for all things classical brought a return to exotic bathing. Following trendsetter Beau Brummell, the Prince Regent installed a bathroom at the new Brighton Pavilion where aristocrats soaked for hours in baths of hot water and milk.

Japanese men and women were unabashed about bathing together until the arrival of the American Commodore Matthew Perry in 1853.

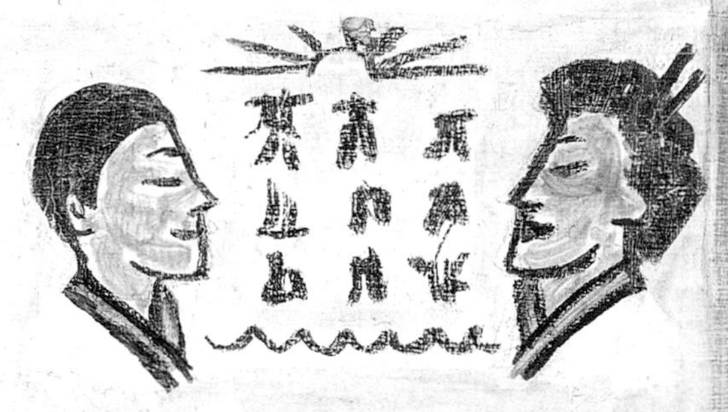

The Americans decreed that men and women should bathe separately. By 1870 a law to that effect had been passed.

After bathing became accepted, baths were still hard to fill until the advent of household plumbing towards the end of the 19th century. Even then, they used so much water that inventors searched for an equally invigorating alternative. The 1883 Berlin Hygiene Exhibition introduced the first hot water shower.

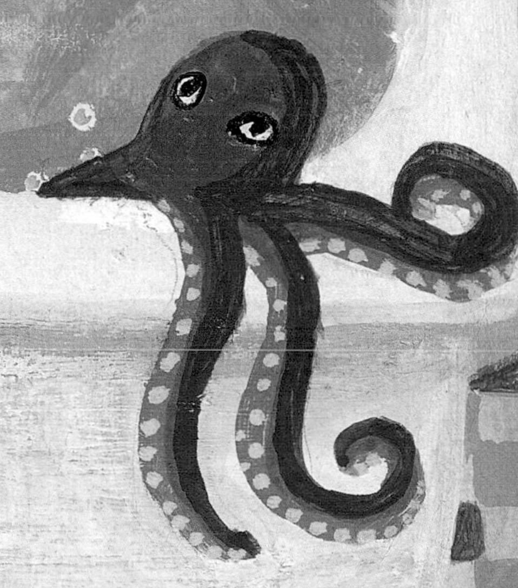

The Japanese are still champion bathers, taking one bath to cleanse the body and a second bath to relax. They love to attain the condition of yudedako, or “boiled octopus”.

LOOFAH

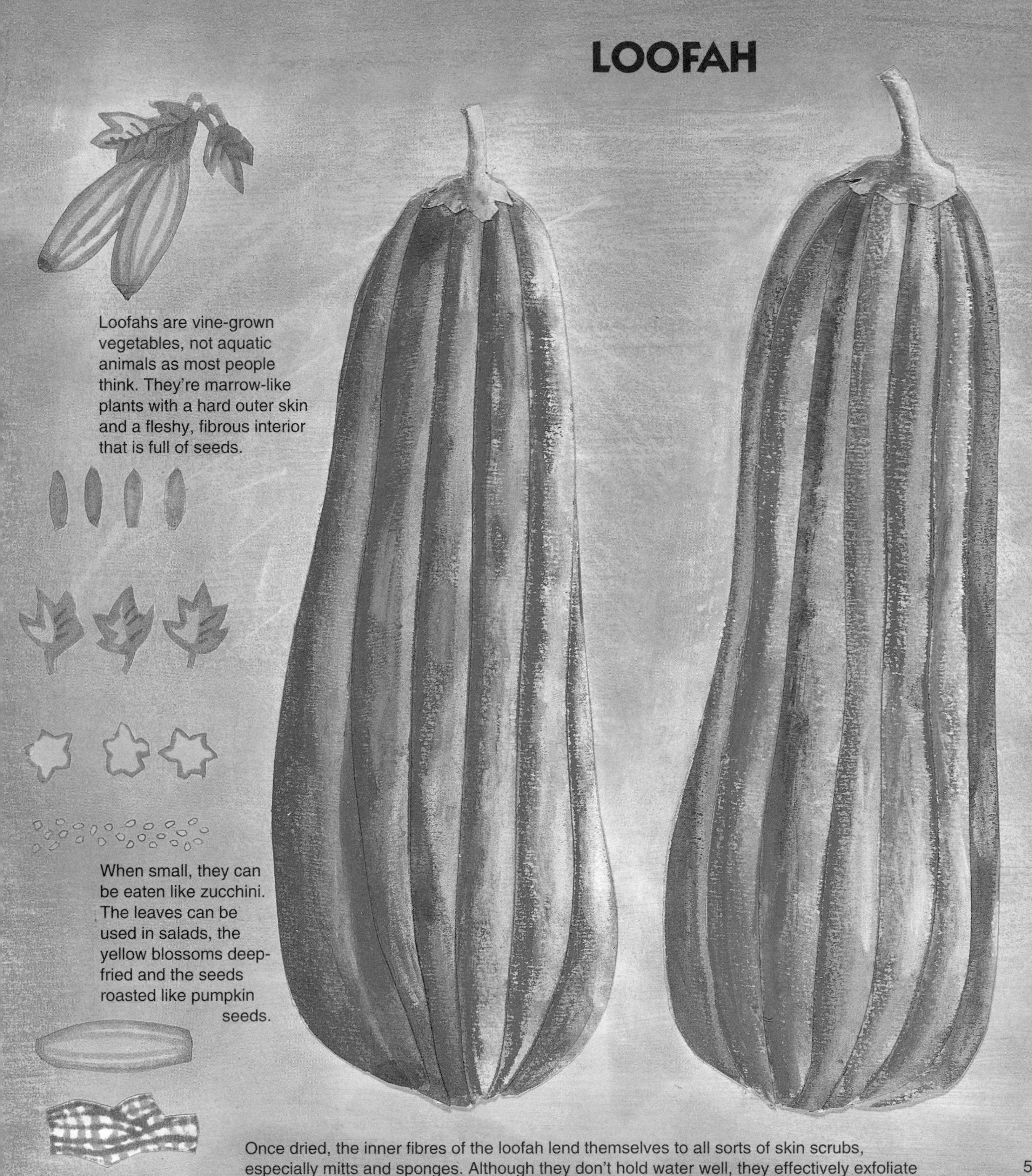

Loofahs are vine-grown vegetables, not aquatic animals as most people think. They're marrow-like plants with a hard outer skin and a fleshy, fibrous interior that is full of seeds.

When small, they can be eaten like zucchini. The leaves can be used in salads, the yellow blossoms deep-fried and the seeds roasted like pumpkin seeds.

Once dried, the inner fibres of the loofah lend themselves to all sorts of skin scrubs, especially mitts and sponges. Although they don't hold water well, they effectively exfoliate dead skin cells and remove dirt and excess oil. They also stimulate blood circulation, which keeps skin looking fresh and healthy.

Why are loofahs better than flannels or wash-cloths?

They dry quickly and they never develop a sour odour. If you can find fresh loofahs you can make your own loofah scrub. For a soft facial sponge, young loofahs (7 to 8in) are ideal.

Slightly larger ones are best for body scrubs, and the biggest of all are great for hard jobs such as pot scrubbing:

1. Dry the fruit on a window sill for two weeks.
2. Cut off both ends of the loofah and shake out the seeds.
3. Soak the fruit overnight then peel away the outer skin. (Soaking in boiling water for ten minutes will make it easier to remove the outer skin and also make the sponge softer.)
4. Wash out the sponge thoroughly, removing any seeds and loose tissue.

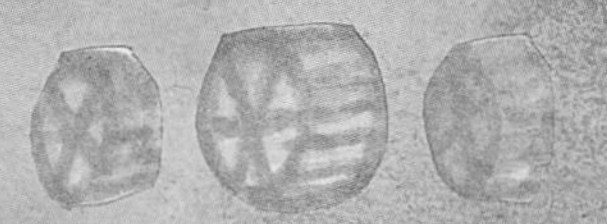

5. Cut the sponge into conveniently sized pieces and leave them to dry slowly in a shady place.

BATH TEMPERATURES

WARM baths both cleanse and moisturise the skin. Get maximum effect by applying a body moisturiser straight after your bath. Physically and mentally relaxing, a soothing warm bath gives you time to be alone. Warm baths also help relieve aches and pains and prevent stiffness after exercising.

OVER-HOT baths are weakening and can dry skin out by washing away too much of natural sebum which helps hold in moisture. Avoid them - they also put unnecessary strain on your heart as it works to dilate blood vessels in order to cool the body. Stick to warm baths for maximum benefit.

COOL baths are ideal for a quick pick-me-up. Try one in the morning to gently wake you and your muscles, or jump in at the end of the day to revitalise your body and get ready for the evening.

COLD baths are only advisable for those in good health, as they can strain the heart. Cold water is a shock to the system - and is most effective when used as a cold plunge after a hot shower.

But if, in contrast to what our ancestors thought, bathing is good for you, it is still possible to overdo it. Though facial and hair treatments work well in the prolonged steam of a warm tub, skin can become over sensitive if soaked for too long. It is sensible to alternate with showers, which are more economical in terms of water and energy and more effective at removing dirt from the skin.

INVIGORATE, EXFOLIATE !

Around 90 per of your household dust is actually dead skin particles! Everyday we shed 4 per cent of our skin cells. Socks alone trap around 190mgs of dead skin daily. It is a natural, regenerative process. If the dead skin is allowed to remain, it settles as a thick layer, especially on areas where there is a lot of friction such as heels, knees and elbows, and is impervious to moisture. The life cycle - the continuous renewal and shedding - of the skin takes between 21 and 28 days. The shorter the cycle, the more glowing the skin appears. In children, the cycle is so fast that their skin is positively radiant. But as we age, the process slows and a grey tone can creep in. It is important to accelerate the renewal process by cleansing the skin of the entire body. That's why exfoliation is your skin's best friend.

Exfoliation involves vigorous brushing, either with the hand, a body brush, loofah or mitt. At its simplest, it means nothing more than brushing the body with the hand after a bath or shower, with sharp movements, always in the direction of the heart. Brush up the arms, up the legs, up over the abdomen and down from the shoulder blades to the chest.

It's even better if you do the same with a more abrasive surface. Scrub gloves and mitts made of rough, stringy sisal are highly effective in stimulating blood circulation, loosening dead cells and leaving the skin soft, supple and glowing. These should only be used on wet skin. The effect of whatever you use - hand or abrasive mitt - can be compounded with an exfoliating gel, cream or scrub.

As well as loosening dead skin, exfoliation also loosens blockages. On the legs, exfoliation can help loosen ingrowing hairs. But though it certainly helps to cut down on winter pimples and grey skin, any serious spots on the body should be left alone. Some may be nervous reactions or caused by any number of irritations. They may even be a sign of another ailment. Ask your doctor to refer you to a dermatologist.

DON'T FORGET YOUR BACK AND SHOULDERS

Most of the year our back and shoulders are given only perfunctory treatment - any blemishes are hidden from sight until the first spell of hot weather appears and our summer clothes come out. Good posture and exercising all year round keep the spine supple and shoulders flexible. Banish dry, flaking skin by exfoliating with a loofah or back brush. A massage is also beneficial - try to find a volunteer. For rough and dry skin, try a salt and oil rub, applied with a loofah or sisal mitt. Dip the mitt in body or olive oil, then into coarse sea salt and rub vigorously over back and shoulders. Rinse thoroughly, rub dry and smooth in moisturising cream or lotion. Result - healthy, glowing skin on your back!

CELLULITE

Cellulite is another term for the ugly, rippled bulges on the thighs, buttocks, stomach and arms. Friction massage, during and after a warm bath, is good for accelerating cell

MAKE YOUR OWN SEAWEED AND LOOFAH SOAP:

Melt a pound of soap flakes in a saucepan over a gentle heat, stirring all the time. Add some pieces of finely chopped seaweed and a few tablespoons of powdered loofah. Take off the heat and, if desired, add a few drops of perfume oil for fragrance. Pour into a mould and leave to dry for a few weeks. Result: a textured soap which makes a great skin exfoliator!

GROWING RATES Nails grow at an average rate of 6mm a month, faster in young people and during pregnancy. Nails on the middle fingers grow quicker than nails on thumbs and little fingers and faster on the right hand (if you are right handed) than on the left.

metabolism and for improving circulation: knead and pinch the fleshy areas and rub vigorously with a loofah, friction glove or body buddy always in the direction of the heart. Coarse sea salt on your massage mitt helps to improve skin colour. Alternate sprays of hot and cold water can also be effective in dispersing cellulite on thighs and buttocks. (For more information, see Massage chapter.)

SAUNAS AND HOT TUBS

The steam heat of a sauna makes for a thorough, deep cleansing of the skin, with the added advantage that increased pulse rate also stimulates the blood supply to skin tissue. And a sauna prepares the skin for massage by easing tension and inducing a relaxed state. The caveat is that a sauna's stimulating effect on the heart makes it inadvisable for anyone with cardiovascular problems.

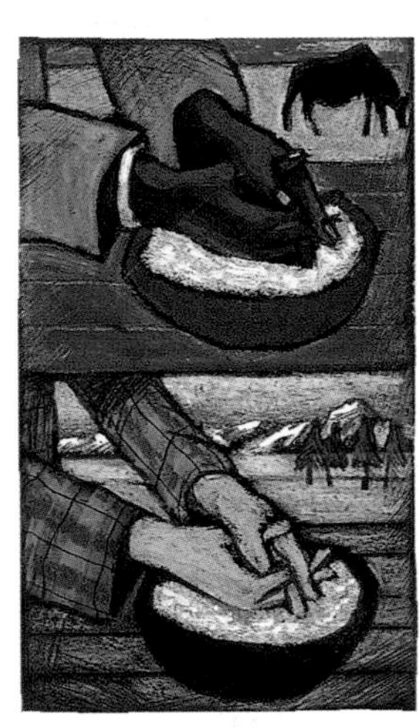

Start using a sauna for just five minutes, building up gradually if you wish. Don't wear jewellery; it will get very hot. To speed up sweating, have a hot shower before going into the sauna and go naked for best results. Or wrap yourself loosely in a towel.

The same kind of benefits can be derived from hot tubs - and the same warning applies. Remember to wash and rinse thoroughly before getting into the tub. And don't stay in for more than ten minutes.

Poorer women in India keep hands soft with curds, bran, oatmeal and almond, just as isolated Scottish crofter women, thousands of miles away, used to rub their hands in oatmeal left over from making porridge to keep them soft and pale.

BODY PARTS

HANDS

Faces are supposed to be the roadmaps of the soul, but soothsayers and mystics look to the palms of our hands to map out our lives. Hands are symbolic, even in the business world where, however much businesspeople might scorn the arcane connotations, a handshake is still a sign of good faith.

The hand is made up of eight bones in the wrist, 14 hinged bones in fingers and thumbs and five metacarpals, which join the bones of the wrist and fingers by ligaments. And there's a whole net of tendons. Our hands are remarkably resilient and indelibly marked. No amount of ill treatment, other than dipping in acid, will wipe away our identifying fingerprints, which are different even on identical twins.

Fingertips are remarkably sensitive. This is why we see safe breakers in old movies sandpapering the tips of their fingers - not in a vain attempt to remove their fingerprints but to sensitise them, because it is there that the sense of touch is at its most acute.

Whereas the face can be surgically altered to give an adult the semblance of youth, there is no widespread cosmetic surgery to keep hands looking younger than they are. Dehydration is the age-old enemy of the hands. True fanatics wear gloves filled with rich creams or gels, even vaseline, to bed. The very best defence for hands is gloves in all weathers and particularly in the washing up bowl. Next best is a rich, moisturising hand cream to protect them from hot and cold water and chemicals, and to guard against painful cracked skin and chilblains.

Today, hands have a new enemy, or at least, one that has been recognised recently. Repetitive Strain Injury (RSI) is caused, as the name suggests, by the constant repetition of actions which freeze the hands in uncomfortable or unnatural positions for long periods of time. Among those most likely to suffer are typists, journalists, musicians and hairdressers. Hand exercises, like those developed for athletes such as tennis players who need strong hands, are thought to help in the early stages. Wooden hand rollers which loosen up gnarled joints and rubber balls can be used.

In any case, finger exercises boost circulation and help keep the hands flexible. Clench the fingers tightly into a ball and then spread the fingers out wide. Or let hands hang limp and revolve each one slowly from the wrist, first in one direction, then in the other.

What always works best for over-taxed hands is care and attention.

DO rub thick moisturising cream into the back of the hands and the wrist. Try Hawthorn Hand Cream or Cocoa Butter Hand and Body Lotion.

DO massage the fingernail bed with enriching wheatgerm or almond oils.

DO gently exfoliate rough patches on hands - these can crack and let in bacteria. After exfoliation, massage with almond oil.

DON'T forget to protect hands with sunscreen.

As well as being the body's busiest appendages, hands can be exquisite adornments. In India and the Middle East, women decorate their hands with intricate patterns of red henna. Rich women show their painted hands as a visible sign of good health. Particularly intricate patterns, often extending up over the wrist and matched by hennaed designs on the feet, signify that a woman is to be wed. Today, in the high-tech cities of the Gulf, women go to the beauty parlour to have their hands painted for special parties.

Peppermint Foot Lotion was created for marathon runners who needed something to soothe and refresh hot, tired feet.

NAILS

Nails need careful attention - not frenzied biting! Some schools of thought say you should never cut them, just keep them neat with an emery board. If you do choose to cut them, you will be continuing a human habit that has existed for so long there are even superstitions about what day is best for a nail trim:

Cut them on Monday, you cut
them for health;
Cut them on Tuesday, you cut
them for wealth;
Cut them on Wednesday, you cut
them for news;
Cut them on Thursday, a new pair
of shoes;
Cut them on Friday, you cut them
for sorrow;
Cut them on Saturday, you'll see your
true love tomorrow;
Cut them on Sunday, and the devil
will be with you all week.

Staining nails for cosmetic enhancement is an old habit. Cleopatra did it. Buffing nails is a rather more recent rite. It became fashionable with flappers in the 1920s who, with their gamine hair cuts and boyish figures, didn't wish to look like painted ladies. In a recent American poll, women who wear nail varnish were deemed less trustworthy than those who don't!

One possibly positive side-effect of wearing nail varnish is that it requires meticulous application, which makes you focus not just on your nails but on the needs of your hands too. But disadvantages tend to outweigh this rather abstract benefit. Nail varnish - and the products used to remove it - can have a terrible drying effect. Low-grade nail varnish removers with the strength of paint stripper are even worse, as these can strip off micro-organisms which are at home on healthy nails. Oil-based removers are preferable.

Another thing to avoid is the metal nail file. Even more threatening implements are the commonly used nail scissors. Never trim cuticles around the nail bed. Instead, soften them with rich moisturiser or almond oil and push them back gently towards the base of the nail for neater-looking nails.

Keep an eye on your nails. They are another of the body's barometers of general health. Flaking nails might be an indication of some far greater imbalance within. Doctors in some countries, including the UK, look at the nails for diagnosis, even for symptoms of life-threatening ailments, including heart disease.

Healthy nails depend on a diet containing adequate proteins, vitamins, essential minerals and trace elements, notably zinc and iodine. They don't depend on gelatine which, despite the persistent myth, does nothing in particular for the nails. Brittle nails can indicate a vitamin A or retinol deficiency. Chlorine in swimming pools and harsh detergents can also be responsible. Hangnails, which can be painful as the lower, sensitive dermis is exposed, may be crying out for rich moisturising. They may also indicate a dietary deficiency of folic acid, a particularly common problem with women. Liver and green vegetables are good sources of folic acid.

FEET

Leonardo da Vinci described the feet as masterpieces of engineering and works of art. They are also the means by which mankind conquered the earth. The ability to stand upright on each foot's 26 bones, 20 finely tuned muscles and 114 ligaments gave us the wherewithal to use what had been our front legs as arms. Our hands made tools and with these we forged our future.

The feet carry priceless information about what might become of us. If one is so schooled, one can read the health of the whole human organism in the feet. A foot massage can be a tonic for the entire body. The feet are

CUTICLE SOFTENER

Blend together 2 tbsp pineapple juice, 2 tbsp egg yolk and 1/2 tsp cider vinegar and soak the nails in it for 30 minutes. Gently push the cuticles back with an orange stick.

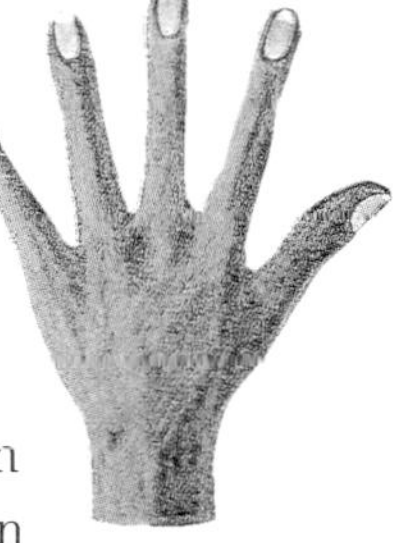

NAIL STRENGTHENER

Cider vinegar - and lemon juice - is good for general health and for strengthening the nails. Three times a day drink a glass of water containing 1 tbsp of cider vinegar or pure lemon juice. Or use the mixture as a handbath.

SIX STEPS TO FABULOUS FEET

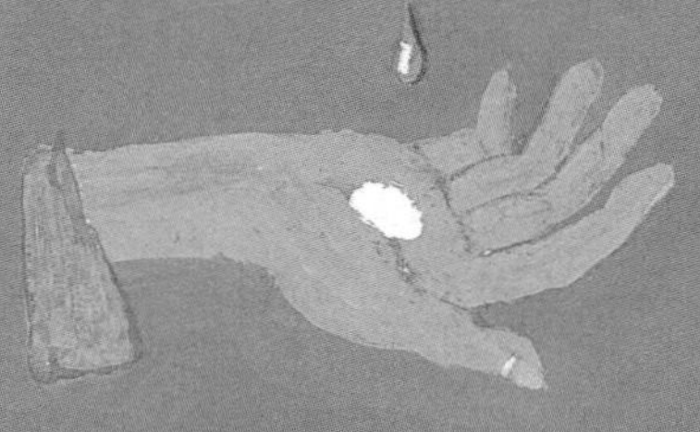

1. After a hard day, take off your shoes and wriggle your toes. Go barefoot - different surfaces stimulate circulation.

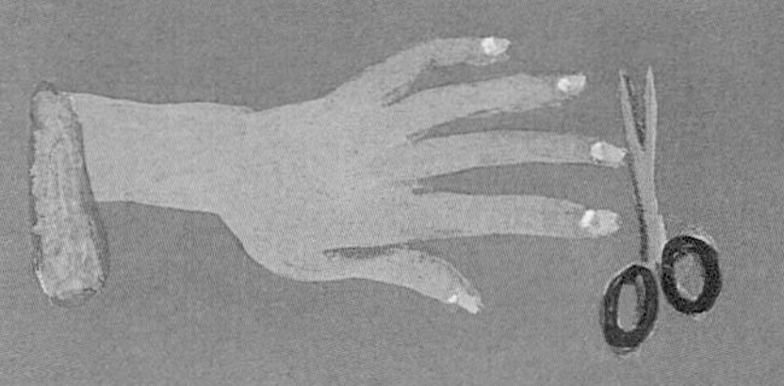

2. Soak your feet in warm water for about ten minutes. Add a few drops of bubble bath or perhaps some almond or lavender oil.

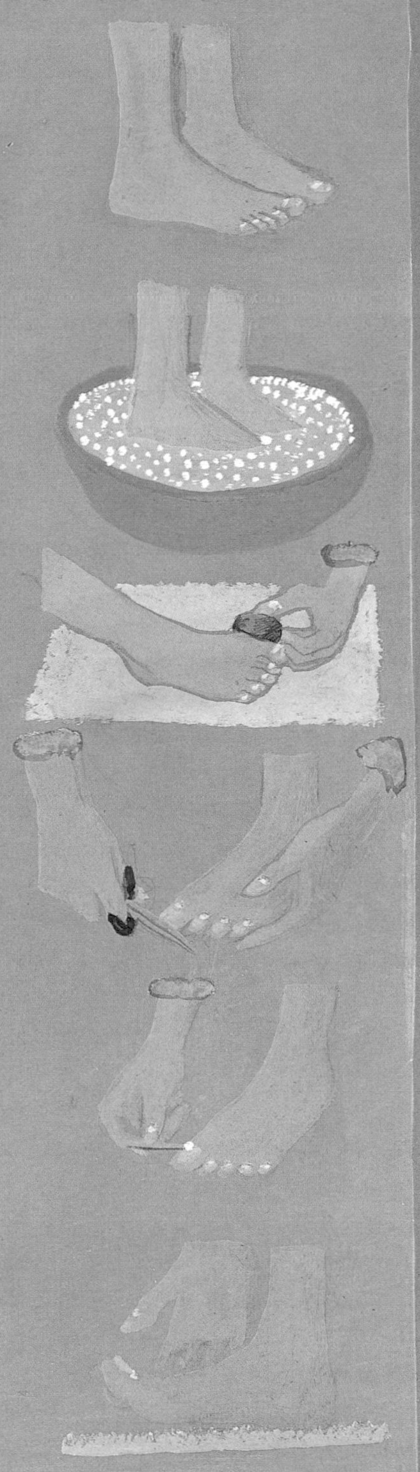

3. While soaking, gently remove any hard skin by exfoliating with a pumice stone. Dry the feet thoroughly, particularly between the toes.

4. Cut nails straight across, taking care not to cut them too short. Smooth sharp corners with the coarse side of an emery board.

5. Soften cuticles with a rich moisturiser or almond oil, and use an orange stick wrapped in cotton wool to push them back gently. Gently buff the nails to make them shine.

6. For a final treat, massage in a moisturising menthol or peppermint-based lotion to cool, soothe and refresh.

SIX STEPS TO GREAT HANDS

1. Exfoliate your hands by mixing a drop of almond oil with a little salt and rubbing it very gently over the hands and nails. Rinse off. Your skin will feel wonderfully smooth.

2. If you need to cut your nails, use nail clippers and snip carefully working from one side to the other. Don't just lop off the tip as this will damage the nail.

3. Get nails into shape using an emery board. Hold the board at an angle to your nail and file from side to centre in one smooth stroke. File in one direction only - this prevents splitting. Never use a metal nail file.

4. Massage a rich hand cream into your hands and nails. Hands have relatively few oil glands compared with the rest of the body, so need help to maintain moisture levels.

5. Soften cuticles with a rich moisturiser or almond oil, and push them back gently with an orange stick covered with cotton wool for neat looking fingers.

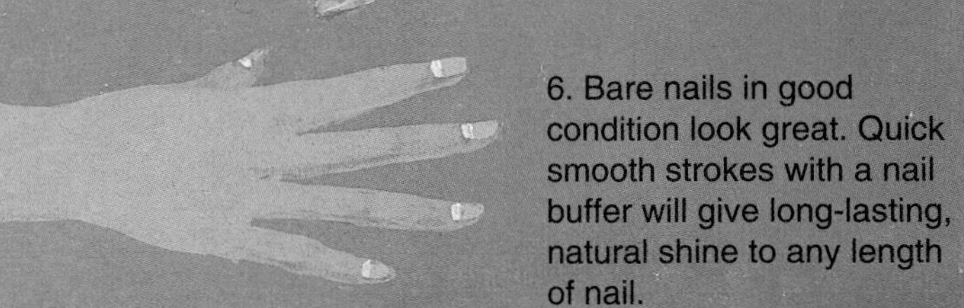

6. Bare nails in good condition look great. Quick smooth strokes with a nail buffer will give long-lasting, natural shine to any length of nail.

the body's shock absorbers, also the point of origin of some back problems and hip pains, even arthritis.

They have also been the focus of much erotic compulsion. In Ancient Egypt, a kiss on the foot was as gallant a gesture as a kiss on the hand to a Renaissance lady. Fragrant women in Turkish harems spelled out erotic messages to the sultan using hennaed symbols on their toenails. Slavic girls would dig up the footprints of lovers from the earth and plant a fadeless marigold in them so that their sweethearts' love would grow and never fade.

But it was in the Far East that the eroticism of the foot reached its extreme. The height of erotic pleasure in Imperial China was the touch of a tiny foot. "Golden lotuses" or "little dumplings" as they were known, brought great pleasure to husbands - and untold suffering to the little girls whose feet were bound as children so that they would never grow more than three inches long. Men never saw their wives' unbound feet, which were encased, even in bed, in delicate shoes. But they loved the tense posture girls had to adopt while walking on their painful stumps. The practice was outlawed in 1928, but there are still old women in China whose feet are so hideously crippled that they have to crawl on their knees.

There may well be a physical foundation for the feet's erotic charge. They have 120,000 sweat glands and the secretion mirrors the secretion of the genital area. The natural odours of the foot are said to be a sexual stimulant.

The smell of the unfettered foot also aids indigenous people in their day-to-day lives. Some Australian Aborigines can tell the identity of individuals who have passed by smelling their footprints and can track other members of their own group, both by the sight and the smell of footprints in the ground. But to most of us, this important odour-producing factor has become nothing but a nuisance.

We can blame our shoes for that. The feet produce an egg-cup full of sweat each day. The bare foot sheds it, the shod foot seals it. But you can help them to health with a few simple steps:

Rub sweaty feet gently with surgical spirit twice a day and dust with foot powder or unscented talc.

DO wash your feet thoroughly.

DO pumice off hard skin and dry the feet carefully to drive out the fungus which likes moist little places between the toes.

DO wiggle bare toes to pep up circulation and guard against chilblains.

DO check athlete's foot by keeping feet dry and powdered and by not wearing running shoes all the time.

DO massage feet regularly with peppermint and menthol-based oils and lotions. Try Peppermint Foot Lotion.

DO have a regular footbath: dissolve Epsom salts or sea salts in warm water and rest the feet for 10-15 minutes, then scrub or pumice, dip in cold water, dry thoroughly and massage in rich lotion or moisturiser.

DON'T wear ill-fitting shoes. Chafing is not only uncomfortable, it can cause corns, the most common foot problem.

DON'T try to treat foot problems yourself. Leave ingrowing toenails, verrucas, corns and chilblains to a chiropodist.

FEET TREATS

- A few drops of lavender oil in a warm footbath eases tension and fatigue. A plunge in cold water afterwards helps revive them.
- Rub soles of aching feet with cider vinegar or lemon juice.
- For a soothing foot balm, stir 1 tsp malt vinegar into a small carton of natural yoghurt and rub over the feet and between the toes; leave for 5 minutes then rinse off with lukewarm water.
- An old-fashioned mustard bath revives cold and tired feet: blend 3 tsp mustard powder to a paste with a little water and add to a bowl of hot water; soak the feet for 15 minutes.
- A foot bath revives tired and swollen feet. Soothe them for 5-10 minutes in warm water softened with Epsom salt, bath crystals, gel or aromatherapy oil, then revive them with a quick dip into cold water before drying, creaming and massaging them.

Why not ask a friend to rub your feet for you, then offer to return the favour. If there's no one around, grab a footsie roller and indulge in a spot of DIY massage.

Pumice Foot Scrub is ideal for cleansing and softening the feet. It contains pumice granules - ground particles of volcanic rock - to exfoliate hard skin from the heels and soles. Revitalising and stimulating rosemary oil invigorates tired feet, while fennel essential oil helps combat foot odour.

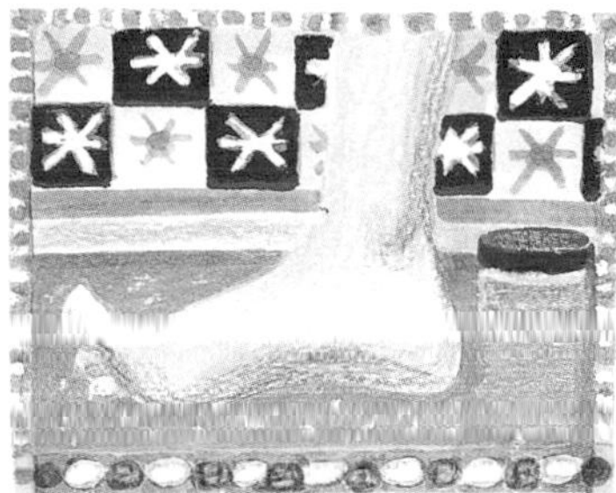

KNEES

Deodorants to make the sweat smell less, or smell better, have been with us since the pharaohs.

Knees vie with elbows as our most neglected body part, so it is no real surprise that one of The Body Shop's favourite treats was formulated with that in mind. Knees love the softening treat of Mamatoto Cocoa Butter Stick. The idea came from Polynesia where women traditionally massage their skin with raw cocoa butter to keep it soft and smooth.

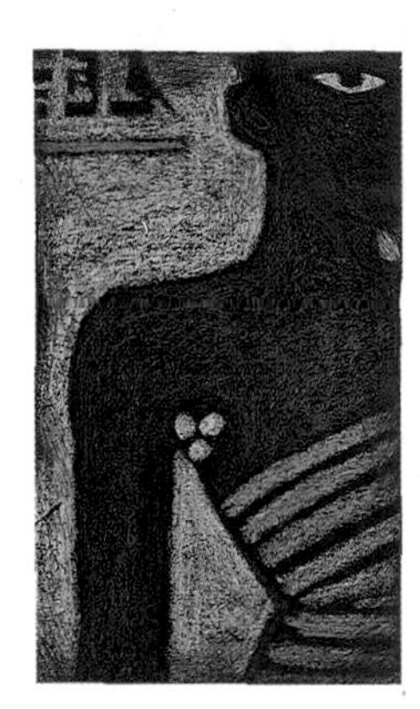

ANKLES

Swollen ankles can be ugly and uncomfortable. The best defence is to put feet up whenever possible and steer clear of tea, coffee and alcohol before and during air flights and menstruation. During pregnancy, it's a good idea to put your feet up supported by a pillow under the ankles a couple of times a day.

The Ancient Egyptians placed little balls of incense and porridge where limbs met to soak up moisture and add perfume.

The simple exercise of revolving ankles first one way, and then the other helps to keep this joint supple. And fill up a footbath higher, so that exhausted ankles don't get left out.

THE BODY'S COOLING SYSTEM

Perspiration serves a valuable purpose - it is the body's heat regulator and one of its essential waste-disposal systems. When the body heats up, the brain orders the sweat glands all over the body to go into action to regulate the internal temperature. The thin film of moisture that covers the skin also protects against harmful ultraviolet light.

Asiatics don't have as many apocrine glands as Occidentals do, and reportedly find Europeans somewhat ripe. This helps explain why Europeans have traditionally scented their bodies, while Asiatics tend to scent rooms.

There are two million sweat glands - eccrine and apocrine - all over the skin. The apocrine glands, the ones that make us smell as they excrete sweat, are chiefly in the armpits and between the legs. They are responsible for that social liability, body odour. Apocrine glands go into overdrive in hot conditions, but other factors, including stress and tension, are also triggers. And sweat isn't just for sunny days. Even in winter, the normal adult excretes around a litre of perspiration per day from all over the body through the eccrine glands.

Sweat glands begin to function at puberty and slow down with age. This is why young children and older people rarely have what we call B.O. During pregnancy and menstruation, women sweat more profusely, and in any case, have more apocrine glands than men, making B.O. a more common condition in women.

PHEW!

When it emerges from the pores, sweat is in fact colourless and odourless. It is only when it is broken down by bacteria - when it sits around on the skin or on clothes - that it may start to reek. Perspiration begins to smell after about six hours and after 24 hours is strong enough to stain clothes permanently. After that, it can become strong enough actually to destroy the fibres of clothing. The worst enemy of costume conservationists is sweat - the concentration of apocrine glands in the armpits means that the underarms of beautiful 18th-century ballgowns held in museums breed bacteria that eat away at these valuable artefacts. Armpits are the costume conservationist's war-zones.

There are three courses of action if you don't like the smell of your underarms. The first, and the most important, is to wash. The other two tend to come in one package - anti-perspirant deodorants. Anti-perspirants incorporate chemicals to reduce sweating and inhibit the bacterial action that causes smell after six hours. Deodorants can also do this, but they mostly do as they say - they de-odourise, or mask unpleasant odour with a perfume.Some people do experience allergic reactions in the sensitive underarm region so it is best to test a small area and, if irritation persists, switch brands to an unperfumed and less irritating formulation.

Hair traps the bacteria which leads to B.O., so if you don't shave, sugar or wax off underarm hair, wash even more thoroughly. If you do remove hair, take care not to apply anti-perspirant or deodorant until at least 12 hours after hair removal, as this can cause discomfort and redness.

Avoid vaginal deodorant. The sweat we excrete from between our legs is similar to that of the underarms, but the genital area is highly sensitive. In the 1960s and 70s, the beauty businessmen decided women should be bothered by their intimate odour and all manner of deodorising potions came on to the market. The result was a huge rise in thrush, due to disruption of the delicate bacterial balance of the genital area.

SWEATHEARTS?

Not that the smell of sweat is necessarily something to be avoided. Some men and women love it. Fresh sweat has long been thought by some to be an aid to attraction. Elizabethans used to give "love apples", which they would first stow in their armpits before handing to their sweethearts. Indeed, some people seem to sweat pure honey. The writer H.G. Wells apparently smelt irresistibly sweet and Marilyn Monroe is said to have exuded her own particular smell that didn't owe much to the Chanel No. 5 she otherwise favoured.

THE BREASTS

Breasts are potent tokens of a woman's aesthetic and sexual appeal. Fashion moves through strange cycles when, at times, it is stylish not to have breasts, but for now, society has accepted the breast. Women are empowered so that they can amplify and reveal them, or cover up and be as low-key as they wish.

We are the only mammals whose breasts remain fulsome when they are not full of milk. And we can alter them - not with operations and surgical incision if we don't want to, but temporarily and for fun with brassieres that can give the shape that nature can't. In the light of implant scares and the frightening statistic that 130,000 women in the USA have breast implants every year, it is encouraging to hear of models now showing up at photo-sessions with silicon pads which they pop into bras if the bigger-breasted look is required. Afterwards, they sling them into their knapsacks again.

Believe it or not, there is still debate as to whether breasts benefit from continual support, but it is an undoubted fact that more women opt for a bra than not. Breasts droop naturally because they have no supporting muscle. They are held in place by the marvellously named "Ligaments of Ashley Cooper".

The key issue if you wear a bra is to make sure it fits. Purists believe you should be fitted for a bra every time you buy one, just as you would be fitted for a pair of shoes. If you cannot afford the kind of stores where a fitting service is available, you should in any case have several different sized bras. You may need a larger bra just before and during menstruation, and of course, you must rethink your underwear during pregnancy, when the breasts can increase in size dramatically. Women experiencing, or having experienced, the menopause, will notice changes in their breasts. This might be the time to be refitted for a bra - you may be surprised to discover you now require a smaller or a larger cup size.

"Montgomery's tubercles" are the small swellings around the areola of the nipple, which are modified sweat glands. These enlarge during pregnancy and lactation and your baby recognises you through the smell secreted by them.

BREAST FACTS AND FICTIONS

• It is normal for one breast to be larger, often markedly. Early on in the short history of breast enlargement surgery, women would complain to surgeons that perfectly matched breasts didn't look natural.

• There is no way, bar surgery and, in some cases, weight-loss, to make breasts smaller. Making them bigger without a bra or an implant is also technically impossible. Exercise won't help because the breast has no muscle of its own but it will build up the muscles in the underlying chest wall, which helps the breast stand out more.

• There is no correlation between size and sexual satisfaction. The breasts change during sex whatever size they are. The nipple becomes erect, the breast swells and in some women, the skin flushes. Post-orgasm, all these changes regress, leaving the breasts tender to the touch.

• The larger breast is no better suited to feeding a baby.

• The often pleasant sensation derived from breastfeeding is natural, therefore no cause for embarrassment or guilt.

• It is not unusual for women to have three breasts. An estimated one in every 200 women have something so tiny it resembles a beauty spot, which might be found nestling in the underarm. It is a remnant of the days when our ape ancestors, like most mammals, had several offspring at once and needed several breasts to suckle their young.

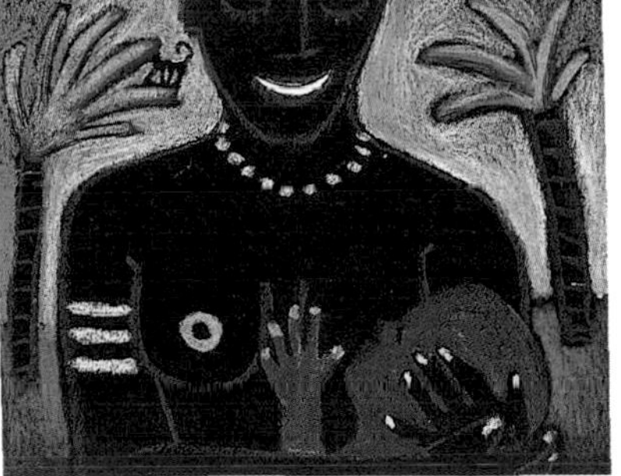

The women of the Taralpe tribe in Brazil traditionally smear their nipples with honey to moisturise them when they're breastfeeding. The Magar of Nepal prefer soothing apricot oil.

BREAST CARE

Whatever your age, from puberty onwards, the breasts need special care. It is essential to get to know the unique form of your own breasts. That knowledge is your best defence against future ills and could even save your life. In puberty, the breasts may ache as they develop and grow. They may also get stretch marks, just as the enlarging

BREAST EXAMINATION

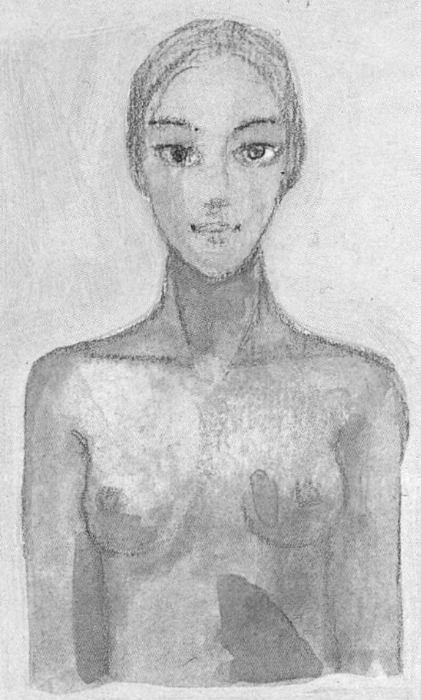

1. Stand naked in front of a mirror in a good light with your hands at your sides.

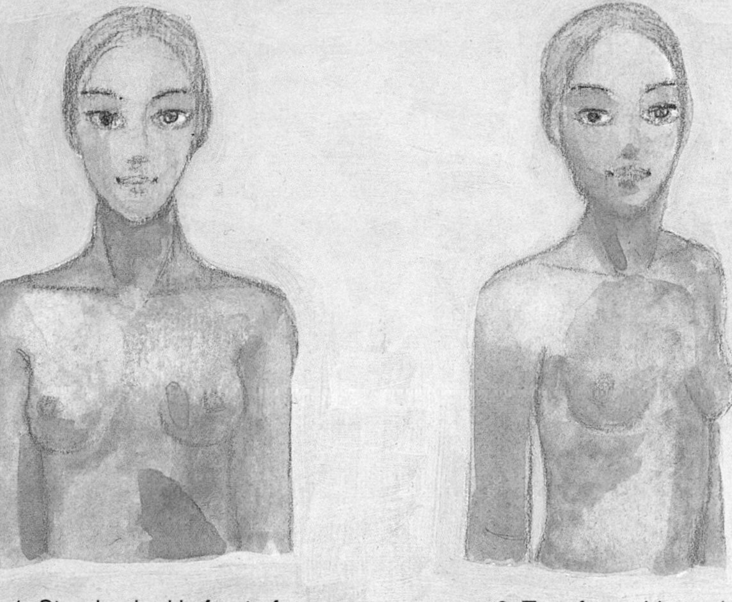

2. Turn from side to side to examine both breasts.

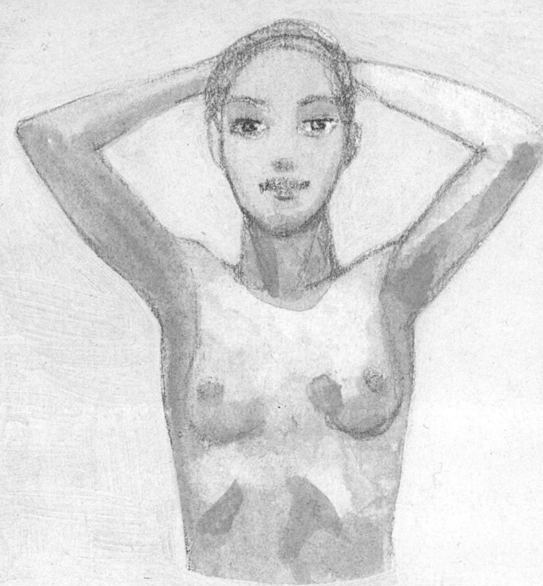

3. Raise your arms above your head and look carefully for any dimpling in the surface of each breast, including under the arm.

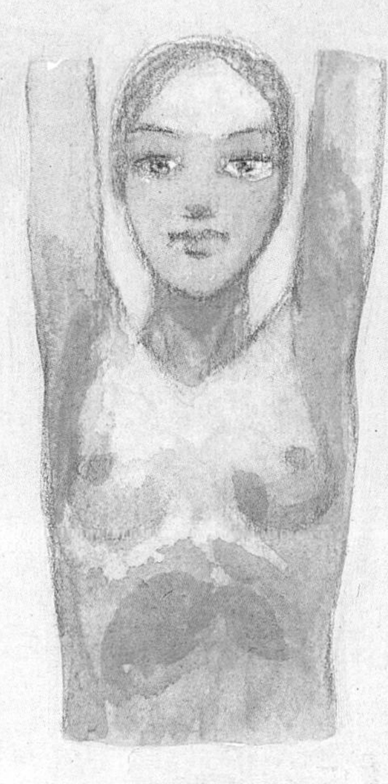

4. Note anything unusual around the nipples.

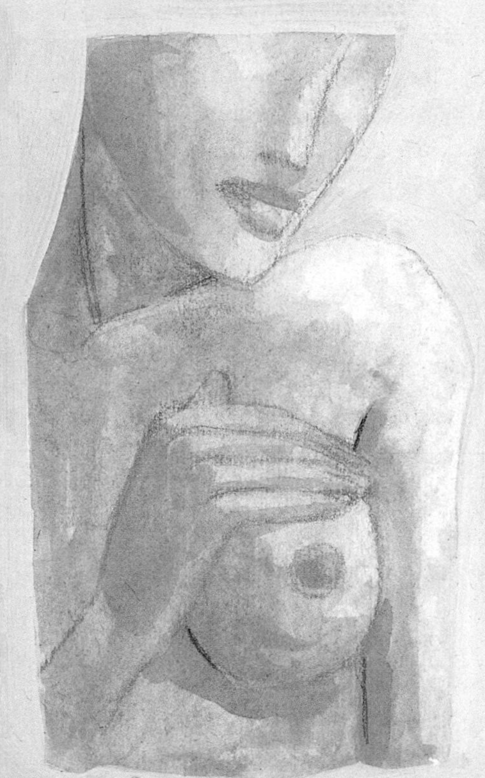

5. Lie down flat on your back. Prop a pillow under the left shoulder and use the fingers of the right hand to examine the left breast.

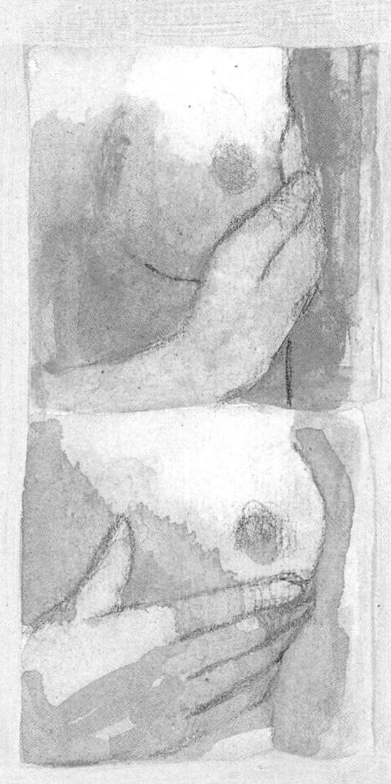

6. Press with the flat of the fingers over the tissues extending into the armpit, where most lumps originate, then move to the upper, outer quarter of the breast before feeling the lower, outer quarter, from the edge to the centre near the nipple.

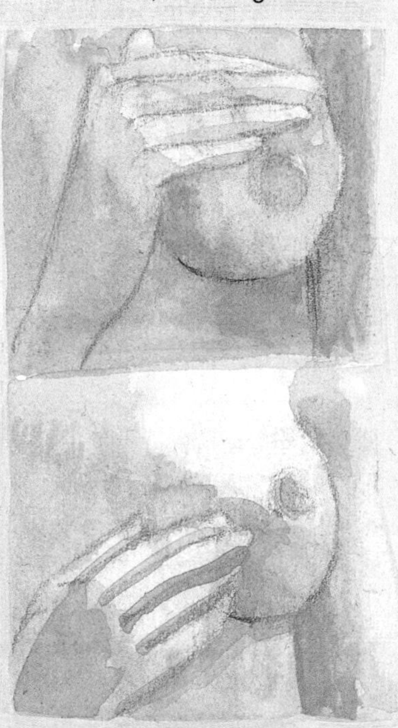

7. Examine the inner, upper half of the breast, pressing it against the rib cage and moving the fingers from the chest bone towards the centre of the breast. Feel over the nipple area, then move to the lower half.

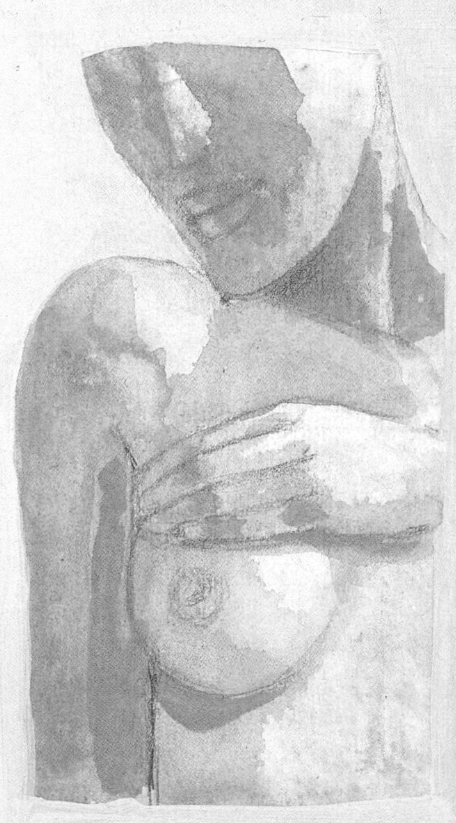

8. Move the pillow under the right shoulder and examine the right breast in the same way.

breasts can do in pregnancy. Apply moisturiser if you want, and relax. These marks fade with time.

Breasts need to be washed and dried carefully. The bigger breasted woman is prone to redness under the bosom, which can be due to moisture or chafing. A dusting with talc can be soothing and preventative. Also caused by chafing is what is known as "jogger's nipple", which occurs in men too. This can be eased with a rich moisturiser: cocoa butter, say, or peanut oil.

A rub, gel, or massage oil containing menthol or peppermint is particularly invigorating for tired legs, whether you're a pregnant woman or a bike courier.

THE IMPORTANCE OF SELF-EXAMINATION

As many as one in every 12 women in the United Kingdom may develop breast cancer. In North America, the ratio is one to ten. These are chilling statistics. Japanese women living in Japan have a far lower incidence of breast cancer, but this changes within a couple of generations of moving to the United States. However, American women moving to Japan appear, in a couple of generations, to reduce their chances of getting breast cancer significantly. This has led some cancer researchers to link consumption of meat and fat and environmental factors to the incidence of breast cancer.

But early detection helps nip this often fatal disease in the bud. Learn to examine your breasts, including the breast tissue that extends under the arms. If you notice discharge from the nipples, or a marked change in shape, you must see a doctor. Don't let the doctor put you off. If you feel he or she is not giving your worries proper attention, demand a referral. It is your body and you should know it better than your doctor does.

The last day or so of her period is the best time for a menstruating woman to examine her breasts - this is when they are smoothest. Don't panic if you find a lump. Not all lumps are malignant - about 80 per cent are caused by other reasons, such as tension which can cause knots in the breasts, just as it does in the back of the neck. But every sign of a lump must be investigated.

It is essential for the post-menopausal woman to continue to examine her breasts and to demand periodic mammography examinations, particularly if there is a family history of cancer.

THE ABDOMEN

The flab factor means the stomach is the part of the body many men and women feel least comfortable with, even though human beings could not exist without fat. Fat transports fat-soluble vitamins A, D, E and K from digestive tracts to body tissue, and it insulates the body. But most of us probably wonder if we really need quite so much insulation.

The best solutions to a rounded tummy are exercise and a balanced diet. But, like the breasts, the abdomen does respond to a bit of pampering. Richly moisturising body butters make the abdominal skin feel smooth and silky - apply them in gentle circular movements over the abdomen and you can also help ease aches that are lurking beneath.

Many women experience a bloated feeling and a swollen abdomen just before and during their periods. This can be due to water retention - it is quite common for the body to store up a couple of kilograms of weight prior to menstruation. Eating sensibly in the run up to your period and cutting down on coffee, tea and alcohol as well as getting plenty of sleep can significantly improve how you feel. Changes also happen to your skin at this time. As well as pimples on the face, you may experience allergic reactions elsewhere. The skin may be puffy and less able to absorb creams. It will return to normal after your period.

CHANGES DURING PREGNANCY

Tremendous changes happen as the abdomen swells with pregnancy. Not only does the body shape change radically, but the skin, all over the face and body, may switch from oily to dry and back again. It may darken, particularly around the nipples, dark lines may appear on the abdomen and freckles and moles can become more pronounced. These are all quite normal and disappear after birth. However, if freckles appear to be growing rapidly, consult your doctor.

Stretch marks are common, but can be minimised by massaging belly and bottom with rich lubricants, like almond oil and cocoa butter.

Bathing in warm, not hot, water, can be relaxing for pregnant women. Hawaiian women are told to let the abdomen sway gently in the water, so the baby becomes loosened and doesn't stick at birth.

WHAT ABOUT...

... BODY HAIR?

Women tend to be smoother skinned than men, which is why some women shave their legs and soften the skin by applying lotions in order to accentuate the gender difference. We remove the hair on our legs in several different ways: shaving, chemical depilation, permanent electrolysis, waxing or sugaring. Each method has its drawbacks. Shaving probably lasts the shortest time, depilation can smell rather pungent, electrolysis is uncomfortable, time consuming and can be expensive, and waxing and sugaring, particularly DIY versions, call for the guts to be able to swiftly pull off wax or sugaring strips against the direction of the hair growth.

The Egyptians removed body hair with a depilatory made from crushed birds' bones, mixed with fly spots, oil, sycamore gum and cucumber which was applied then stripped off like wax.

There's nothing like a foot massage or a pedicure to make you feel fabulous, especially if you've been on your feet all day.

... SHAVING?

Unless you use an electric razor, use shaving cream or soap to soften the hair and prevent the razor from snagging the skin. Always shave in the direction of hair growth to prevent hair from growing in. If you cut yourself while shaving in the bath, get out quickly as hot water increases the blood flow. When the bleeding stops, smear the area with wheatgerm oil. Shaving is quick, cheap and efficient; it does not increase hair growth but the skin will feel stubbly. Always moisturise the legs after shaving.

Regrowth occurs between one to four days later. Never shave on your face, the bikini line or round the nipples.

... WAXING?

Waxing can be carried out at a salon or at home - depending on your pain threshold! If you opt for home waxing, melt wax over a gentle heat and leave to cool to a bearable temperature. For the legs it is easiest to apply the wax to strips of gauze cut to the length of from knee to ankle; lightly dust the legs with talcum powder, smooth down the strips in the direction of hair growth and rip them up from the ankles to the knees. Waxing is unsuitable for delicate areas such as the face and breasts but is OK for legs, underarms and the bikini line. Regrowth takes about four weeks.

... SUGARING?

Sugaring is the method of hair removal most popular in North Africa and the Middle East. It has been winning fans in the West because its results are claimed to last longer than the more commonly used wax. Supporters also agree that sugaring is less painful than waxing. And cotton sugaring strips can be handwashed and reused over and over.

To sugar:

1. Warm sugaring in a basin of hot water until it is thin enough to spread.
2. Apply in the direction of hair growth to clean, dry skin, that has been lightly dusted with talc.
3. Cover with cotton strips.
4. Grit your teeth and pull the strips against the direction of hair growth. Legs should stay hair free for several weeks.

... VARICOSE VEINS?

Those with any varicose veins should avoid sugaring and waxing and may find the razor less aggravating. Varicose veins are unsightly and can pose serious health hazards. They can show up during pregnancy or of their own accord at any time. Unfortunately, they are caused by gravity. The blood vessels in the legs are under continuous strain because the blood flow back to the heart operates against gravity; if the valves in the veins fail to work properly, the veins begin to bulge where the incoming and backflowing blood meets. They become blue in colour and twist into permanent knots which can, in severe instances, cause ulcers and thrombosis. You cannot prevent varicose veins, but you can stop them from getting worse.

DO get plenty of exercise. Any exercise that involves the legs, such as walking, swimming or cycling, is especially recommended for easing discomfort.

DO eat healthily - foods high in fibre such as whole grains and raw vegetables help counteract constipation which can increase the discomfort of varicose veins.

DO give your legs a regular massage, massaging, as always, up towards the heart.

SKIN-CARE GUIDE

SKIN TYPE	DRY	SENSITIVE	NORMAL	MATURE	ACNE PRONE
SOAP	Aloe Soap	Aloe Soap	Any Glycerine or Textured Soap	Aloe Soap	Vitamin E Soap Wheatgerm Body Bar
BATH / SHOWER	Orange Cream Bath Relaxing Bath Oil Reviving Shower Oil Bath Oil	Bath Oil Foaming Bath Oil	Any Fruit Bath and Shower Gel Milk Bath Aromatherapy Relaxing Bath Oil Reviving Shower Oil	Orange Cream Bath Oil Relaxing Bath Oil	Any Fruit Bath and Shower Gel
EXFOLIATION	Rice Bran Body Scrub Skin Sponge	Rice Bran Body Scrub	Loofah or Skin Sponge Marmalade Body Scrub	Rice Bran Body Scrub Sponge	Skin Sponge Marmalade Body Scrub
SPECIAL TREATS	Massage Oil Rich Massage Lotion Mango Body Butter Cocoa Butter Stick Cocoa Butter Hand and Body Lotion Aromatherapy Massage Oils	Unfragranced Lotion Baby Lotion Aloe Gel	Relaxing Moisture Cream Cocoa Butter Hand and Body Lotion Avocado Body Butter Aloe Lotion Dewberry 5 Oils Lotion White Musk Lotion Ananya Lotion	Cocoa Butter Hand and Body Lotion Mango Body Butter Cocoa Butter Stick	Aloe Gel Unfragranced Lotion

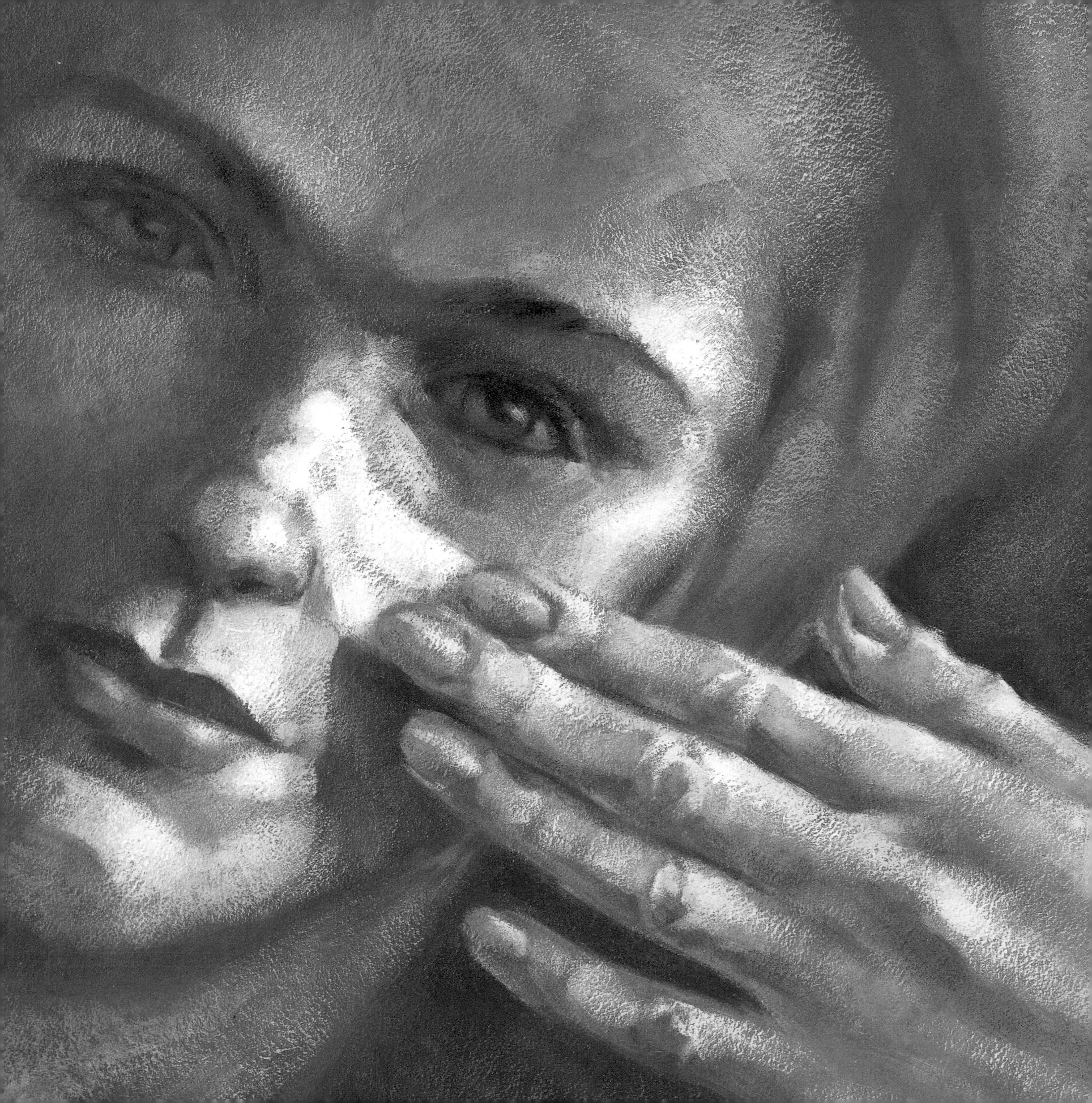

FACE

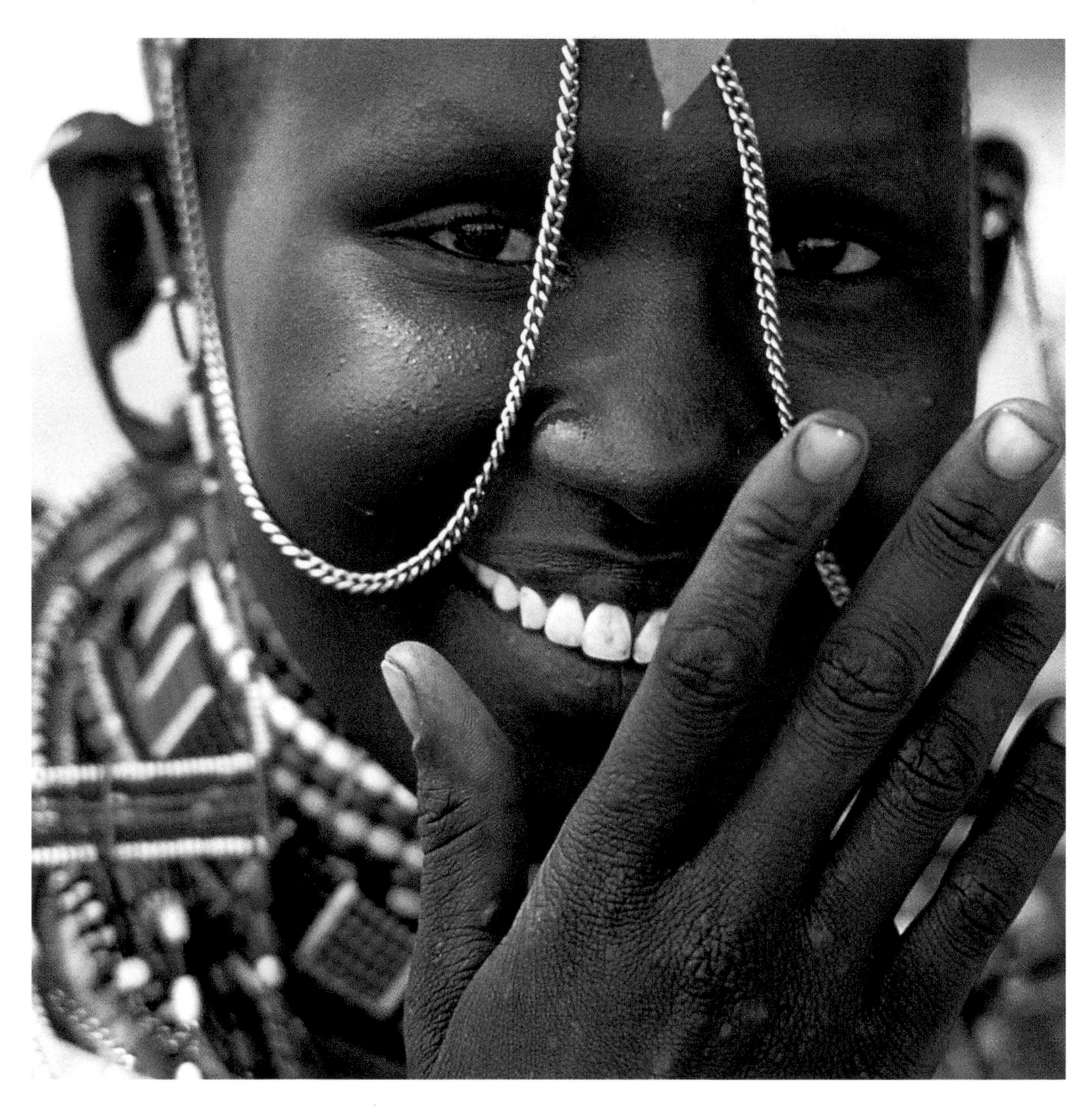

The Maasai in Kenya believe that true beauty is defined by your attitude to life rather than your physical assets.

face

Whether we like it or not, the face provides those around us with information on our sex, age and health as well as our emotional well-being, long before we choose to open our mouths and talk.

The face is capable of around 7,000 different expressions. The main expressions of emotion such as love, fear, anger and sadness appear to be universal. Studies designed to test how tribal and industrial cultures interpret facial expressions show little variance. We all seem to agree on what we mean when we smile or grimace, regardless of our culture.

We certainly get a lifetime's worth of practice. Psychologists have found that babies can discern distinct emotions in a mother's face just 36 hours after birth. By the age of two weeks, they can tell the difference between their mother's face and a stranger's. One of the reasons for this proficiency lies in the brain, which sets aside a section specifically for recognising faces.

The art of reading what's in a face is an old one. As early as 2,000 BC Babylonian diviners were interpreting the meaning of a newborn's head for society at large. The tendency to leap to conclusions based solely on a person's face was turned into an art form in the 17th century, when divining someone's personality by their facial characteristics became a popular pastime. People would read the moles on a face or the lines in a forehead and then make a character assessment. In the 19th century a popular science was phrenology: the diagnosis of a person's mental ability according to the shape of their skull and face.

The face is the body's communications centre, not only housing the eyes, nose and mouth (with the ears close by), but revealing our thoughts and feelings to strangers with flushes, blushes, frowns and smiles.

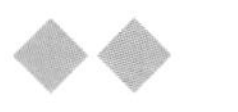

All over the world, ideas of what is considered beautiful are as different as night and day. And the face is often the starting point. What is beautiful in one culture, can be quite the opposite in another. Take the Nuba of Southeastern Sudan, for example. The process of meeting Nuba standards of beauty begins at birth. The top of a baby's skull is rubbed with oil and then with either red or yellow ochre, depending on its kin group. Later, when the child reaches puberty, scars are cut into the face. They are primarily for reasons of beauty, but the scars above the eyes are also considered to enhance eyesight, while those on the temples inhibit headaches. Contrast this with Western society's view of beauty based on young, smooth, wrinkle-free skin - an ideal perpetuated by the mainstream cosmetics industry which builds a dream of perfect skin that lasts forever. The time has come to redefine beauty and to question the cosmetics industry which presents us with a huge variety of disguises, encouraging us to present a standardised version of ourselves by redrawing our features, redefining our shapes, evening out our blemishes. The ideal of beauty before us is a mask behind which we can hide. The cosmetics industry survives on our feelings of inadequacy.

Beauty is personal and individual; it is also holistic. Taking care of your health and skin is far more important than trying to change a feature that doesn't quite match up to current trends. Beauty begins with fitness and well being - you cannot expect a handsome painting if you maltreat the canvas.

Jojoba oil is great for dry skin. Cleanse face and moisten with warm water. Smooth on a few drops of oil and splash with cold water. Pat dry with tissues.

The Suya of Brazil use ear plugs and lip discs to emphasise the aspects of the face they find most important. For the Suya, to hear something well is to understand it intellectually. The ears are pierced at puberty, which is the time of life when children are expected to become rational beings - truly to understand their world and make moral judgements. Lip discs reflect the importance of speech to the Kayapo Indians of Brazil. Male babies have their lips pierced soon after birth with discs that get progressively larger. Within the men's house it is the ability to speak eloquently in public which denotes power and influence.

A sparkle in the eyes, or a clear complexion immediately denotes health to an observer. In fact, the skin's condition is a combination of many factors ranging from the immutable - including our sex, genetic heritage, the hormonal changes we experience throughout our lives and, if we are women, our monthly menstrual cycles - to the variable.

While we cannot alter the kind of skin we were born with and the hormonal programme that will decide whether or not we are likely, among other things, to suffer from acne, we can all alter our diet. The old adage that you are what you eat is truer than many of us would like to admit. Many of us could also change the stress levels experienced on a day to day basis and our environment.

The skin on the face and hands is exposed to the elements more than skin located elsewhere, which explains why it ages more quickly. The effects of increasing levels of pollution, especially in the cities in which many of us live, contribute to the skin's texture and lack of clarity. So too do cigarette smoke and central heating and air conditioning systems that dry the skin out. In an age when air travel means many of us can switch continents and weather systems with ease our skin bears the brunt of climactic changes as it veers from hot to cold, and from wet to dry.

YOUR SKIN AND . . .

... THE SUN The sun is the worst factor in skin damage. The face, neck and hands are first to show signs of ageing because they are most often exposed to the sun. The sun damages elastin and dries out the skin every time it is exposed. Damage is cumulative - it happens every day and you have to pay sometime. However, proper skin care can ensure you pay later rather than sooner. A broad spectrum sunscreen is essential every day - no matter what the weather.

... TOBACCO Smoking hastens skin ageing: the skin of smokers is known to wrinkle and age years sooner than that of non-smokers. The act of puffing encourages wrinkling around the eyes and mouth, while benzopyrene, a substance present in tobacco smoke, inhibits the body's absorption of vitamin C, thus damaging healthy collagen. So add cosmetic damage to the health risks as one more very forceful reason for giving up smoking.

... POLLUTION City air is also detrimental to healthy skin. The dirt, smog and grease of the city must be kept at bay with a regular and effective cleansing routine.

... ALCOHOL Alcohol contains none of the vitamins or minerals essential for cell growth. It robs the body of B vitamins, and ruptures blood vessels causing a network of broken veins on the face. Cut it down - or out!

... LIFESTYLE Too little sleep equals tired grey skin: maximum cell renewal goes on while you sleep. Living life in the fast lane can also play havoc with the appearance of your skin. So can negative emotions such as fear, anger or anxiety. That's why we often have an outbreak of spots when a big day is approaching. Try to learn to relax and take time for yourself - it will show in your skin.

For some people, the skin is almost like a litmus test, informing them by its reactions when they are heading for a sensory or emotional overload. That's a valuable warning sign, especially in an age when we are more sensitive than ever to the ways in which the nervous system suffers at the hands of outside stimuli.

Now how would you go about addressing such a warning sign? Perhaps by making sure you eat well, getting plenty of sleep, maybe exercising regularly and, in the long term, learning how to handle stress better. The skin is clearly a good teacher. And by understanding how it works and how to look after it, you are clearly doing your whole system a big favour.

Watch for fresheners or toners that list alcohol as an ingredient. It may be an effective astringent, but is harsh and unsuitable for sensitive or dry skin.

THE BASICS

STRUCTURE

We've already analysed the structure of the skin in the previous chapter, and established that everyone's skin is basically the same. But despite this essential similarity, the skin tends to work in different ways on different people. Some have extra eccrine glands on the forehead, causing them to sweat more profusely; others may experience an excess of sebum along the T-zone (the forehead, nose and chin area); still others may not produce quite enough. So everyone's skin type and needs are quite different. Not only do women experience hormonal changes during their adolescence and menopause that alter the texture of their skin and its sebum production, many also witness changes on a monthly basis that are tied to their menstrual cycles. Skin is also affected by the seasons, adapting naturally to the weather.

Though the main difference between darker skins and paler ones is the amount of activated melanin present, colour can affect the assessment of skin types. Black skins tend to look oilier simply because oil reflects better off a dark surface. Darker-skinned people may therefore assess their skins as oily and choose cosmetic formulations that are too harsh and degreasing. If you have dark skin and experience an irritant reaction from preparations for oily skins, change to a gentler formulation for normal skin and see if the condition improves.

SKINTYPING

Traditionally, types of skin have been divided into three groups - dry, normal and oily - to help identify general characteristics and focus on a proper skin-care regime. Many people do not fall into any one of these groups, but have a combination skin. More importantly, perhaps, the skin rarely remains in the same condition for long everyone's skin type changes from time to time. Do not think of your skin type as etched in stone and be prepared to tailor your skin-care regime as required. By ignoring a change in the skin's condition, a problem can be exacerbated.

Skintyping is based on measuring the amount of sebum, the natural oil produced in the the skin. A normal skin will produce just enough to protect the uppermost layer - the stratum corneum - and keep it supple without interfering with the natural process of shedding dead skin cells.

Oily skin, typified by a greasy film on the surface, is caused by overproductive sebaceous glands and often by an excessive number of sebaceous glands in the T-zone. These produce a thick acidic coating which can clog pores and encourage the development of blackheads and acne.

In dry skin, which often appears rough and flaky, the "cement" that holds cells together sometimes fails to break up on time, causing dead cells to stick to the skin's surface and curl at the edges, encouraging moisture loss from the underlying layers of cells. Dry skin can also suffer from a lack of sebum production, which creates further moisture loss.

The Egyptians and Mesopotamians, were famous for their cleanliness. They used scented oils to cleanse their faces, but relied on a blend of bullock's bile, ostrich eggs, oil, dough, refined natron, hantet resin and fresh milk when it came to problem complexions.

THE DAILY GRIND

Finding the right skin-care regime is a combination of focusing on the right products for your skin type and choosing those you enjoy using. Remember, as your skin and environment change over the years, so should the skin products.

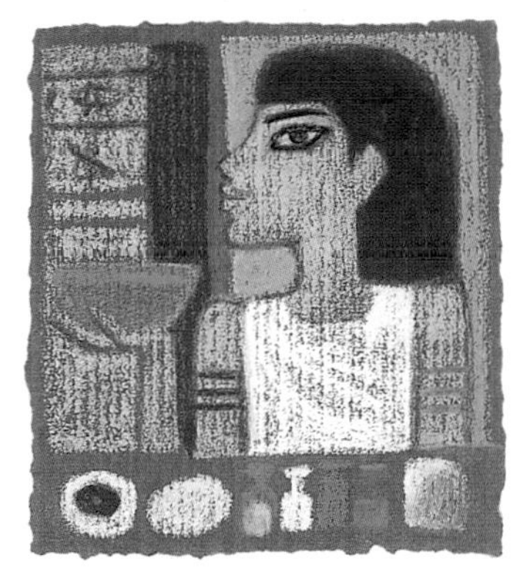

Today there are as many kinds of products as there are types of skin. Every skin-care guru, actress and supermodel has a patented formula for perfect skin, usually within a magic bottle. The reality is a lot simpler - and a lot cheaper!

Despite advertising campaigns to the contrary, there are no instant solutions for problem skin. The only way to improve your skin is to treat it well. Three simple steps - cleansing, toning and moisturising twice a day, every day - will help keep skin healthy and protect it from the stresses of daily life. But remember, because skin renewal takes between 21 and 20 days, you must follow a new skin care routine for at least three weeks before results can be seen.

STEP 1 - CLEANSE

To the uninitiated, dirt is dirt: the end result of a hard day's work. In fact, it is a mixture of sebum, dead skin cells, dirt, dust, salt and urea produced by sweat, bacteria and make-up. Without thorough cleansing, it would take about 25 days for this mess to wear off, never mind the additional dirt built up over that period. No wonder cleansing is probably the one beauty ritual that has been faithfully stuck to through the ages.

Unless skin is thoroughly cleansed every night, it will look dull and lifeless, and will be more prone to spots and blackheads from clogged pores.

Water alone cannot clean the skin. It needs a detergent of some sort to form an emulsion that will lift dirt up off the face so that it can be wiped or washed off. The key to effective cleansing is getting the balance right. Too strong or abrasive a formula will strip the skin of its acid mantle, too mild a product won't do the job properly.

Skin-care products were popular in post-Roman Britain even when cosmetics were banned, while facial ointments of hog's lard, honey and beeswax were used to uncertain effect in Elizabethan times. Even women in the 20th century have used deadly compounds in a vain attempt to improve their skin. Klintho Cream used in the early 1900s in the United States was banned by the government because it contained mercury.

WASHING WELL

• Avoid using very hot or very cold water on all skin types as extremes of temperature can damage tiny blood vessels and help to cause thread veins.

• Face flannels may also prove too abrasive and irritating as they can retain some of the detergent silicates with which they were laundered unless rinsed very thoroughly.

• The best way of washing your face is to use your fingers, a well-rinsed sponge or a soft complexion brush. Black skins shed their outer layers slightly more quickly than white ones, and they particularly benefit from a gentle but thorough scrub with a soft complexion brush.

SOAP

Soap use can be traced to before AD 200. Essentially a combination of animal or vegetable fats combined with alkali, salt and water, soap is designed to strip the skin of all dirt and oil. Unfortunately, it is also harsh and alkaline. Though the skin will eventually return to its proper pH, that can take between a few minutes and several hours, leaving the skin more susceptible to attack from harmful bacteria. To make such an effective cleanser less abrasive, soap has been host over the years to other ingredients designed to soothe or calm the skin.

Superfatted soaps, for example, contain extra fat to help protect dry and sensitive skin, while oatmeal is sometimes included for its soothing properties. Face soaps often incorporate milder ingredients, such as glycerine and vitamin E to keep the skin from reacting, while "soapless" soaps, such as those made with milk and cornstarch, are specifically designed for sensitive skins. Oily skins may benefit from gentle soaps, although it is important not to stimulate overproduction of sebum by stripping the epidermis bare of its protective coating.

Opinion has varied over the years on the importance of water in the cleansing ritual. For many, the appeal of soap as a cleanser is connected with the invigorating, pleasurable action of flushing the residue from the face with water. Washing with warm water will help to loosen dirt more quickly. If you do use a soap bar on the face, make sure it is gentle and that you rinse carefully with water before applying a moisturiser. (Remember - avoid water that is very hot or very cold.)

CLEANSING CREAMS

The first recorded cleansing cream was created by the Greek physician Galen in AD 150. A simple formulation of beeswax, olive oil and water or rose water, it was described as a cold cream because it conveyed a cooling sensation when applied to the face. Cleansing creams and cold creams are oil-in-water emulsions which clean the skin by dissolving the detritus in oil, which is then removed by wiping it off the face. Make-up should always be removed with a cream or lotion make-up cleanser. Most make-up is wax or oil based and needs a wax/oil combination to remove it. However, as it leaves a greasy film on the skin, this too must be thoroughly removed. People who clean their skins with soap and water are following an excellent routine, provided they first cleanse off their make-up with a cream or lotion.

WASH-OFF CREAMS AND GELS

Wash-off cream lotions and gels combine the deep cleansing properties of creams with the efficiency and revitalising effects of soap-and-water rituals. Water based and made with synthetic detergents that emulsify on contact with the skin, they are designed to wash off with ease. These cleansers treat the skin gently, leaving much of the acid mantle (the mixture of sebum and water) intact, and usually irritate the skin less than soap. Soapless formulations are ideal for people who like to use water on their skin as part of their cleansing routine but are unable to use soap.

In Finland, smart Scandinavians use Honeyed Beeswax, Almond and Jojoba Oil Cleanser on their faces to protect them from the cold.

THE NATURAL CLEANSING DEBATE

The use of natural ingredients, especially fruit or alpha-hydroxy acids, as active cleansers is a current focus in skin-care research. Used in effective concentrations, they are excellent exfoliants. The Body Shop's founder Anita Roddick noticed a variant of this principle at work in Sri Lanka, where she saw women massaging their faces with fresh pineapple. Further research revealed that the pineapple contained an enzyme called bromelin which encourages dead skin cells to slough off. This gentle exfoliation helps to speed up the process of cell renewal, leading to a healthier skin tone. That's the secret behind Pineapple Facial Wash.

STEP 2 - FRESHEN

Despite appearances that suggest the contrary, no two skin fresheners are ever alike. Distillations and infusions of natural ingredients ranging from cucumbers and tomatoes to honey and elderflower, as well as flower waters and toners have been used for centuries to refresh the skin. Although some simple waters, such as rose water, are used as ingredients in other products, many can be used on their own, bringing their own special properties to the three-step skin-care process. Often used to double-cleanse the skin, ridding the epidermis of excess oil or the final traces of grime and make-up, fresheners can also soothe and soften the skin, especially in combination with gentle oils. Elderflower water, for instance, soothes and tones the skin. The Body Shop adds castor oil to its Elderflower Eye Gel to soften and protect the delicate skin around the eyes.

TIP: QUICK SPRITZ

Cool down with refreshing cucumber water in a pump spray bottle. Keep it in the fridge and use it on your face for a quick pick-me-up on a hot day.

Some fresheners with astringent properties are thought to shrink pore size. Be warned - no product can close them completely. Pores on the face tend to be larger than pores elsewhere on the body because the sebaceous glands are larger. Excess sebum production during the teenage years and the development of blackheads can also stretch pores which cannot return to normal. Astringent fresheners only mask their size by slightly irritating the skin cells around the pores and encouraging them to inflame, thereby making the neighbouring pores look smaller. Unfortunately this effect is cosmetic and does not last.

Cosmetics queen Harriet Hubbard Ayer wrote in 1899, "The longer I remained in the laboratory manufacturing cosmetics, the less I felt the average woman should use them, and the more respect I had for scrubbing brushes, soap and water, without other aids, at least for women under 30."

STEP 3 - MOISTURISE

A moisturiser forms a protective film over the skin - holding the skin's natural moisture in. Moisture is the most important aspect of skin care and keeps skin smooth and supple.

THE KEY TO HEALTHY LOOKING SKIN

Each cell in our body is 80 per cent water, while the moisture content of the air we breathe is only 1 per cent of its total. Humans are therefore constantly losing moisture to the atmosphere; our only protection is the epidermis and its acid mantle.

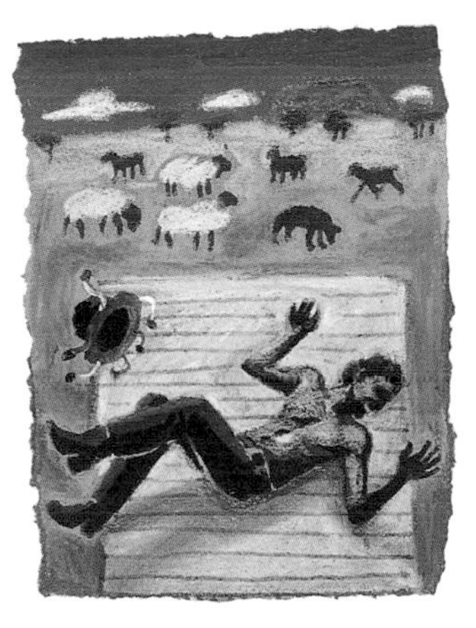

Lanolin straight from the sheep has remarkable skin-softening properties - it is rumoured that sheep shearers in Australia roll on the shearing table at the end of the day.

Moisturisers are particularly important for people with dry skin who suffer from low sebum production. If the body is not able to produce an effective acid mantle (a thin film of oil and sweat), the skin will be left unprotected, allowing the skin cells on the surface to dry and curl at the sides, encouraging even more moisture loss from the layers beneath. Adding a topical moisturiser creates an artificial barrier that combines with the sebum on the skin and keeps the moisture where it belongs.

Many moisturisers also have a cosmetic effect. When the moisture content in the epidermis is enhanced, skin cells tend to swell, helping to plump out fine wrinkles and making the skin look fresher and younger.

TIP: SEALING IN THE MOISTURE

Apply moisturiser to slightly damp skin in order to seal in water. Never forget the throat in all face treatments - the neck shows the same signs of ageing as the face.

Not everyone needs to wear a moisturiser all the time, or indeed all over their face. It is important to treat the parts of the face individually. An oily T-zone, for instance, may not require an extra layer of protection while its neighbouring cheeks may be significantly drier. Do remember that sebum production slows down during the cold winter months, often requiring a switch to a richer moisturiser. People who live and work in moisture-sapping artificially heated and air-conditioned atmospheres are prone to dry skin and will notice that their skin needs an extra boost of moisture to maintain its balance.

Plain water is great for healthy-looking skin and pores, and a flower water is even more refreshing. Strong jets of water, for example showers or jacuzzis, are both cleansing and relaxing. But remember, those with sensitive skins should avoid very hot or very cold water because extremes of temperature can burst blood vessels and cause thread veins.

Apply moisturiser using gentle upward and circular movements on the forehead, from chin to eyes, and up the "smile" line from mouth to nose.

Many different ingredients have been used since Galen combined beeswax, olive oil and rose water for his cold cream. Lanolin - an oily mixture extracted from a sheep's fleece - is similar in structure to human sebum and has been used to great effect for years, as have a variety of vegetable oils from almond to jojoba. Avocado oil, rich in vitamins B,C and E, has good skin penetration properties and is therefore an ideal base for moisturisers for both oily and dry skins.

But whatever the ingredient, the premise remains the same: to combine oil or fat with water in a compound that will spread on the face and lightly coat the skin.

FACT: JOJOBA OIL - THE COSMETIC OIL OF THE CENTURY

Though it was technically neither an oil nor wax, spermaceti, obtained from the sperm whale, was a great skin softener. First used in cosmetic creams in 1780, it caused the indiscriminate slaughter of thousands of whales until the sperm whale was declared an endangered species. In the late 1970s, jojoba oil was found to have similar qualities - but with one vital difference. Jojoba oil is extracted from the nuts of the jojoba shrub which grows wild in the arid deserts of Mexico and the Southern United States. Just one acre of jojoba bushes yields the same amount of oil as 30 sperm whales. Jojoba oil is also much better for cosmetic purposes because it is self-adjusting and suitable for all skins. That's why Jojoba Moisture Cream is a superb light moisturiser which is readily absorbed into all skin types.

A LITTLE EXTRA HELP ...

When choosing the moisturiser that is right for you, don't get lost in the sea of miracle claims and false promises - more have been made in this area of the cosmetics industry than in any other. Read the labels carefully and decide what you want out of your moisture cream. Here are some ingredients that play an active role in making the skin look good:

• Natural moisturising factors or NMFs are a collection of compounds (found naturally in both the epidermis and dermis) that improve the degree of moisturisation in the cells by helping to hold water inside the epidermis. Adding manufactured NMFs to a moisturiser can improve the formula's efficiency considerably.

• Vitamin A is one of the most important vitamins for healthy skin. It is particularly useful for relieving dry skin because some experts believe it reduces the hardening and flattening of skin cells in the epidermis. The Body Shop Carrot Moisture Cream contains beta carotene, a natural source of vitamin A which helps keep skin healthy and supple.

• Vitamin E, commonly recognised as a free radical scavenger, hinders the oxidisation process in the skin which can harm the cell structure and speed the ageing process (for more on this, see the Ageing chapter). Vitamin E is used in the medical world in the treatment of herpes and burns and can also help the skin absorb other ingredients. We used it in our Vitamin E Cream and Rich Night Cream with Vitamin E to promote healthy skin and leave it soft and supple.

NIGHT CREAMS

Night creams are often richer formulations of a regular moisturiser with a high oil content designed to replenish the skin while it is not being assailed by pollutants on all sides. As the skin tends to grow more quickly and does

DIY FACIAL

You will need: Cream or Liquid Cleanser, Boiled Water and Bowl, Cotton Wool, Tissues, Facial Scrub, Face Mask, Moisturiser, Towel

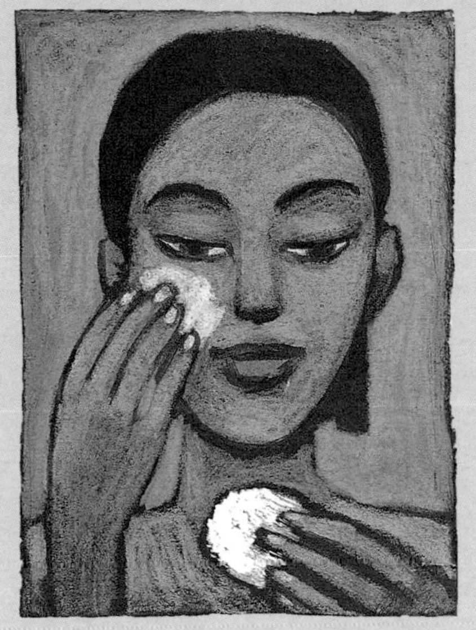

CLEANSE
Massage in cleanser using firm, circular movements over your face and neck. Blot off with a tissue or gently wipe with cotton wool.
Be careful not to drag skin around the eyes.

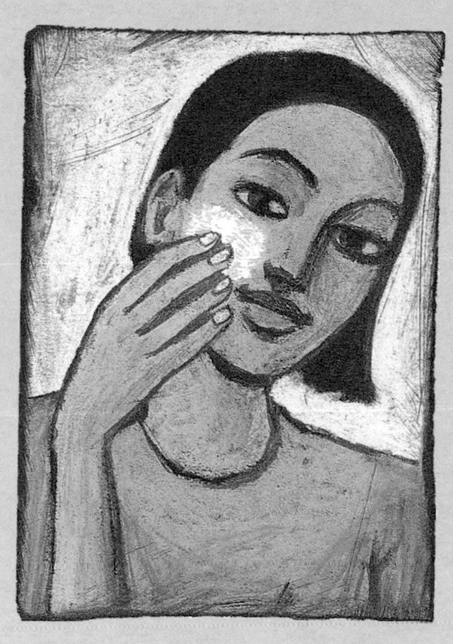

SCRUB
Exfoliate or scrub your skin to slough off dead skin cells and leave a healthy glow. Gently rub a facial scrub over your skin, avoiding the delicate eye area, then rinse off and pat dry.

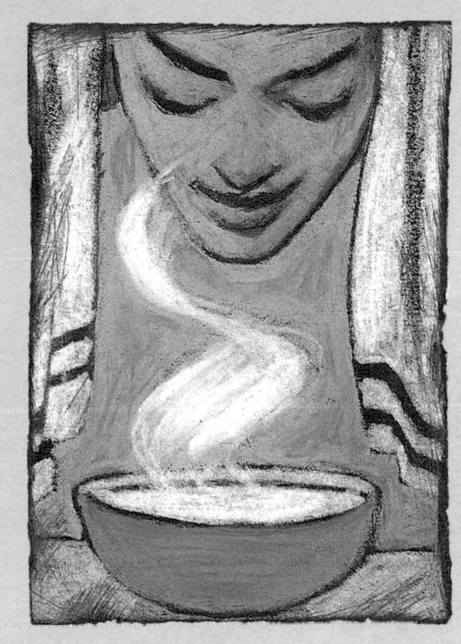

STEAM
Steam to open up pores and release grime and make-up. Pour boiled water into a bowl, hold face about 10 inches over it and cover head with a towel. Wait 5 minutes for dry skin, 10 for oily skin. Pat face dry with clean tissues.

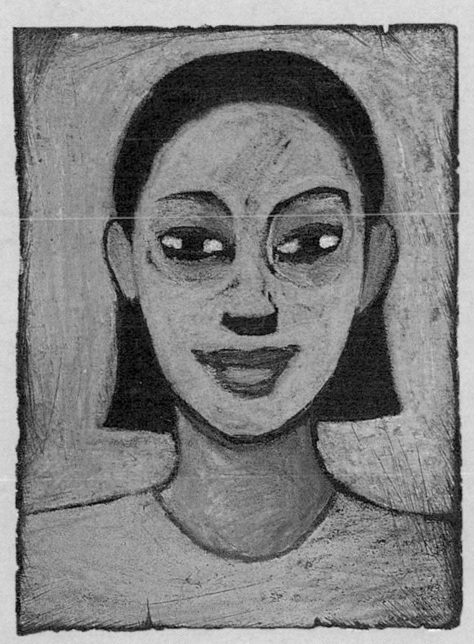

MASK
Choose a face mask to suit your skin: deep cleansing for normal to oily; hydrating for dry and sensitive. Smooth on the mask, avoiding the eyes and mouth.
Leave on for recommended time. Rinse off.

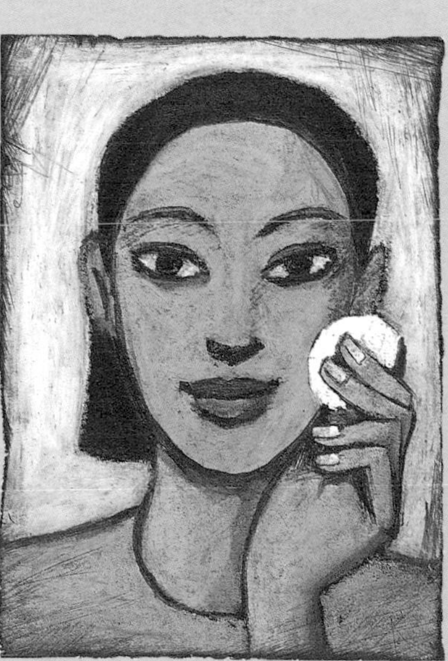

FRESHEN
Gently smooth cotton wool soaked in skin freshener over your face to take off the last traces of your face mask. Leave to dry.
Your skin will feel cool and refreshed.

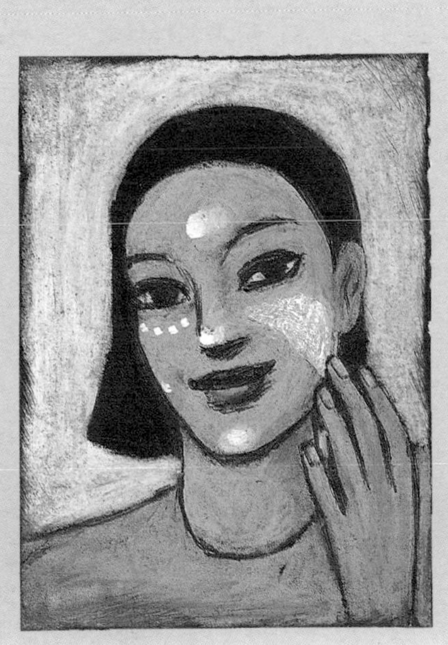

MOISTURISE
Moisturisers act as an effective barrier to cold weather, the wind, pollution and central heating and help prevent the skin's natural moisture from escaping. Dot moisturiser sparingly on your face and neck and gently rub in.

BLUE CORN

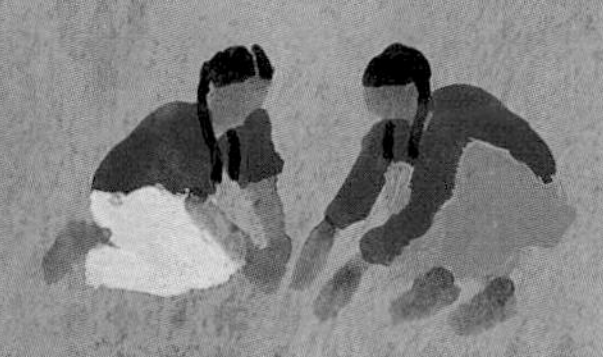

For the Indian societies who live along the Rio Grande in Arizona, New Mexico and Utah, maize has been the main crop for centuries.

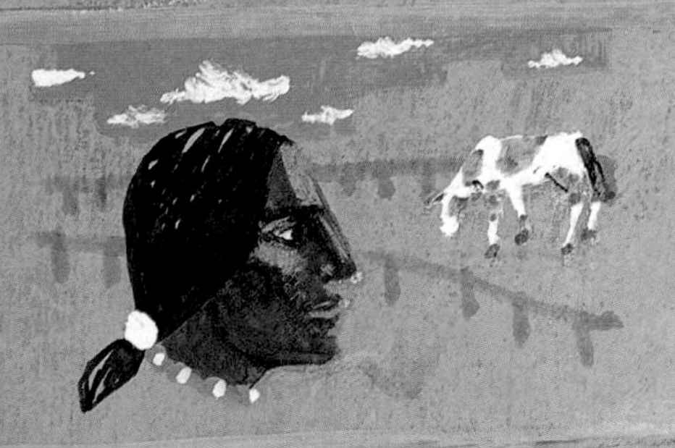

The Body Shop's Blue Corn is grown and ground by the Santa Ana Pueblo Indians of New Mexico. In the 1980s, the Tribal Government committed to a long term plan to restore the tribe's agricultural traditions. The result was a tribal farm sited on 100 acres of prime land where the Indians grow alfalfa and vegetables, as well as blue corn.

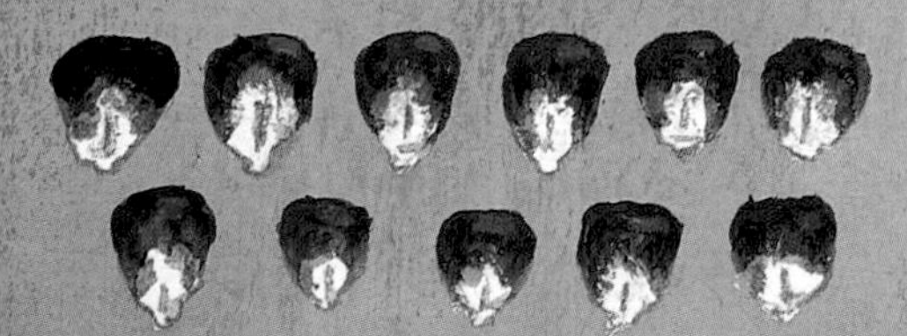

Kernels of blue corn are roasted, then ground to a powder (atole) which is the basis of The Body Shop's Blue Corn Scrub Mask. The proteins extracted from blue corn form a light moisturiser ideal for oily skins.

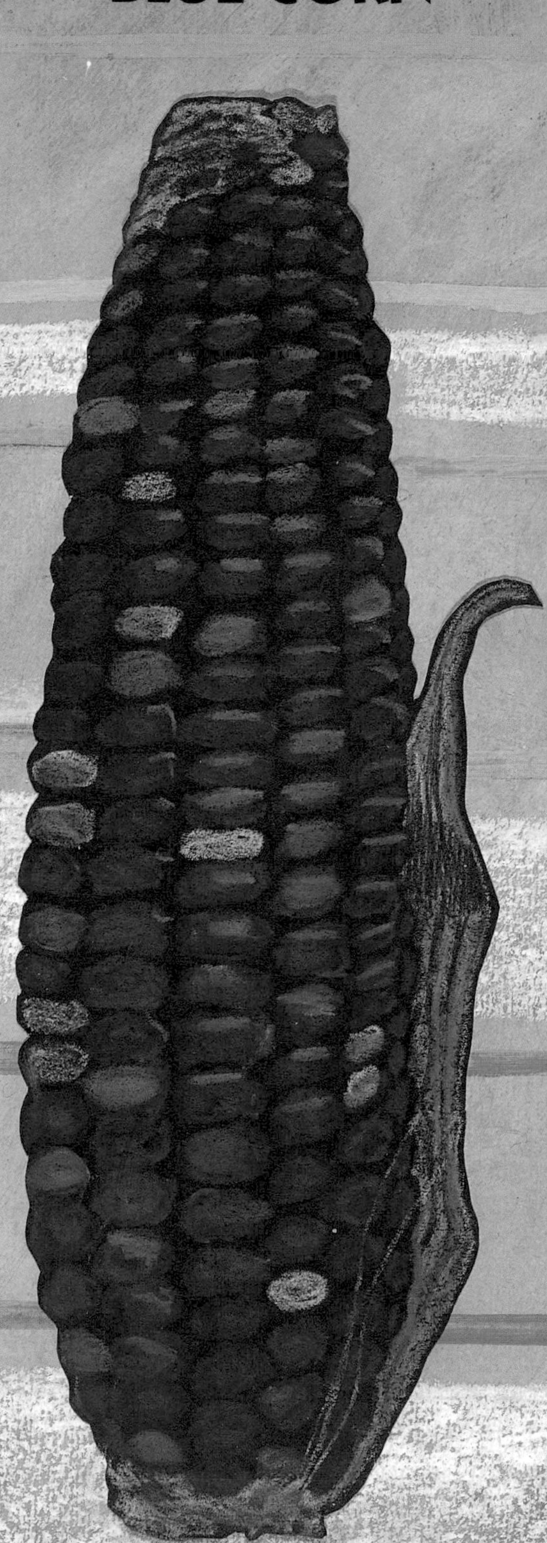

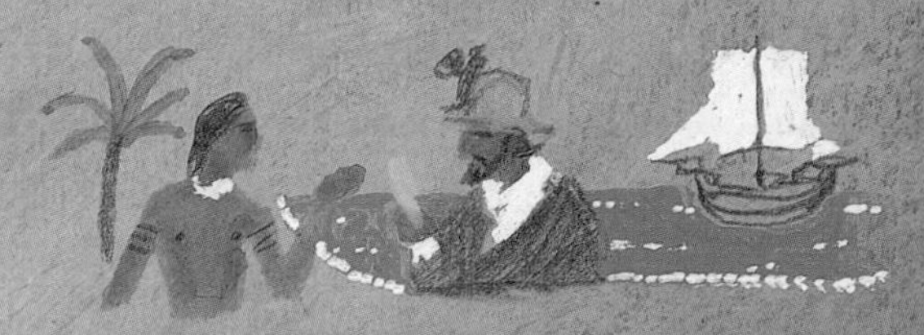

Christopher Columbus was introduced to corn in the late 1400s by the Indians in Cuba, and he in turn introduced it to Europe on his return.

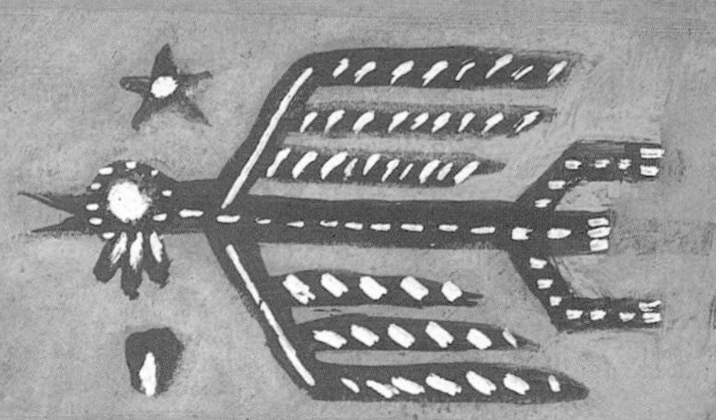

According to legend, the Navajo discovered corn when a turkey hen came flying from the direction of the morning star and shook from her feathers an ear of blue corn.

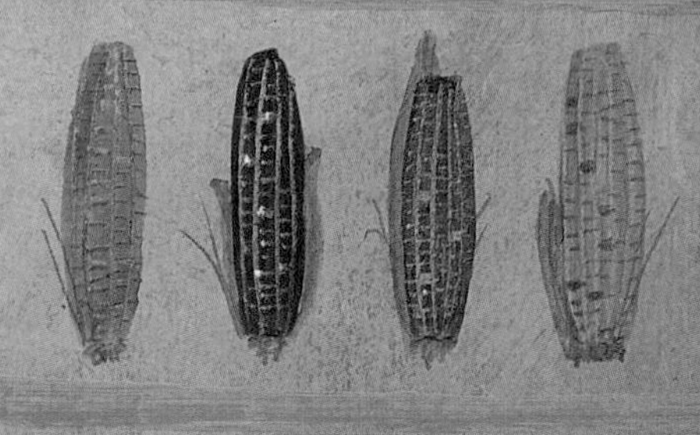

Blue corn is central to the Hopi creation story. When people came into the world, they all chose various colours of corn. The Hopi chose blue, the shortest, most resilient kind, meaning that they would endure while others fell by the wayside.

most of its repair work at night it makes sense to provide a moisturising product when the skin can use it most effectively. However, although particularly useful for drier or older skins, these creams should be used with care by those with oilier skin. Rich Night Cream with Vitamin E is an ideal evening moisturiser, or use a regular moisturiser enriched with a natural oil, such as wheatgerm, carrot or jojoba.

To get the most from a scrub, try a facial steam first. Cover head with towel, lean over a bowl of hot water for 5 minutes. Camomile in the water will relax you.

RECIPE FOR GREAT LOOKING SKIN ...

- Drink lots of water to flush out your system. Use only sparkling or still mineral water or diluted fruit juice.
- The much maligned face flannel is an effective and inexpensive exfoliating tool. But make sure your flannel is scrupulously clean and free from any washing detergent.
- Keep your skin protected against the sun and wind. Always use a broad spectrum (UVA and B) sunscreen, no matter what time of year; cloudy days can be deceptive and the sun always damages your skin.
- Always keep skin well moisturised in cold weather to prevent drying and chapping.
- Watch out for central heating, it can dry out the air and lift moisture from the skin. Keep the thermostat as low as possible and place small bowls of water by the radiators to act as humidifiers.
- Do not wear make-up all the time. Your skin needs fresh air and a constant mask of make-up stops dead cells flaking off easily.
- Take lots of exercise - this keeps the circulation working well and the skin well fed and glowing.
- Make sure you have enough sleep. Apart from making you feel good - and when you feel good you look good - cell division and skin tissue renewal is most active then.
- Keep alcohol intake to a minimum. Alcohol dehydrates your whole body.
- Try to avoid touching your face when you have blemishes - this spreads bacteria and hinders natural recovery.
- Try to relax - tension can make skin oilier and screwing up your face spreads wrinkles. Remember, it takes far fewer muscles to smile than it does to frown!

MORE THAN BASIC

EXFOLIATION

A simple and effective beauty treatment, exfoliation artificially encourages the gentle removal of surface skin cells. The body sloughs off up to 500,000,000 dead skin cells daily as part of its 28-day cycle - by actively assisting this process we help cell renewal.

Exfoliating actually lifts off the top layer of dead skin cells, dirt and sebum, revealing a new layer of skin cells beneath. This stimulates the blood circulation in the dermis, which in turn feeds the newborn skin cells more efficiently and rids the area of waste products. As the skin ages, the production of new cells slows down, often leading to dull skin tone and uneven texture. Removing the top layer of skin can accelerate cell production and help smooth the surface layer.

TIP: CLEANSE 'N' SCRUB

Add The Body Shop's Japanese Washing Grains to a cleanser to make it more exfoliating; it's particularly good with Honey and Beeswax and Almond Oil Cleanser. It's ideal as a deep cleansing scrub for sensitive skin.

TIP: GRAPEFRUIT AND OATMEAL SCRUB

Blend the juice of a grapefruit with three to four tablespoons of oatmeal into a fine paste and smooth it onto the face. Leave for 15 minutes and remove with warm water, working the scrub over the face. Rinse off with cool water.

THE EXPERT OPINION

Regular exfoliation has become the siren call of anti-ageing experts and dermatologists alike. Until recently, exfoliation was recommended for use once a week only for those with dry skins. Some experts now believe that regular exfoliation every other day not only encourages cell renewal, but may solve the root problem of dry skin, which is that the skin is unable to slough itself off because the "intercellular cement" will not break down. Regular exfoliation regardless of skin type also thickens the epidermal layer, creating a better skin tone.

Shape a piece of cheesecloth or butter muslin to fit face and front of neck, cutting holes for eyes, nose and mouth. Immerse it in warm oil - jojoba or apricot kernel - or honey for dry skins. Try milk or iced astringent lotion such as Orange Flower Water or White Grape Skin Tonic for oily and dull normal skins. Place mask over face and neck, with eye pads over eyes and leave for 10-20 mins. Carefully peel off mask and wipe skin clean. Spray face with freshener and let it settle for a few minutes before applying make-up.

SKIN-AGEING PROFILE

The basic principles of skin care don't change over the years. But to maintain a glowing, healthy complexion, you must adapt to your skin's needs as it grows older. Simply assess them and adapt your routine as necessary.

TWENTIES

• Damage done early on prepares our skin for later life. It is vital in our teens and twenties to protect the skin from sun. Always use a broad spectrum sunscreen in the daytime.
• Establish a skin-care routine in this most stable of skin years. Cleanse, freshen and moisturise, twice a day, everyday. Ensure you always remove make-up thoroughly to give skin a chance to breathe.
• Exfoliate twice weekly; skin at this age doesn't need it more often.
• Ensure you eat a good diet and find time to relax. The hectic twenties can play havoc with your skin.

THIRTIES AND FORTIES

• Make moisturising a priority - fine lines start to appear in your thirties. Skin tends to get drier so you may need to switch to a richer moisturiser.
• Don't forget your neck - use moisturisers and gels to keep it soft and smooth. Remember, the neck shows signs of ageing too and needs protection.
• Cell renewal slows down so regular exfoliation is important to banish the dead skin cells which make skin look dull and lifeless.
• Avoid sunbathing and use a broad spectrum sunscreen all year round.
• Remember an active lifestyle is the key to clear skin, vitality and a supple body.

FIFTIES, SIXTIES AND BEYOND

• Skin gets thinner as we advance in years. Use a night cream to help prevent skin drying out and use a rich moisturiser every day.
• Rethink your make-up and avoid frosted eyeshadows and too much powder which settles into, and enhances, wrinkles.
• Keep the neck and under eye area soft and supple with creams and gels.
(See Ageing chapter for more information on skin ageing.)

Many of us gently exfoliate when washing our face with a face cloth, by using a mildly astringent freshener, or by selecting a cleanser with natural bromelin enzymes. Choose your exfoliating agent carefully, taking into account your skin type and sensitivity. Acne-prone skins should be very careful about infecting acne sites and should choose a gentle scrub, perhaps one based on oatmeal.

FACE MASKS

Face masks have been called on since time immemorial to perform minor miracles on the face. Perhaps because most masks seal the whole face at once in an opaque covering, they have always been thought to have transforming and reviving powers.

Multipurpose beauty aids that not only deep-clean, soothe and soften the skin but can provide quick psychological boosts on demand, masks are the ultimate face treat. There are two kinds of masks, moisturising masks that follow in honey's footsteps, usually formulated in gels or creams, and masks that "deep clean" the pores. The kaolin or fuller's earth used in many of these masks work by drawing grease and dirt away from the face with surface tension created between the occlusive masks and the skin.

MASKS FROM YOUR KITCHEN ...

• Fine ground oatmeal plus witch hazel makes a great absorbent mask for oily skin.
• Moisturising and soothing honey is good for dry skin. Mix with a selection of egg yolk, almond oil, milk, avocado oil or wheatgerm oil for an effective dry skin mask.
• Normal to oily skin reacts well to a face mask made of egg white plus 1/4 teaspoon of lemon or cider vinegar.
• Yoghurt, fresh or sour cream and butter all make excellent bases for masks for dry and dull skins. Mash fresh peeled apricots with a little olive oil and cream, or squeeze ripe strawberries and a small lump of butter to a paste. Mashed peaches, bananas or grated apples can be mixed with honey, cream or yoghurt. Rinse off with cool water.

NATURAL OILS

Natural oils were the first cleansers and moisturisers used on the body. So important were they in dry, hot climates that when Egyptian labourers working on a necropolis at Deir el-Medina went on strike in the 11th century BC, one of the reasons given was that they had no access to the oils and unguents needed to moisturise their skin and protect it from the drying effects of the sun. In fact perfumes and oils were not considered a luxury but a necessity in Egyptian times, and while a wealthy woman might employ many attendants to help her in her toilette, everyone had access to the oils, creating a demand great enough to create the first skin-care industry.

Oatmeal and ground almonds are good exfoliators. Mix with a natural oil and rub over your face for healthy, glowing skin.

Natural oils are fairly similar in structure to components of human sebum, making them highly compatible with the skin. Often neglected because people are unsure about how to use them, natural oils are in fact one of the simplest, easiest to use and effective skin-care preparations available. They are also the most natural. Despite the assumption that layering oil on oil might clog the epidermis's pores, natural oils are efficient cleansers and moisturisers, combining easily with the sebum to dissolve dirt and loosen dead skin cells.

NATURAL FACE TREAT

Natural oils are the ideal ingredient in a facial massage to stimulate circulation and make skin more supple. Wheatgerm oil, or carrot oil are great for very dry skin, while sweet almond or jojoba oil suit normal or sun-dried. Massage gently for about fifteen minutes. Next take a teaspoon of Japanese Washing Grains, apply to the face and gently rub in circular motions. Wipe off the oil and grains and hold your face over steaming water for five minutes. Dry and apply Honey and Oat Scrub Mask. Remove the mask and freshen up with a spray of Honey Water.

WHAT TO DO ABOUT...

SENSITIVE SKIN

The beauty industry catchphrase "sensitive skin" is a bit of a misnomer - with thousands of nerves placed in the dermal layer, no skin is anything but sensitive. Many women, however, think their skin really is especially sensitive, though whether this is a result of their feelings about their skin or a reaction to its real physical state is debatable.

In fact, the term "sensitive" covers a broad spectrum of problems ranging from excessive flushing caused by thin skin, to acne cosmetica, caused by a reaction to some ingredients used in moisturisers such as petroleum jelly, fatty acids and benzophenone, to phototoxicity, a reaction to certain ingredients used as scents in some products, which is triggered by exposure of the skin to sunlight.

While most of these conditions are rare, no product can be completely non-allergenic - someone somewhere will always have a reaction to one of the ingredients in any given product. Any product that describes itself as hypo-allergenic is simply announcing that it does not contain ingredients known to be likely to cause allergies or that those ingredients are in it at a level too low to cause reactions. Most allergic reactions are triggered by the perfume used, for example, to mask the smell of some ingredients or preservatives needed to keep a product bacteria-free.

There are two kinds of substances which can harm the skin: irritants, which affect the skin on first and repeated contact, and allergens or sensitisers, which encourage the body to build up antibodies to a given ingredient before causing a reaction on reapplication. Allergic reactions are essentially a defensive mechanism by the body which, for some reason, has identified an ingredient as hostile. Redness, swelling, heat and pain and dry flaking skin are the result of histamines released by the body to protect the skin.

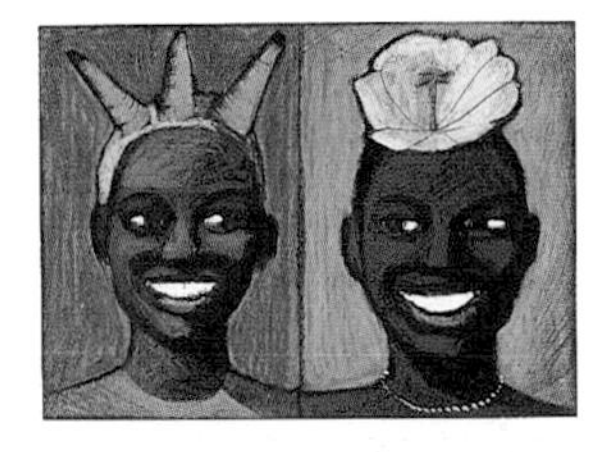

Like any allergy, an allergic reaction to an ingredient in a skin-care product or cosmetic can be due as much to a change in weather or diet as to the ingredient itself. You are twice as likely to be allergic to something or other three days before the start of the menstrual period. And allergic reactions are more likely in winter.

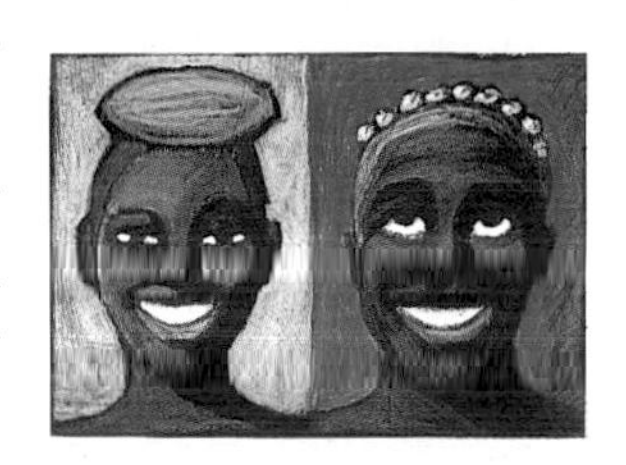

HOW TO USE NATURAL OILS:

- **Sweet almond or jojoba oil makes an effective cleanser regardless of skin type - massage gently into face and remove with a warm cloth.**
- **Wheatgerm oil is the richest natural oil - use as an under eye cream, a night cream or with Rich Night Cream with Vitamin E for very dry skins.**
- **Carrot facial oil is ideal for dry skin. Add it to a moisturiser for a rich night cream, or to washing grains for an excellent scrub.**
- **Add a few drops of evening primrose oil to the bath water for an allover body conditioner, or mix a few drops with your body lotion, moisture cream or aloe gel to keep skin supple.**

STRUCTURE OF THE SKIN

• Skin cells are formed in the basal layer, where they are fed by the blood system in the underlying dermis.

• Each time a new layer of cells is created, it pushes the maturing cells up a level. From the time these cells reach the second layer, the stratum spinosum, they start to die.

• At the stratum granulosum, an insoluble protein called keratin enters the cells, displacing the nucleus and other cell contents and causing the cells to flatten and harden (a process called keritanisation).

• The dead cells eventually fit together rather like fish scales to create the outermost layer, the stratum corneum (also called the horny layer), from which they are naturally sloughed off.

• The hair follicles and nerve endings found in the dermis make it one of the body's sensory centres. The muscle arrector pili contracts with cold or fear, giving us the sensation that our hair is standing on end.

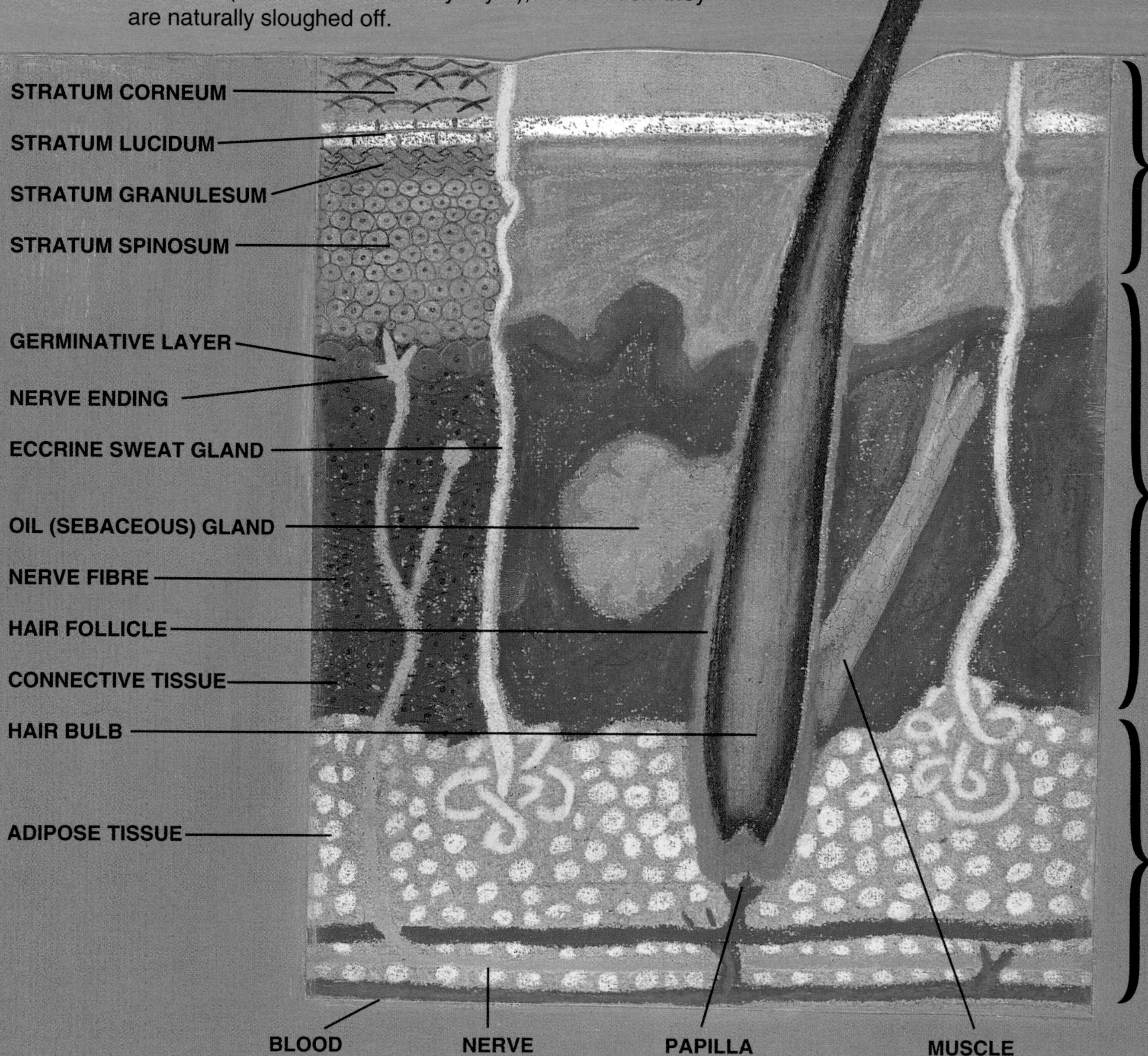

EPIDERMIS about 0.2 mm thick, contains no blood vessels and is made up of five cellular layers.

DERMIS about 1.8 mm thick, made up of blood vessels, nerve endings, sweat and oil glands and the lymphatic system which helps feed and keep clean newborn skin cells. Home to two kinds of sweat glands, apocrine and eccrine, which help clean pores and control the body's temperature. In the dermis,connective tissue (fat globules interwoven with collagen and elastin fibres) gives the skin its firmness and elasticity.

SUBCUTANEOUS TISSUE insulates the body with layers of muscle, veins and fat cells (adipose tissue).

If you think you are suffering from an allergic reaction:

DO wash the product off your face with cold water.

DON'T be tempted to soothe the skin immediately with another cream, and certainly not an antiseptic one. The skin will be hypersensitive until it has calmed down and it can often take a week or two before this happens.

DO use as little as possible of any skin protective cream during the calming down period. Camomile aromatherapy oil is ideal for helping to soothe sensitive skin (but not for use by epileptics and women in the first three months of pregnancy).

Very often people who experience a tightening of the skin after cleansing suspect they too have sensitive skin, while they may have simply been following the wrong skin-care routine. Those who are particularly interested in gentle products should choose items tailored specifically for sensitive skin. If you do have an allergy problem, full ingredient listings, already available in North America and currently being introduced in Europe, are designed to provide you with the information you need before purchasing a product. The Body Shop has full ingredient listings on products so customers are aware of what they are putting on their skin and hair.

Try a dab of Sage and Comfrey Blemish Gel for isolated spots. Infusion of comfrey soothes and conditions; astringent witch hazel curbs the urge to pick spots.

ACNE

Acne has long been considered a teenage affliction - 80 per cent of all teenagers are affected - but acne can, and increasingly does, affect the skin at any age. It is hardly surprising then that in a culture which places such an emphasis on physical beauty, acne can be emotionally crippling. Studies in the United States have shown that acne sufferers have scored significantly poorly in tests for anxiety, depression and well-being, even in comparison with patients suffering from debilitating diseases.

Acne is traditionally triggered by the onset of adolescence in both sexes when a male androgen hormone called testosterone is secreted by the adrenal glands. Although testosterone is present in the body to encourage growth, it has the added effect of over-stimulating the sebaceous glands on the face. Adding insult to injury, there is often rapid generation of cells in the walls of the hair follicles at around the same time. As the follicle walls thicken with cells, the sebum's natural pathway to the surface is blocked, inevitably causing an outbreak of some sort, be it pimple, cyst, whitehead or blackhead.

GENTLY DOES IT

If blackheads and spots look ready to pop out, try emptying the pore by gentle squeezing. Steam your face first to relax and soften the skin. When using a blackhead remover, place the tiny hole at one end over the pore and press gently until the blockage is eased out. Alternatively, cover your fingertips with tissues to prevent breaking the skin and gently press.

Blackheads - or comedones - are non-inflamed lesions which occur when sebum and skin cells combine to form a plug in the hair follicle which turns black when exposed to the air. Whiteheads are also non-inflamed lesions, but they are quickly covered over by skin, forming small white bumps on the surface. Sebum production in mature blackheads soon slows down, but in whiteheads it does not, leading to further problems below the surface of the skin. As the sebum increases it often bursts into the dermal layer, causing a pimple which is signalled by an irritated red surface on the epidermis and an accumulation of white blood cells at site to deal with the intrusion. Acne on its own is not considered an infection, but the irritated sites are often invaded by harmful bacteria that add further to the skin's problems.

BANISHING BLACKHEADS

Smooth sweet almond oil over the affected area and apply hot towels on top. This will soften deeply imbedded blackheads and will help loosen them enough for you to push out with a tissue, cotton wool or blackhead remover.

Although teenagers are the main victims of acne, some people do experience recurrences for years afterwards. Diet and stress are often considered important factors in

Wash your face with clear glycerine soap and gently massage it with one teaspoon of caster sugar; rinse thoroughly. Spots seem to beat a retreat within 10 days.

acne cases and to a degree this may be correct. Without a doubt, the quality of diet is reflected in skin tone. But the development of acne remains largely an issue of excessive sebum production caused by the hormonal pattern we inherit from our parents. Although we cannot control our hormone production, we can alter our diet and follow a gentle skin-care routine.

Until recently, received thought on the subject encouraged sufferers to strip away all facial oils to minimise comedogenic activity. Unfortunately, all this does is stimulate the sebaceous glands, creating an endless cycle of sebum production. By gently washing dirt away without affecting the acid mantle, it is possible to cleanse the skin without triggering an increase in sebum. Double-duty ingredients that calm and absorb oil, such as oatmeal, are extremely useful. Try gentle washing two or three times a day and avoid touching the face to keep bacteria to a minimum. Although sufferers rarely seek medical advice, accepting acne as an insoluble problem, persistent cases can be successfully treated by dermatologists.

Puffy eyes can be caused by a number of things: lack of sleep and fresh air, a bad diet, smoky atmospheres, or even sinus problems such as hay fever. Soothing eye gel, cooling and refreshing cucumber slices, raw slices of peeled potato, lukewarm camomile tea bags, or cotton wool pads soaked with herbal infusions (iced witch hazel is especially good) can help reduce puffiness and refresh eyes.

THE EYES

Some parts of the face are more equal than others, requiring extra special treatment. The skin around the eyes is a case in point. The thinnest and most delicate skin on the body, it has no sebaceous glands and is one of the first areas of the face to show signs of stress and age through wrinkles, shadows under the eyes, swelling and bags.

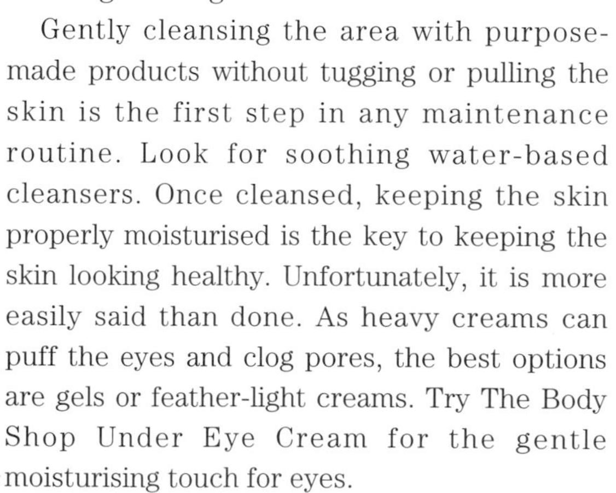

Gently cleansing the area with purpose-made products without tugging or pulling the skin is the first step in any maintenance routine. Look for soothing water-based cleansers. Once cleansed, keeping the skin properly moisturised is the key to keeping the skin looking healthy. Unfortunately, it is more easily said than done. As heavy creams can puff the eyes and clog pores, the best options are gels or feather-light creams. Try The Body Shop Under Eye Cream for the gentle moisturising touch for eyes.

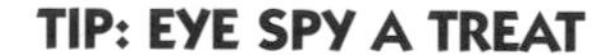

TIP: EYE SPY A TREAT

Wheatgerm oil, the richest of natural oils, is a perfect under eye treat. Like all other natural oils, its chemical structure is similar to sebum and contains vitamins A, B, C and E to firm and tone the skin.

CONTACT LENSES

DO insert lenses before applying make-up.

DON'T apply hand cream just before inserting the lenses and never use oils around the eyes when wearing them. Both will form a film over the lenses.

DON'T use lash-building mascara - the fibres may become trapped between the lenses and eyes when wearing them and cause irritation.

LIPS

Despite our obsession with decorating our lips, we tend to treat them cavalierly, conditioning them only in winter. Placed in a vulnerable position on the face and yet surprisingly poorly protected, our lips require constant care. They have a very thin stratum corneum which allows the capillaries in the dermis to show through, creating their typical red colour.

As lips have no sweat glands, few sebaceous glands and few melanocytes, their only protection from outside aggressors is saliva, a double-edged sword because the constant evaporation of moisture on the lips leads to chapping, cracking and, ultimately, bacterial infection. The best protection is a lip balm designed to seal the moisture in used at least twice a day. Try The Body Shop Lip Balms in a variety of lip-smacking, mouth-watering flavours to keep lips soft, smooth and protected.

Because the lips are particularly vulnerable to skin cancer, a good sunscreen is essential in any product that will be worn outside. In the United States a connection has been established between lipstick use and the fact that fewer women than men suffer from premalignant lesions and cancer of the lower lip. Lipstick can clearly work as an effective sunscreen. The Body Shop Honey Stick Lip Balm has an SPF of 15 to protect lips from the damaging effects of the sun.

Cold sores are the lips' other major affliction. Although there are 50 different types of herpes, the strain that most commonly affects the face is Herpes Simplex Type 1, more often known as cold sores. Contracted by touching someone who has an active lesion, the virus manifests itself on the face through small blisters that can develop on the lips, nose, chin or cheeks. Once the first set of sores is healed, many people never display signs of the virus again, although it remains dormant in the nerve cells. For those who do suffer from recurrences, their appearance can be maddeningly difficult to explain, with reasons varying from stress and exposure to sun to menstrual cycles. Though any serious outbreak should be monitored by a dermatologist, camomile and eucalyptus aromatherapy oils can help soothe the irritation (not recommended for epileptics or women in the first three months of pregnancy).

Chew sticks from the Peelu or Toothbrush Tree have been used in Africa for centuries to clean the teeth and tongue.

TEETH

Our teeth are constantly on show - so it's vital that they're kept in the best possible condition. Good teeth and a healthy mouth can be almost anyone's, as long as you follow a thorough dental care routine - and the earlier you start, the better.

Humans develop their first set of teeth during the first two years of life, with the second set pushing through at about six years, when our baby teeth fall out. We don't get another chance. Our adult teeth should last throughout our lifetime - and they will if cared for properly. Good toothcare starts with regular and thorough cleaning of the mouth and regular dental check-ups, also, by reducing intake of sugary food and drinks. Fluoride too, is an essential part of any early preventative campaign.

Ninety five per cent of British adults have some degree of gum disease. It is caused by plaque, a soft sticky film made of bacteria that coats the teeth. Bacterial toxins in plaque inflame the gums, causing them to bleed and swell; a condition called gingivitis. If not treated, the next step could be periodontitis, inflammation and recession of the gum tissues which can lead to loss of the supporting bone and eventually the tooth itself.

Make sure you practice good dental hygiene. Toothpaste can only give full protection if used as part of a complete dental care routine. When choosing a toothpaste, bear in mind that many on the market contain artificial sweeteners (saccharin), colours, flavours and preservatives - none of which are necessary in dental care. Try natural toothpastes instead - go for ones which contain fluoride. They may taste slightly different because of unfamiliar natural flavourings but a little perseverence is well worth it. You'll soon come to love their clean, refreshing taste!

Run out of toothpaste? Try these natural ingredients on their own or with water for quick cleaning:

- **Slices of fresh strawberry rubbed over teeth remove stains.**
- **Rub fresh sage leaves over teeth and gums.**
- **Shift brown stains by rubbing lemon peel over the teeth and rinsing with water.**
- **Sprinkle half a teaspoon of bicarbonate of soda on a damp toothbrush and brush to remove stains.**
- **Freshen breath by chewing parsley or watercress.**

THE ROOT TO CLEAN TEETH STARTS HERE ...

FLOSS teeth first. Even the most careful brushing cannot remove plaque lying under gums and between teeth. Wrap the floss around the tooth in a v-shape and slide it down into the gum crevice and back again. Repeat all round the mouth.

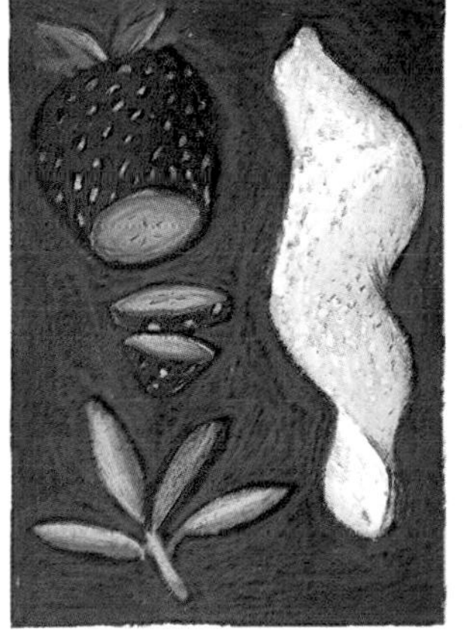

BRUSH regularly (ideally after every meal) with a good toothbrush with firm nylon bristles that are soft enough to flex over surfaces and reach into crevices. Place the brush in your mouth at gum line at an angle of approximately 45 degrees and rub gently but firmly backwards and forwards over the teeth.

ALWAYS replace your toothbrush as soon as the bristles start to wear out.

GARGLE with an effective mouthwash - it can prevent bacterial growth.

EAT a healthy balanced diet - make sure you get enough protein, which is essential for healthy teeth and gums. Eat plenty of crunchy fruits and vegetables and cut down on sugars, the prime cause of tooth decay. Try not to eat anything between meals to minimise the time the mouth is in an acidic state.

HAVE your teeth professionally cleaned and polished by a dental hygienist or dentist at least twice a year. This will remove any tartar build up and check for signs of impending gum disease.

MAP OF THE FACE

WHAT SKIN TYPE ARE YOU?

DRY SKIN: Normally fair and sensitive, finely textured and often lined with a low level of sebum production. Can be attractive and delicately textured during youth but may develop wrinkles and lines at an early age if not kept supple. Increased by wind, extremes of temperature and air conditioning.

NORMAL SKIN: Clear, with a fine-grained texture, soft, supple with a smooth velvety feel. No areas of excess oiliness or dryness. Can become drier with age.

OILY SKIN: Sallow, looks shiny, greasy to touch, has a coarsely-grained texture with the pores often visible. Subject to infection because excess sebum clogs pores (blackheads and spots are common). Tends to develop wrinkles less readily than other types.

COMBINATION SKIN: Common skin type - oily central panel (forehead, nose and chin) with dry cheeks. Oily skins often become combination with age. To keep oiliness and dryness under control, the skin needs to be cared for as two distinct types - oily and dry.

T-ZONE The oiliest section - the central panel from the forehead down to the chin, where the sebaceous glands are concentrated. Combination skin means an oily T-zone and dry cheeks. Adapt your skin-care routine to cope with this.

WRINKLES Young skin is like a firm new mattress, plumped up with moisture and kept springy by collagen and elastin. As time passes, these substances lose their strength and skin surface becomes worn and irregular like an old mattress.

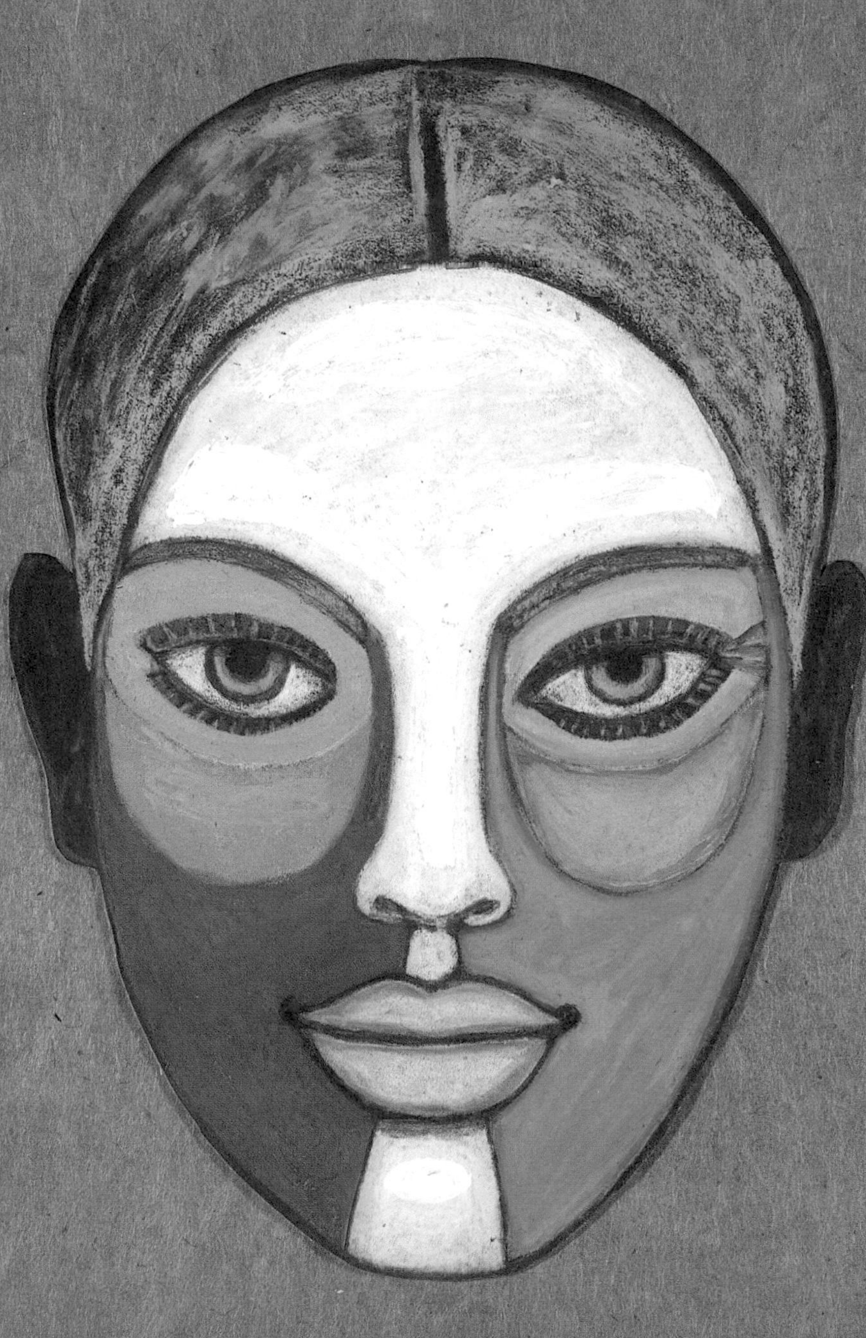

EYELASHES Your eyelashes protect eyes from dust particles and act as a frame for your eyes. Regular applications of castor oil will slowly improve lash condition. Curl clean lashes, before applying mascara.

EYEBROWS Keep eyebrows well defined and shapely to balance your face and give it character. Keep them neat by regular plucking. First cleanse, then brush brows up with an eyebrow brush or a toothbrush. Use clean tweezers and start from inner corner, following the shape of the brow and plucking from underneath only in the direction of hair growth. Taper the curve gradually, following the line of the brow to the other corner of the eye. Brush back into shape.

UNDER EYES The skin around the eyes is the thinnest and most delicate on the body - it has no sebaceous glands and is quick to show signs of stress and age. Gently cleanse the area, keep it properly moisturised and don't drag or pull the skin around the eyes - ever.

LIPS Lips need lots of protection - they are thin-skinned (the stratum corneum allows the capillaries in the dermis to show, creating their red colour)and have no melanin (protective tanning pigment). Protect them with a lip balm or lipstick during the day.

SKIN AGEING Up to 90 per cent of the changes in our skin that we think of as getting older - wrinkling, dryness, blotching etc - are in fact sun damage. It can be avoided.

SKIN-CARE GUIDE

SKIN TYPE	TEENAGE/ BLEMISHED	DRY	NORMAL	OILY	MATURE/DRY	MATURE/ NORMAL	MATURE/OILY
CLEANSER	Pineapple Facial Wash Oatmeal Cleansing Gel	Honeyed Beeswax & Almond Oil Cleanser Orchid Oil Cleansing Milk	Orchid Oil Cleansing Milk Glycerine & Oat Facial Lather Cucumber Cleansing Milk	Passion Fruit Cleansing Gel Pineapple Facial Wash	Honeyed Beeswax & Almond Oil Cleanser Orchid Oil Cleansing Milk	Orchid Oil Cleansing Milk Milk Protein Cleansing Bar Cucumber Cleansing Milk	Passion Fruit Cleansing Gel Pineapple Facial Wash Aloe Soap Vitamin E Soap
FRESHENER	Elderflower Water Cucumber Water	Honey Water	White Grape Skin Freshener	Cucumber Water	Honey Water	Honey Water White Grape Skin Freshener	Cucumber Water
MOISTURISER DAY	Vitamin E Cream Oatmeal Moisturiser	Aloe Vera Moisture Cream Neck Gel	Jojoba Moisture Cream Carrot Moisture Cream	Vitamin E Cream Unfragranced Lotion	Aloe Vera Moisture Cream A Moisturiser with added Wheatgerm Oil	Vitamin E Cream Jojoba Moisture Cream Carrot Moisture Cream	Vitamin E Cream Carrot Moisture Cream
MOISTURISER NIGHT	Vitamin E Cream	Rich Night Cream with Vitamin E	Aloe Vera Moisture Cream	Vitamin E Cream	Rich Night Cream with Vitamin E Carrot Moisture cream with added Carrot Oil	Carrot Moisture Cream	Carrot Moisture Cream
EXFOLIATOR	Blue Corn Scrub Mask Japanese Washing Grains	Pineapple Facial Wash Glycerin & Oat Facial Lather	Glycerin & Oat Facial Lather	Blue Corn Scrub Mask Japanese Washing Grains	Honey & Oat Scrub Mask	Japanese Washing Grains mixed with Passion Fruit Cleansing Gel	Blue Corn Scrub Mask Japanese Washing Grains
MASK	Blue Corn Scrub Mask	Peanut & Rosehip Face Mask	Peanut & Rosehip Face Mask Parsley & Mint Face Mask	Parsley & Mint Face mask Blue Corn Scrub Mask	Peanut & Rosehip Face Mask	Peanut & Rosehip Face Mask	Parsley & Mint Face Mask

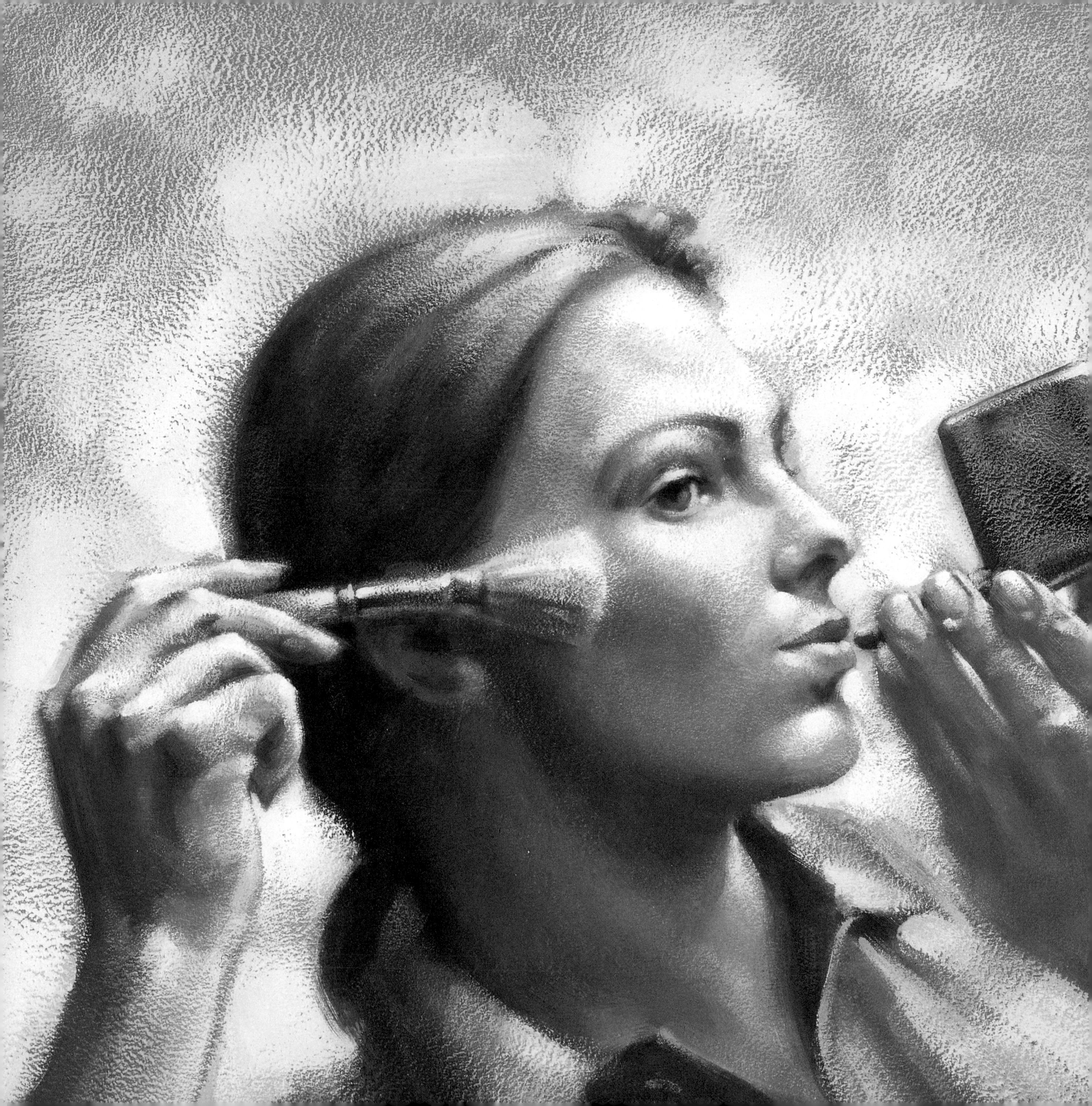

COLOUR

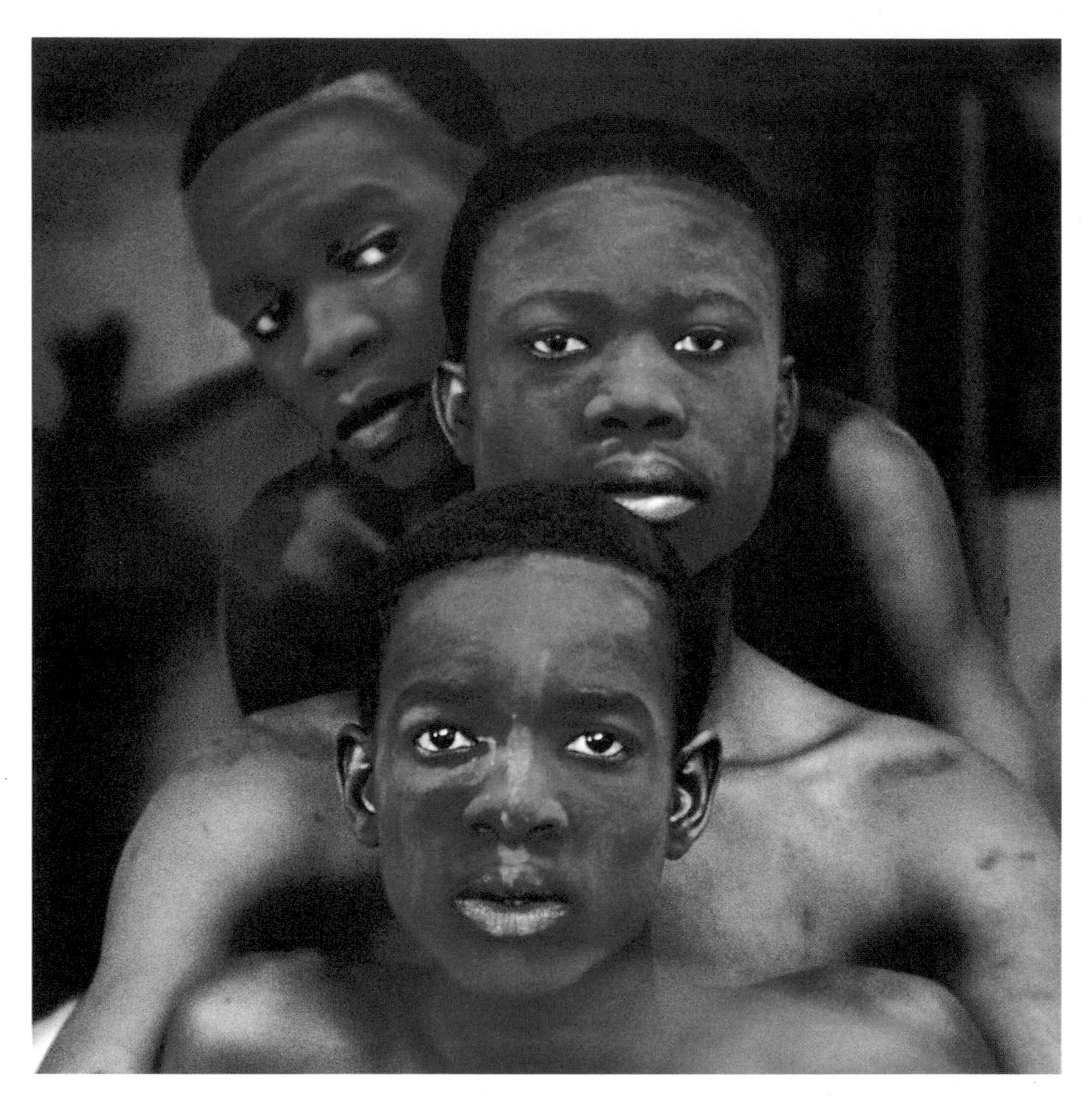

The Kota in the Congo paint their faces to mark the transformation from boy to man - the unearthly blue represents the ghost of the childhood that has passed forever.

colour

Wanting to wear make-up is just as much a part of human nature as decorating the clothes that we wear for warmth and protection. Today cosmetics are sometimes considered a symbol of late 20th century excess, but they have been used for thousands of years by men as well as women. The basic idea - the application of colour to the face is so simple that it has remained the same from culture to culture down through history. It's each individual's reasons for wearing make-up and the results that introduce a wealth of differences.

At various times in centuries past, colour cosmetics have had a bad reputation in the West. Reams have been written by disgruntled men on the subject, and their use has become, at times, a moral issue. They were banned by pious early Christians who felt they had been worn to garish excess in the Roman Empire. Their use for trapping a man into marriage was banned by an act of British Parliament in 1770. By contrast, many indigenous cultures embrace the application of colour to the body, not only as a form of decoration but as a means of communication. In Southern Sudan, for example, the Nuba apply colour in intricate facial designs to denote their clan, family, and age.

In the West, make-up is also used as a form of subliminal communication, though the signals are a little harder to grasp.

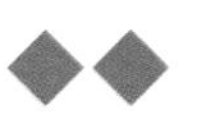

The need to transform and uplift ourselves is part of human nature. Psychological research shows that women feel better about themselves when they wear make-up. When you look good, you feel good!

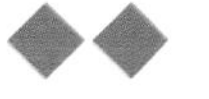

Still, even if we don't display our family history on our faces, we do use cosmetics as a kind of language, wearing different kinds of make-up for different occasions, professional, festive or casual. Punk make-up of the 1970s may have been effective in displaying feelings of alienation, but more typical make-up tends towards the conservative. Its use in our own culture is mostly by women to create an image or establish a mood that helps to clarify to others who we are.

For many, make-up serves as a public mask, and the time it takes to apply is a rite of passage between the private and the public self. People who are shy often take refuge in elaborate make-up, with its power to transform. Our habit of making-up might also be a way of participating in the collective identity. In other words, a particular way of wearing make-up can signify that we are part of a particular group. Unfortunately as make-up practices aren't codified in our society we tend to impose our own interpretations on their use, some of which can be wrong. Studies have shown that men tend to see women who wear pink lipstick as gentle while women who wear bright red lipstick are perceived as dominant. As often as not, this isn't the case.

It is because of baseless interpretations, such as the correlation of good looks and talent, that make-up has come in for a lot of criticism over the past few years from those who feel it may not be politically correct to decorate the face. In some ways make-up is the perfect product for a consumer society: it profits by an appeal to our emotions. But if we do react to cosmetics in such a crass way, surely it is due to the dress-for-success society we live in and not the fault of the make-up itself. For the Nuba, to be bare faced is to be anti-social. The only time the Nuba appear without their complex and highly personal facial designs is when they are working outside their community where different values apply.

Language can indicate the importance of a colour to a culture: the Japanese traditionally had no word for the colour blue.

One American university study, designed to monitor the importance of looks in the job market, discovered that while appearance might not affect whether a person was taken on or not, it could affect the amount of pay he or she was offered, in some sectors of the market by up to 20 per cent.

OLD HABITS DIE HARD

Why do we wear make-up? Certainly not because of the cosmetic advertising that assaults us at every turn these days. It is an instinctive habit, and one that is difficult to break. In fact, it is almost possible to say that we have been decorating our faces and our bodies forever. Cosmetic use may date as far back as one-and-a-half million years ago, when Homo Erectus discovered red ochre in Africa. This iron oxide was probably the first "cosmetic" to be smeared over the skin. Its natural properties as a disinfectant, sunscreen and deodorant proved useful as humans migrated north.

Other specialists believe that cosmetics were originally used for three different purposes: for camouflage in the wild; as a means for hunters to scare their prey (which may explain why in some cultures it is the men, i.e. the hunters, who wear the make-up in the family); and as a way of animating their gods in ritual ceremonies.

As the use of ritualised make-up passed into daily life, specific types of decoration come to represent particular experiences, a practice which is still evident in some cultures today. For the Maasai of East Africa, make-up is an intrinsic part of the rite of passage by which young Maasai men pass from warrior to elder status. To the nomadic tribes of Africa, the pursuit of beauty through elaborate decoration, scarification, and make-up is their greatest form of personal expression in a changing world. In the Kenyan Samburu tribe both sexes spend hours beautifying themselves with jewellery, oils and make-up while the Woodabé of Niger and Northern Nigeria, consider beauty an inherent part of their lives and their value system, alongside such ideals as happiness and freedom.

Finally, sexual attraction cannot be ignored as a factor in the popularisation of cosmetic use. From the young woman in Victorian times using a little surreptitious rouge on her cheeks to the Woodabé man enhancing the best face he puts forward to potential marriage partners, the urge to make oneself sexually attractive is undeniable. To be considered beautiful and highly prized isn't a bad way to succeed in a world where only the fittest survive.

PERMANENT EFFECTS

While the Western world concentrates on temporary cosmetic use, some native peoples permanently decorate their faces through scarification, tattooing and the addition of ear plugs and lip disks. Often, the exaggeration of body parts is designed to express their importance. The Suya of Brazil, who pierce their children's ears at puberty, consider ear plugs a symbol of the importance of hearing in their culture, which to them is akin to knowledge. To the Kayapo in the Amazonian rainforest, the lip disks they wear are a reminder that the ability to speak well is a sign of power in their society. Not so in Africa however, where the women of the Kichepo tribe in Southeastern Sudan began wearing lip plates in the 19th century to emphasise their "otherness" and thus dissuade slave traders from taking them from their homes.

TATTOOING

Tattooing, the permanent deposit of dye under the skin, has been practised all over the world but seldom for the same reasons. To the ancient Britons, for instance, tattooing was part of their defence and they decorated themselves with animal designs to scare off intruders. This practice didn't die out completely in the British Isles until Norman times. In other cultures, tattooing served as a form of permanent communication, even a sort of uniform. The Polynesians, for example, believed that without the tattoos that listed their rank and family history, a man was not a true human being. In Japan, tattoos around the eyes and the forehead have served to identify criminals although, conversely, in other cultures they have been used as a form of protection against evil spirits.

This form of decoration has had several waves of popularity in Western culture. When Captain Cook returned home from Tahiti with the tattooed Prince Omai, it created a flurry of activity amongst members of the aristocracy (even crowned heads were said to have suffered the needle). More recently, tattoos have been used as antisocial stigmata by sectors of society who felt the need to declare their outlaw status. It is this tough-guy patina that has won the tattoo its current chic-ness among rock stars, Hollywood celebrities and a horde of teens looking for trouble.

A HISTORY OF COSMETICS IN TWO-AND-A-HALF MINUTES

Trends in make-up have veered just as wildly over the years as trends in fashion. Like an elaborate game of swings and roundabouts, our ideal of beauty changes, moving from the natural through to the excessive with familiar regularity. Certainly, make-up is an accurate reflection of its time; the recent interest in "naturalistic" make-up is surely tied in with consumer concern for the environment and related green issues, but it is just as surely a reaction to the appetite for artifice that preceded it.

The first recorded use of make-up in Western cultures comes from Ancient Egypt. As a nation, Egyptians were known for their cleanliness and the women, especially those from Thebes, were famed for their beauty, anointing themselves regularly with a variety of oils, unguents and cosmetics. The eyes were the centrepoint of a fantastical make-up that some specialists suggest was inspired by magic and ritual symbolism. Eyes were a symbol of both good and evil in ancient cultures, and also the symbol of the Egyptian sun god, Ra. This explains, perhaps, why priests manufactured cosmetics in their temples. The temple of Edfu - built by Ptolemy III in 237 BC - still has some of the formulae on its walls. Suffice to say that Egyptian eye make-up, called kohl, emphasised the eyes magnificently, with eyeliner lining the eyes and eyeshadow of varying shades swathing the eyelids in colour that was often swept towards the temples. Made of a variety of powdered substances, including malachite, galena, copper oxide and iron, kohl was worn by men, women and children, not merely for decorative value, but to protect the eyes from disease and to cut down on the sun's glare. Egyptian women were also fond of rouge and lip colour, although the oldest known lip salve, dating from 3,500 BC, is Mesopotamian.

The Egyptians were instrumental in introducing neighbouring nations, including the Greeks, to the wonders of cosmetics through their trade links. But although it was the Greek physician Galen who developed cold cream, a skin-care standby, cosmetic use remained at a minimum until Roman women picked up the habit from the Greeks. The Romans adored cosmetics and became excessively fond of them. Eyeshadows, powders, and lip tints were used with abandon, along with burnt cork to coat the eyelashes. Small wonder then that when the Roman Empire collapsed, making-up was marked as a pagan indulgence and cosmetics use fell into disrepute, with pale natural complexions becoming the ideal of beauty.

One innovation of the Elizabethan era was the application of an egg-white face glaze designed to protect the skin and the make-up from the fresh air.

NATURAL WAS NEVER ENOUGH

The Middle Ages are commonly thought to have been make-up free, with women preferring to improve their paler-than-pale complexions naturally. But "natural" methods actually ranged from the obvious - avoiding the sun or plucking the brows - to the arcane - shaving the hairline to create a perfectly oval face (the ultimate sign of beauty) and being bled every so often to maintain the requisite pallor.

Cosmetic potions also played a supporting role, with items ranging from ceruse, a corrosive white lead powder (destined to destroy generations of women's faces, and cause the occasional death), to delicate rouge, lip rouge and even eyeshadow in shades of purple, brown, grey and green. Their use varied from country to country and from place to place. Prostitutes in 6th century Spain favoured pink paint (rouge generally remained the cosmetic of choice for prostitutes), while their social betters opted for white powder.

Face patches - tiny bits of black silk, velvet or leather cut in the shape of stars, moons, suns, even love birds - were the last word in the 17th century, used by one and all to highlight best features and disguise the scarring effects of smallpox. The only people who were lucky enough to avoid this disfiguring disease were milkmaids who were rendered immune by a version of smallpox they contracted from the cows they milked. Patches were worn to excess, sometimes up to a dozen at a time, much to the exasperation of Oliver Cromwell who banned their use in England. The practice was resumed after the Restoration.

The Italians were particularly passionate about decorating the face, and their unique styles were imported to England around the time of Elizabeth I's coronation and introduced to France by Catherine de' Medici. Both women encouraged the use of cosmetics in their courts, and launched their subjects into ever more vigorous attempts to bleach their skin, brighten their cheeks and redden their lips.

OPEN SECRETS

Western culture has been on a fashion see-saw ever since. Although the look remained generally pale until the 20th century, blusher has come and gone time and again in various intensities, in various places on the cheeks, and indeed in various countries with regularity. "Any woman in Paris who neglected to wear rouge was assumed to be English", said Horace Walpole on the subject of French maquillage in 1781.

After the powder and rouge excesses of the previous two centuries, the Victorian age was one of cosmetic restraint. Various powders from talc to rice powder and vegetable rouge were tolerated, but only in the name of heightening natural beauty. Artifice was unheard of in polite society, although the benefits of cosmetics for fading complexions was discussed in books and practised, discreetly, behind closed doors. By the early 1900s, cosmetics were once again becoming an open secret, popularised by actresses, written about and advertised in magazines. The advent of the First World War sent a lot of women into the factories, providing many of them with a disposable income for the first time. Fashion, and all its beauty accoutrements, suddenly became accessible to more than the privileged few.

PLUS CA CHANGE...

The wholesale changes in society after the First World War affected the way women wore cosmetics and thought about their looks. Suntans became fashionable for the first time, and sporty, active good looks won the day over more contrived efforts. As women cropped their hair, focus was placed squarely on the face and cosmetics became more important - there was a definite difference between boyish good looks and gamine style. The lipstick, which had been invented around 1915, came into its own as the variety of colours available increased. Rouges varied in shade from pink to mauve and powders came loose or in compacts. Eyebrows were plucked and filled in again with eyebrow pencils, and eyes were coloured, lightly for the most part. In 1925, American women spent almost a billion dollars on cosmetics. The beauty race was in full cry.

Influences in make-up and beauty changed as well. With the advent of film, movie stars became role models. In the 1930s, Garbo, Dietrich, and Jean Harlow inspired thousands of imitators. By the 1940s make-up was less delicate, lips were large and well defined, brows were arched and thicker.

The focus moved back to the eyes in the 1950s when eyeshadow and eyeliner came into their own. Matched by a strong lip, the look was arch, and often contrived. The 1960s saw a colour revolution as icy shades and pastel tones competed with heavy black eyeliner on the eyes (which were never complete without false eyelashes), while lips disappeared completely or shone in a frosted halo of pink. The 1970s left off where the 1960s began, focusing on shine and shimmer, multicoloured eyeshadows and glossy lips.

The speed of life these days has affected beauty trends, which trip over each other in their efforts to create something new. The result is a layering of ideas that ensures that virtually anything goes. Perhaps the trend that underlies all others is a kind of tolerance for make-up that would probably be more familiar to the Ancient Egyptians than our great-great-grandparents.

COLOUR

As babies, we learn to distinguish colours at the same time that we learn to use our sight. Although we start off by focusing on brightly coloured objects, by the time we have matured, most of us can detect about 200 different shades. Most adults the world over tend to list their favourite colours as blue, red, green, violet, orange and yellow. Red and yellow, however, have a special resonance for some native peoples. Anthropologists relate this to the importance of the sun as a sign of warmth and safety.

In Western cultures at least, choosing colour is supposed to be a decision that reflects our personalities and our moods. Unsurprisingly in our consumer driven society, an entire industry has blossomed in the past few years devoted solely to guiding the colour-challenged

FACES OF THE 20TH CENTURY

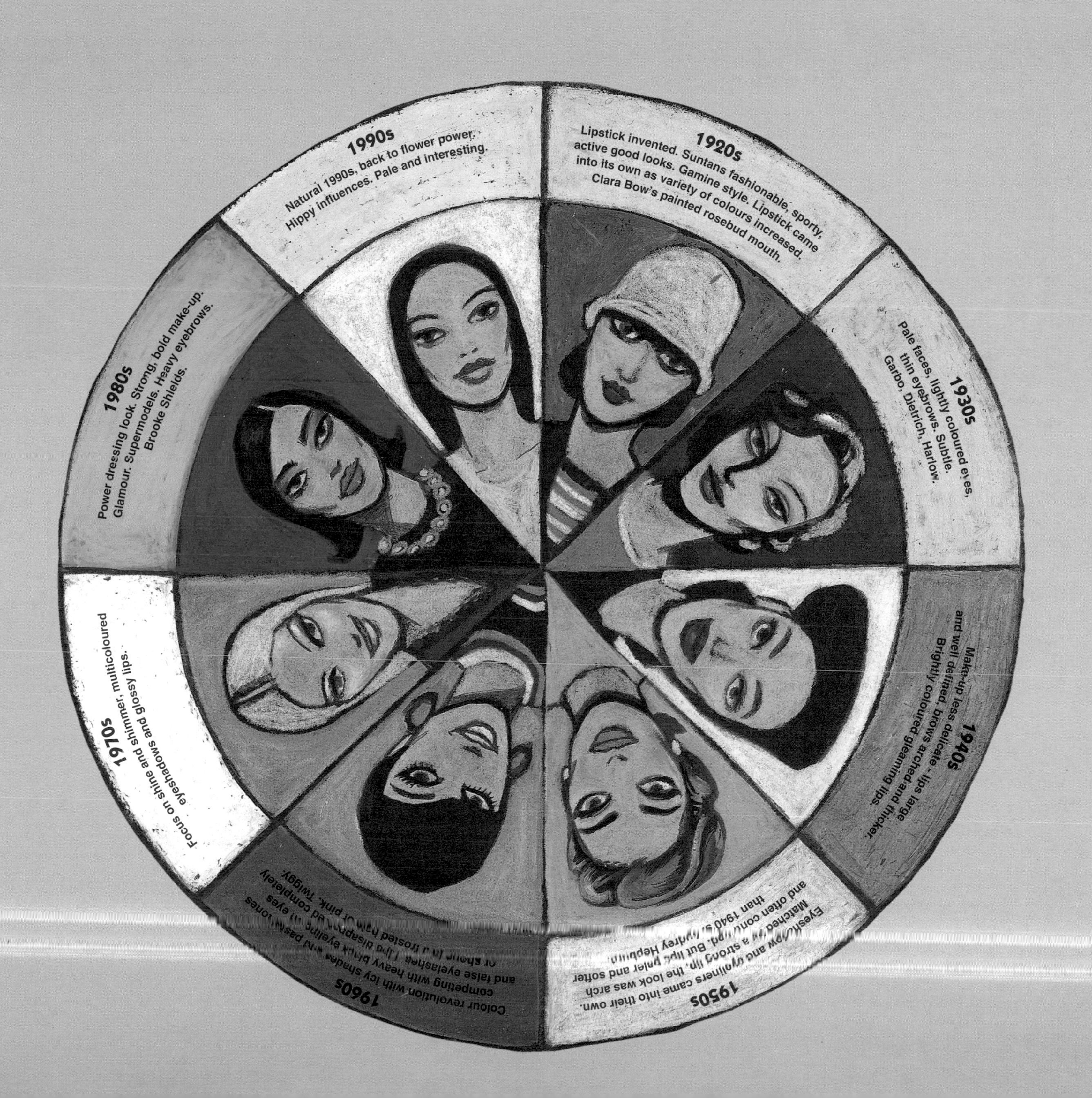

.8 per cent of men are colour blind, while less than .5 per cent of women suffer from the condition. Colour blindness is usually an inherited trait although it can be contracted through various eye diseases. Most people who suffer from the affliction have difficulty distinguishing between green and red, with a smaller percentage finding it difficult to identify blues and yellows correctly.

towards the right purchases. Over the years we have been advised to choose the colours we wear on our faces depending on our skin's undertones, our eye or hair colour, the clothes we wear, or a combination of these. Colour psychologists suggest that our choice of colours can reflect our moods; orangey lipsticks suggest a sense of optimism; brown tones, traditional values; and red, strength. Deeply reflective people may favour darker tones like emerald green over lighter colours, and extroverts, who require lots of external stimulation, will opt for stronger shades. Wearing particular make-up colours may not actually affect our own moods, but it can outwardly project our emotions and feelings.

CHOOSING YOUR SHADES

Of course fashion has always played a role in the kinds of colours we like. What is "right" for one season may be out the next. There has been a discernible move overall in the past few years towards a new level of naturalism in cosmetics, especially for more mature women who aren't quite as subject to fashionable fancies. Browns and pinks vye for popularity in light, sheer textures that let the skin tone show through. But equally, for those who willingly surrender to the modeish dictates of the day, strong colour periodically exerts fascination.

Although there is no deep significance in selecting make-up colours, finding the right shade can be the trickiest part of a make-up purchase. With the vast variety of shades now available in every kind of product, the consumer is likely to suffer from sensory overload.

DO match your foundation to your skin tone.

DO be aware that not every colour is for everyone. No matter how good it looks in the package, it can tell a different story on the face. Grey eyeshadows, for example, darken the skin's colour and can create a heavy-lidded effect on the eyes for those with tired or sallow skin. Fern greens and lavenders are far more flattering to older skins and brighten the eyes as well.

DO try to coordinate your make-up with your clothes. Peachy make-up probably won't suit a burgundy outfit, and a rich blue-red lipstick won't take too kindly to an orange suit.

DON'T put too many colours on the face at the same time. They simply detract from the main attraction - you.

TRANSFORMERS

The humble lipstick has a lot going for it as a quick pick-me-up. Nothing changes the face more strikingly, or more quickly than a switch in make-up, especially lip colour. The proportions of the face change, the focus changes from the eyes to the mouth, and the colour itself can give you a lift.

Manicurists, hairstylists and cosmetic counters are often the first line of defence for women in need of a boost in morale. While such notions of beauty may seem trivial, in fact an interest in the way we look is often considered a sign of recovery in those who are ill — people who don't feel well don't take care of their appearance. By applying a lipstick, and in essence, trying to recreate our public face, we are making the decision to re-enter the healthy world. To this end, The British Red Cross regularly sends volunteers into local hospitals to offer patients neck and shoulder massage, face cleansing and make-up applications. In North America, cosmetic companies have banded together to offer helpful advice to women undergoing cancer treatment, providing information on how to alter their make-up habits to compensate for changes caused by chemotherapy and radiation. In Britain, The Body Shop's cosmetics division Colourings works regularly with the visually impaired and the severely disfigured, teaching them how to apply make-up, which for many is a key to feeling a part of the larger community.

PUTTING IT ON

Times have changed since Nero's empress Poppaea required the help of one hundred slaves for her daily ablutions. Although ritual remains an important part of making up (remember watching your mother prepare for a night out?) few of us have the time to spend whole days covered in beautifying masks. Still, the act itself remains essentially the same.

The point of make-up in the western world has always been to heighten reality, drawing attention to our features without creating the abstract designs of other cultures. Poppaea used chalk and deadly white lead as we would a foundation, just as she rouged her cheeks and highlighted her eyes in the same ways that we do today.

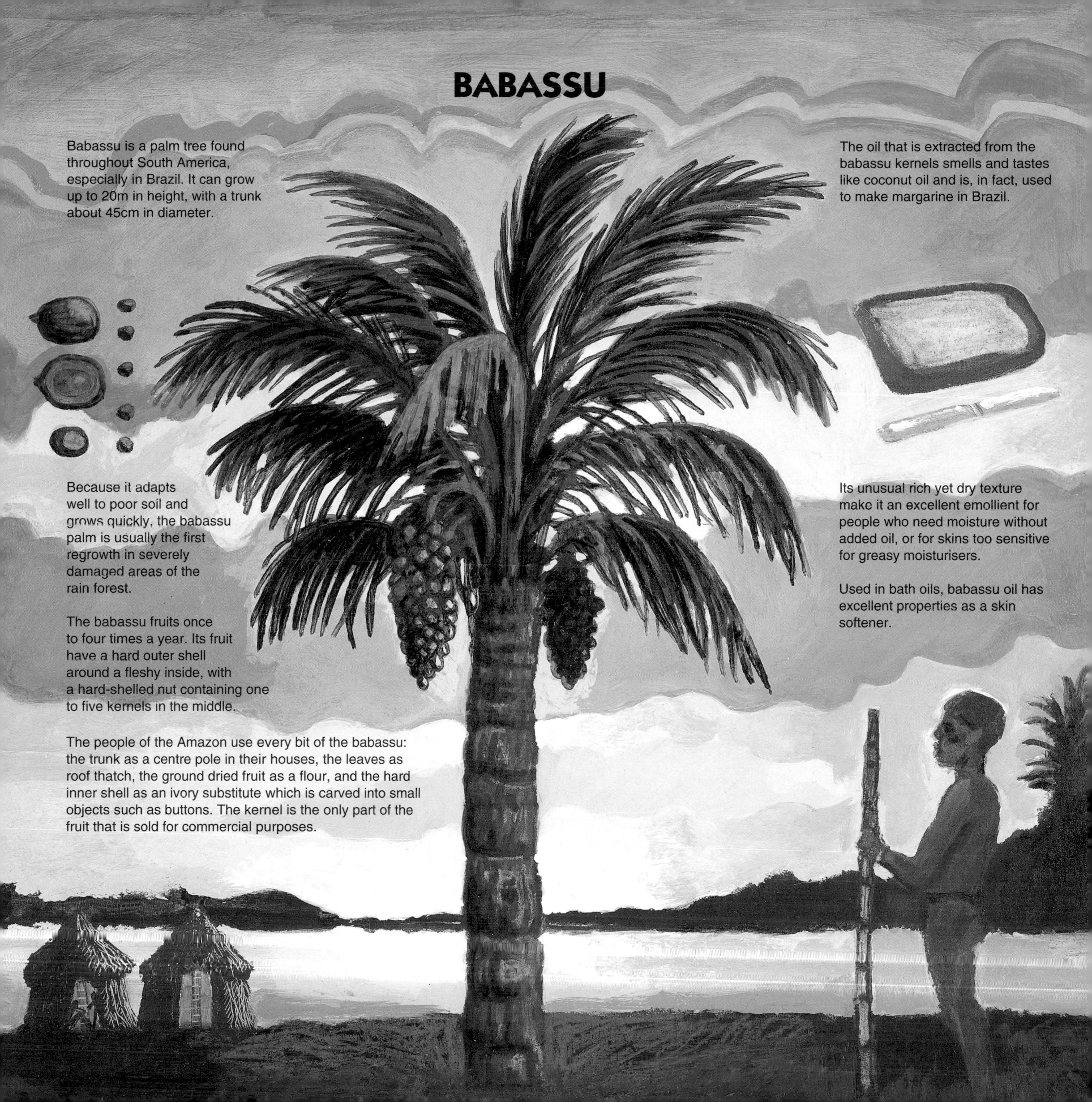

BABASSU

Babassu is a palm tree found throughout South America, especially in Brazil. It can grow up to 20m in height, with a trunk about 45cm in diameter.

Because it adapts well to poor soil and grows quickly, the babassu palm is usually the first regrowth in severely damaged areas of the rain forest.

The babassu fruits once to four times a year. Its fruit have a hard outer shell around a fleshy inside, with a hard-shelled nut containing one to five kernels in the middle.

The people of the Amazon use every bit of the babassu: the trunk as a centre pole in their houses, the leaves as roof thatch, the ground dried fruit as a flour, and the hard inner shell as an ivory substitute which is carved into small objects such as buttons. The kernel is the only part of the fruit that is sold for commercial purposes.

The oil that is extracted from the babassu kernels smells and tastes like coconut oil and is, in fact, used to make margarine in Brazil.

Its unusual rich yet dry texture make it an excellent emollient for people who need moisture without added oil, or for skins too sensitive for greasy moisturisers.

Used in bath oils, babassu oil has excellent properties as a skin softener.

Brush care is all-important. Always keep your tools clean by washing them regularly with a mild shampoo, and rinsing them well in lukewarm water. Condition brushes made of natural hair with a tiny dab of conditioner and rinse again. Squeeze gently and allow the brushes to dry naturally.

To cover a spot: load a brush with concealer, paint over the spot, then dust with powder. Or turn it into a beauty spot or freckle with a smudge of matt shadow.

Decades, even whole periods of history, are recognisable by their beauty trademarks. But luckily no single beauty look is de rigueur anymore. With the variety of cosmetics on the market, and the freedom to dress as we please, make-up has become very much a part of our own identity. If we choose to put on a face that would rival Cleopatra's, or wear the lightest of make-up, or even none at all, it is hardly grounds for comment. Still, many of us fall into beauty ruts, relying on the same colours and the same techniques year in and year out, living in our own beauty time-warp without really thinking about it. Updating the colours you use and keeping a lookout for new formulations can keep you up-to-date with new beauty ideas.

Today, the variety of cosmetics is vast, varying not only in colour, but in texture, and weight. Foundation is available in a liquid, or powder formulation, or mixed in with moisturiser. Eyeshadow is by turns matt or pearlescent, opaque or sheer enough to let your own skin tone show through, and may even contain conditioners to keep the skin protected and hydrated. There are few hard and fast rules about applying make-up: it all depends on how much time you have and the kind of look you are out to achieve. Still, here are some basic guidelines that can ease the way.

FIRST THINGS FIRST

Before putting on any kind of make-up it is wise to cleanse and moisturise the skin. Not only will this create a clean, smooth canvas on which to work, but skin that has been hydrated is less likely to absorb whatever moisture the make-up contains, bringing on a disappearing act before the day is half-way through.

Make sure you apply your make-up in even, daylight conditions if possible. Make-up changes drastically in different types of light, so a look that appears soft and sultry in the amber glow of evening is likely to be harsh and unflattering in the light of day. Apply your make-up in unforgiving daylight and it should look good no matter where you end up.

BRUSHES

Application is half the battle, so having the right brushes is just as important as having the right make-up. Don't worry about having a full professional set, but do try to have a few key items:

- A blusher/powder brush distributes make-up evenly on the face and helps to blend it in.
- Lip brushes are useful for adding definition to the lips, filling in thin lips, or creating a more even, longer-lasting colour.
- There are a variety of eye make-up applicators available, from sponge-tip applicators to brushes designed to blend eyeshadow in. Choose those you are most comfortable with.
- Sponges and puffs are generally useful for blending and finishing looks.

THE BASE

We've come a long way from the chalk and white lead concoctions popular for hundreds of years. Foundations not only colour the skin, but many products now contain extra ingredients to protect and moisturise. They are also manufactured in a variety of textures, from matt to glowing, and from heavy opaque coverage to sheer.

Colours are not only likely to vary from dark to light these days, but also from pink to yellow. People with yellow undertones in their skin will find that pinky foundations will look mask-like on them, while foundations with yellow tones should blend right in. Matching foundations accurately is particularly difficult for people with Asian or Afro-Caribbean skins. These skin colours often have a variety of undertones making it a little more difficult to find the right colour. Some darker foundations formulated with the same ingredients as paler foundations will also cast an ashy shadow on the face, due to a surfeit of titanium dioxide in the product.

CONCEALER

Concealers, in essence extra-thick foundations that come in a stick form, are perfect for masking dark shadows under the eyes or camouflaging broken capillaries. Use sparingly, applying dots of concealer where needed and blending lightly with the fingertips. To mask spots, apply concealer lightly after applying your base. For port wine stains or birth marks, try a concealer with double-density pigment.

By removing dark shadows around your eyes with concealer, you will automatically make them look brighter.

FOUNDATION

When applying foundation, remember a little goes a long way. The point of most foundations is to even out skin tone, not to create a thick mask, and as you are more than likely to layer translucent powder and blusher on top, a light touch is essential.

• Apply foundation outwards from the centre of the face, using a damp sponge or your fingertips to smooth it across the skin. Careful blending is the key, especially around the nose and mouth where foundation can cake. Blending properly along the jaw and hair lines also helps to avoid harsh demarcation lines.

• Not everyone needs complete coverage. For a more natural look, apply foundation only where it is needed, often in the T-zone area, or to camouflage blemished skin. Tinted moisturisers are perfect for low maintenance skins that simply need a hint of colour along with a daily dose of moisturiser.

FIX IT

Once the base has been applied let it stand for a moment before applying a layer of powder. Often forgotten by people who are attracted to colourful or gimmicky products, translucent powder is an all-purpose basic, and an important tool for every professional make-up artist. A light wash of powder not only sets the foundation, soaking up oil, but it will help in blending blushers and eyeshadows as well. By creating a uniform surface, powder also helps bounce light evenly off the skin, creating the illusion of an ultra-smooth finish.

To match any kind of foundation to your skin colour, apply a drop to the jawline and blend lightly. Choose the colour that blends best with your natural skin tone.

BLUSHER

Blusher is the ultimate victim of fashion. Trends in lip colours and eyeshadows may vary, but colour is always in evidence in some way on the lips and eyes. Blusher, on the other hand, is the only cosmetic that disappears completely from time to time - and when it turns up again, it isn't always used in the same place. In the 1970s the only way to wear blusher was as an angry stripe of purpley brown painted from temple to lip. Then it was ostracised, only to return as a discreet wash of pale colour.

CHOOSING COLOUR

Simply put, there is nothing better than blusher to make you look healthy. Choose a natural shade that flatters the skin tone, and apply with a fat blusher brush to the apples of the cheeks.

• Blend carefully to avoid looking like a china doll, and for an especially understated look, dust the edges of the blusher with translucent powder.

• Dusting blusher on the eyelids and lightly on the corners of your forehead can create a flattering all-over glow.

• Gently colour coding your blusher to your lipstick will help to avoid colour disasters - a rich blue-red lipstick and a peachy blusher, for example are not a match made in heaven. Working with shades in the same colour family is probably not only the safest kind of colour match, but also the most sophisticated. And today there are even three-in-one eye, lip and cheek colours that can be used in all these areas.

• Always apply blusher after the rest of your make-up, that way you can see how much colour you need.

CHOOSING TEXTURE

Of course, choosing the right colour is only half the decision. Weighing the pros and cons of powder blusher versus cream, and tinted versus allover colour is the other half. Finding the right formulation is largely a question of deciding what you are comfortable using. A

In a hurry or need a quick touch up to your make-up during the day? Reach for an all-in-one face base - a mixture of powder and foundation in one easy application.

TOOLS OF THE TRADE

Quality brushes and applicators - and a little bit of practice - will allow just about any make-up user to achieve better looking results. Using the correct applicator will give a smoother finish and create a make-up that lasts longer, so saving time in the long run.

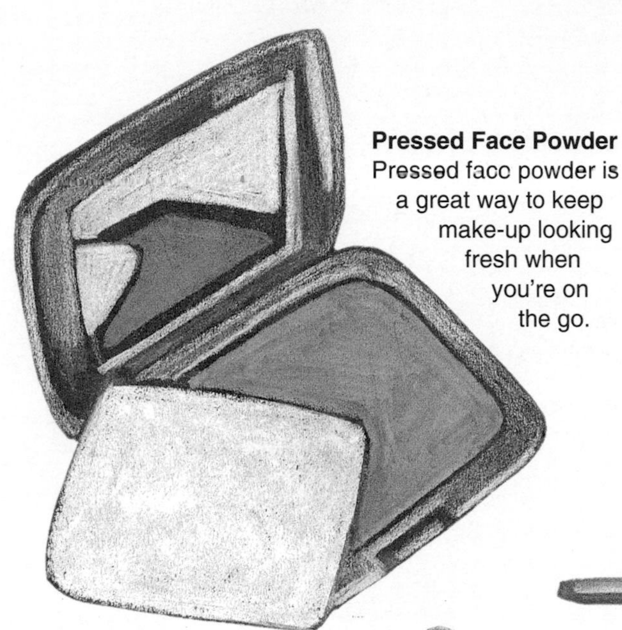

Pressed Face Powder
Pressed face powder is a great way to keep make-up looking fresh when you're on the go.

Pencil Sharpener
Designed to work with all pencils, this sturdy double-bladed sharpener won't split or snap the pencil tip. Use regularly to keep cosmetic pencils sharp and accurate.

Foundation
The quickest way to even out skin tones and create a smooth base for any make-up. Look for one that not only goes on evenly, looks natural and lasts, but also offers the skin sun protection and perhaps a moisturising treatment too.

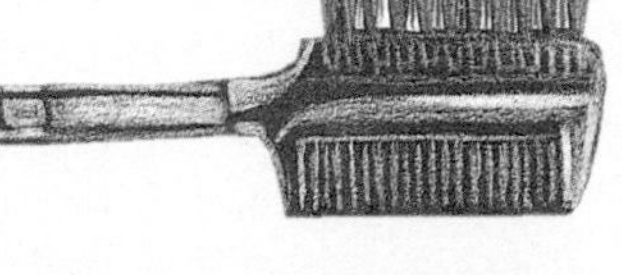

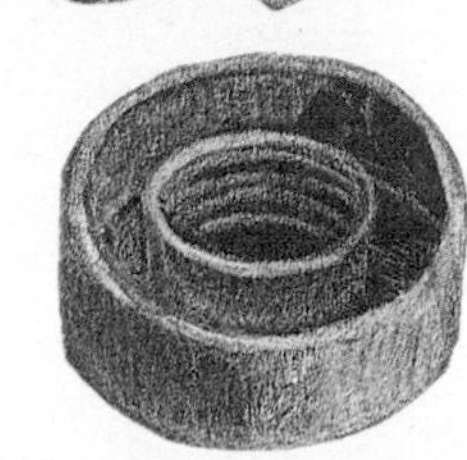

Brow & Lash Brush/Comb
Use one side to exile clumpy mascara forever by combing through the lashes after every coat of mascara. Use the other side to sweep brows tidily into shape, after applying Brow & Lash Gel.

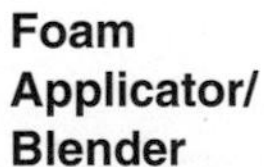

Eyeshadow Brush
A small, soft-haired brush for applying eyeshadow. Eyeshadow has a softer look when applied with a brush than when it is applied with a foam applicator.

Foam Applicator/ Blender
Originally designed for applying eyeshadow, this applicator gives a stronger depth of colour to eyeshadow than when it is applied with a brush.

Lip/Concealer Brush
Applying lipstick with a lip brush will give you a smoother, better looking and longer-lasting finish and, on average, 20 more applications than when it is applied straight from the stick!

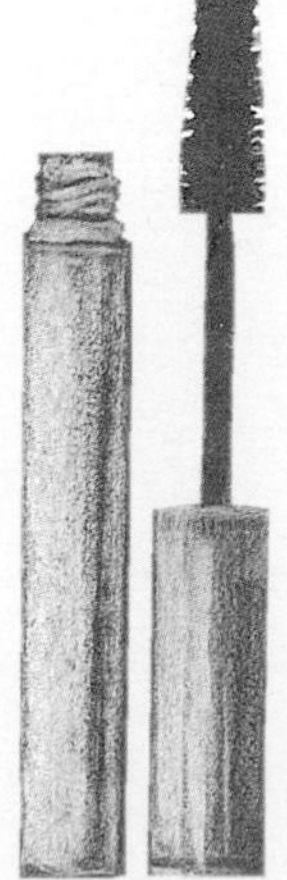

Mascara
Use mascara to lengthen or thicken the look of the lashes. There are two types of mascara: water-resistant and waterproof.

Eye definer
Also known as eye liner or eye pencil, it's a great way to add definition to the eye. Look for an eye definer that is firm enough to prevent smudging but won't drag the skin on application. And remember to apply along the outer third of the eye only.

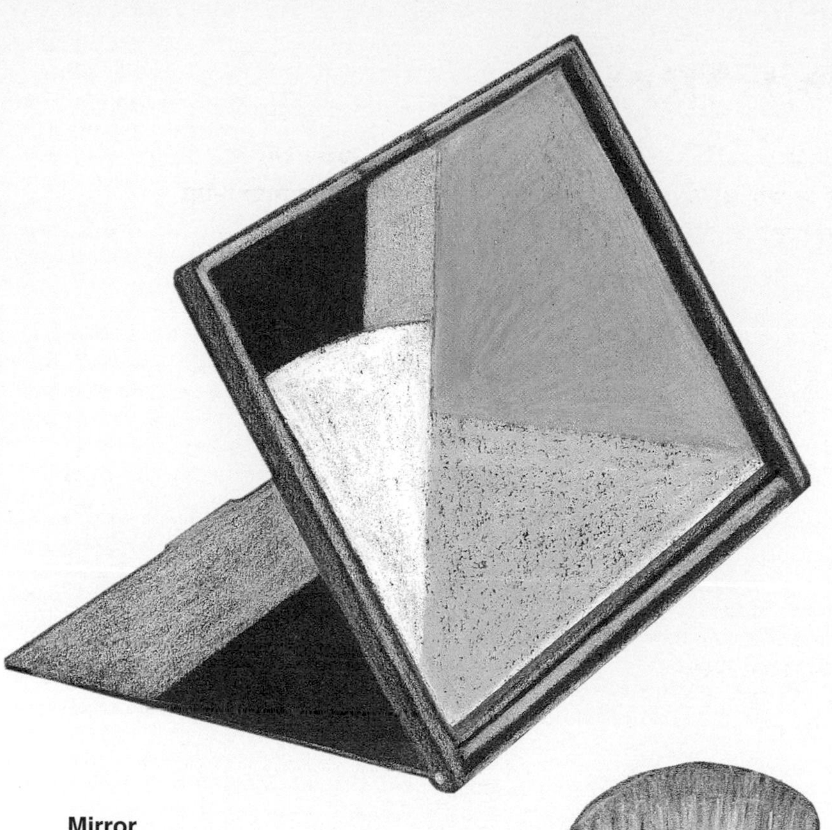

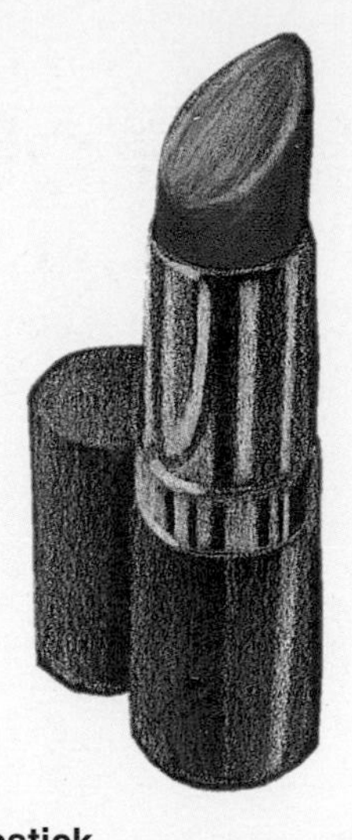

Make-Up Sponge
Forget messy fingers! A slightly dampened make-up sponge will apply any type of foundation more evenly in the most difficult nooks and crannies, such as around the nose and the corner of the eyes.

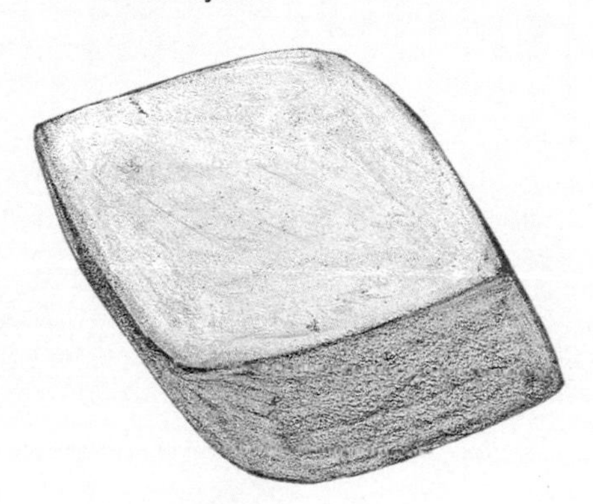

Lipstick
Worldwide the most popular item of make-up. Choose a lipstick not only for colour and price but for it's durability, texture and the moisturising and protective benefits it can have on your lips.

Mirror
A good sized mirror is essential when applying make-up. Look out for one that can be your everyday make-up mirror and double up as a portable mirror too.

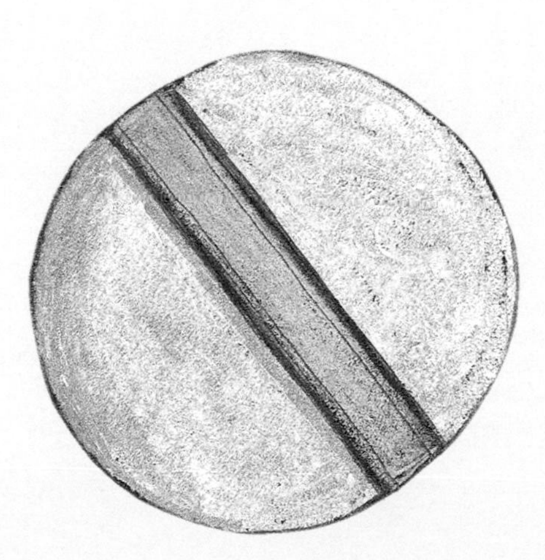

Powder Puff
Ideal for the application of loose face powders. If you have only ever applied face powder with a brush, you'll be pleasantly surprised by the tidy application and better finish achieved with a Powder Puff.

Powder/Blusher Brush
An essential in any make-up kit. Great for applying and blending all types of powder blushers, cheek colours and bronzing powders. Can also be used to dust off excess powder.

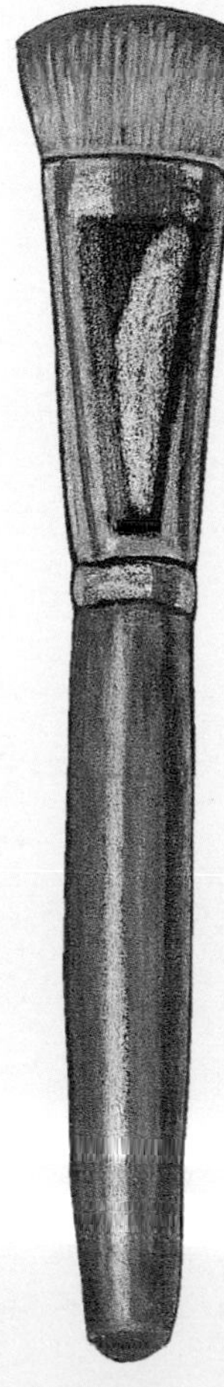

Foundation Brush
If you have a very blemished skin, you'll know that conventional methods of foundation application can still leave your skin looking red and patchy. This unique brush has been specially designed to "paint" on our Extra Cover Foundation and "blank out" very blemished skin.

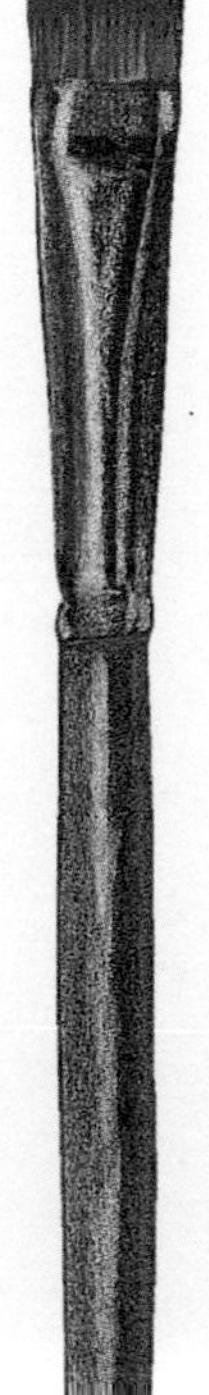

Eyeshadow Blender Brush
Whether you are wearing one single eyeshadow or graduating several colours into one another it is probably impossible to blend eyeshadow too much!

fairly new innovation is the use of all-over bronzing powders to highlight the entire face. A by-product of our new caution about suntanning, these powders offer a golden glow without ultraviolet after-effects. As always, use a light hand, and blend carefully to avoid stripes of colour.

Socialites in Ancient Egypt shaved their eyebrows and applied false ones. Eyebrows that met in the middle were the most popular look - if nature wouldn't oblige, women joined their brows with a kohl pencil.

When deciding where to put colour on your eyes, remember this rule: light colours bring forward, dark colours push back.

EYES

Mute testament is still borne to the status the eyes have enjoyed through the ages in the amount of make-up paraphernalia devoted to them: liquid eyeliners, pencil eyeliners, eyeshadows, cream shadows, eyeshadow pencils, mascara, and eyebrow definers all compete for attention.

EYEBROWS

Although we often think solely about decorating the space between the eyelashes and the eyebrows, the brows themselves are an important feature, creating the perfect frame for the eyes. Like everything else in beauty, eyebrow shapes flit in and out of fashion. Eyebrows that met in the middle were considered a sign of beauty in Roman times but have had little fashion credibility since (with the exception of Mexican artist Frida Kahlo). The thick Brooke Shields-style brows of the 1980s have been getting thinner over the past few years. Look at Madonna's brows, shrinking from the mildly hirsute to the all-but-gone.

Grooming the brows to create a clean line is the best approach as over-plucking can be disastrous and create even more problems with regrowth. Tidy up the brow area by removing stray hairs from under the brow, but if you want to experiment with a more exaggerated look, consult a professional make-up artist or a cosmetician. To hide any imperfections or define the brow shape use an eyebrow make-up or a soft eyebrow pencil. For a natural look, slick on some brow and lash gel to keep them in shape.

USING EYESHADOW

• To get the best out of any eye make-up it is wise to start with a light base of foundation. This creates a smooth, evenly coloured canvas for the products to cling to. Applying a pale, almost skin toned eyeshadow before adding extra colour will add depth to any look, and will make shadow easier to blend. From there it is really up to you. Although multicoloured eye make-up was the fashion for years, choosing a single shade or two complementary colours may be a more sophisticated alternative.

• When applying eyeshadow, build the colour up gradually. Start by stroking colours lightly from the centre of the lid to the outer corner. Deepen the colour on the outer corner and brush one or two strokes across the whole for a pale wash of colour.

• For a more dramatic effect, stroke on colour like eyeliner then smudge it lightly upwards from the lashes. Liquid eyeliners and eye pencils define the eyelids offering everything from a retro to a smoky look, while eyeshadow itself can be used to rim, shade, or highlight the brow bone. Eyeshadow can be used to soften the effect of eye pencils and fix the colour for a long-lasting look. Many eyeshadows have a bit of pearl in the formulation to give the product a little slip, and help it blend on the eye without looking cheap and cheerful. Pearl also helps refract the light, making the eye look smoother.

• Remember that a little colour goes a long way. Try depositing some colour on the eyelid and blend gently inwards and upwards to create a gradation of light colour.

• People with darker skins should look for eyeshadows with a higher pigment content to ensure that the colour is visible. But this doesn't mean sacrificing a light texture or easy application. There are new products that offer both sheer washes of colour and stronger, more vibrant looks.

DON'T FORGET LASHES

• A quick curl of the eyelashes helps open the eye, creating the illusion of being wide awake.

• Applying eye definer to the inner rim of your lower lashes will always make the eyes look smaller. Instead, apply it underneath your lower and above your upper lashes.

• Apply at least one coat of mascara, double at night, to frame the eyes and show off the lashes. Subtly coloured mascaras flatter the eyes and add a gentle boost of colour to any make-up look.

• Avoid smudging by applying mascara to the upper lashes of both eyes, before moving onto the lower lashes.

LIPS

Of all make-up habits, the application of lipstick has always been the most public. Witness the after-dinner freshen-up - a sensuous ritual that is tolerated just about everywhere. Lipstick is also the one luxury that we allow ourselves when we are depressed, or money is tight, which probably explains why lipstick is most cosmetic companies' top-selling product.

> ***Lip colour helps alter the shape of the mouth - so choose carefully. Pale colours add fullness, dark ones slim down and bright ones emphasise.***

The secret to making really long-lasting lipstick has recently been cracked. One Japanese company has a lipstick so durable it had to create another product to remove it! But here are a few suggestions for making just about any lipstick last:

DO use a base. Apply a light coating of foundation and define their shape by lightly lining the lips with a lip pencil that matches the lipstick. You can even use lipliner all over as an extra base. Then fill in with your chosen colour, either with a lip brush or with the tip of the lipstick, making sure to cover the surface evenly.

DO remove excess by blotting with a tissue. Then place another tissue over the lips and brush a little translucent powder on top to set the lipstick. Remove and carefully reapply another coat of lipstick. Blot again.

LIP TIPS

• Applying lipstick with a lip brush not only means it will last longer, but you can get up to 20 extra applications out of it!

• Lining lips gives them an even shape, and can also help stop the lipstick creeping into any fine lines around the mouth.

• Many women prefer a little shine in their lipsticks as it makes the lips look fuller and lighter. If you prefer a sheerer, more natural look, start with a base of lip balm, add lipstick then a tint or a gloss. Rub with a finger to blend.

• Make your lips look fuller by applying a little highlighter to the cupid's bow before applying your lipstick.

MAKE-UP FOR MATURE SKIN

Just as skin-care needs differ quite radically from our early twenties to early forties, so do make-up requirements. Here are a few points to bear in mind to keep mature skin looking its best:

• Avoid dark colours around the eye area.

• Avoid pearly shades of eyeshadow as these can accentuate the fine creases around the eye.

• Try matt, soft shades of eyeshadow and lipstick.

• Avoid heavy, creamy foundations and concealers as they will give the face a mask-like appearance.

• The Body Shop's Continual Eye Colour is a perfect example of a long-lasting matt colour.

• Use products which add a little definition to the face, eyes and lips. For eyes, mascara and eyebrow make-up are a must. For lips, a lipliner is essential and will make lipstick last longer and look better.

• Try using a natural cream blush as opposed to a more colourful powder blush.

• Select colours which won't look too harsh: try using brown or blue mascara instead of black.

• Use products which will create a softer make-up look: try using an eyeshadow pencil instead of eye definer

• Treatment products can be particularly beneficial. Colour balance fluids are a good example of a product which makes the complexion look and feel better.

WHERE MAKE-UP IS GOING

• Cosmetics companies will gain an environmental conscience, with more refills available.

• The raw materials used in cosmetics manufacture will become more refined (e.g. smaller particle pearl) leading to finer textures.

To set make-up:

• Powder sets base make-up - it also reduces shine and disguises large pores.

• When all make-up is applied, set it with water. Spray the face with spring water from a plant-misting bottle, then blot once with a tissue. Your make-up will stay put for longer.

• On hot days, keep your spray in the fridge for a cooling spritz. You can even add a drop of rose or lavender essential oil for extra refreshment.

HOW TO APPLY MAKE-UP STEP-BY-STEP

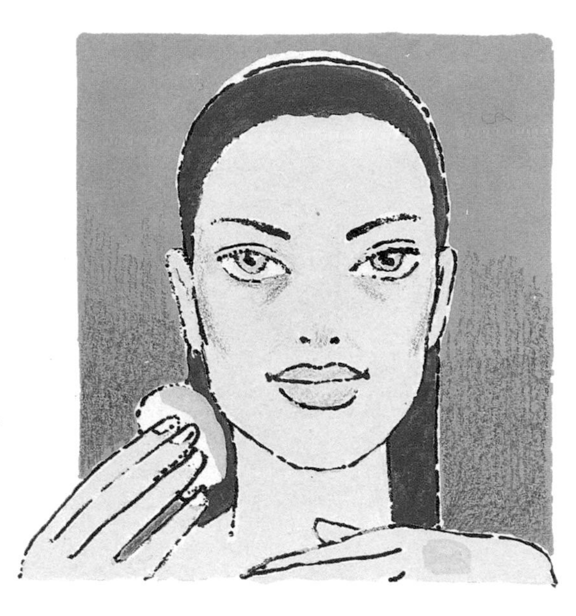

1. Use foundation to even out your skin tone. Apply with a sponge, rather then the fingers for smoother coverage. Start at the centre of the face making downward strokes remembering to cover the eyelids and the edge of the lips lightly.

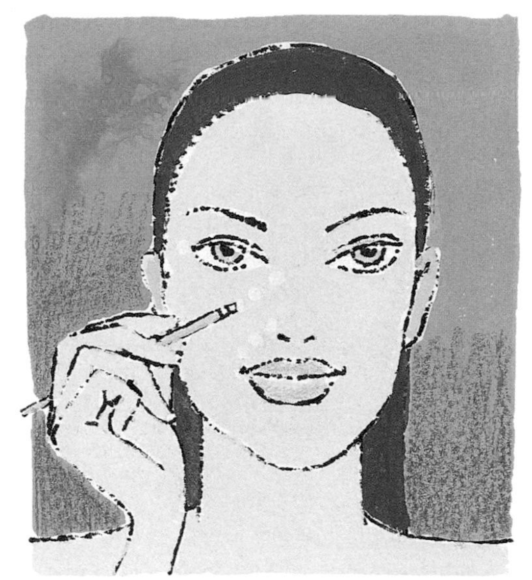

2. Concealer will disguise dark circles under the eyes and a host of minor blemishes. To avoid a caked affect, apply sparingly with a brush and gently blend it over blemishes with a foam applicator.

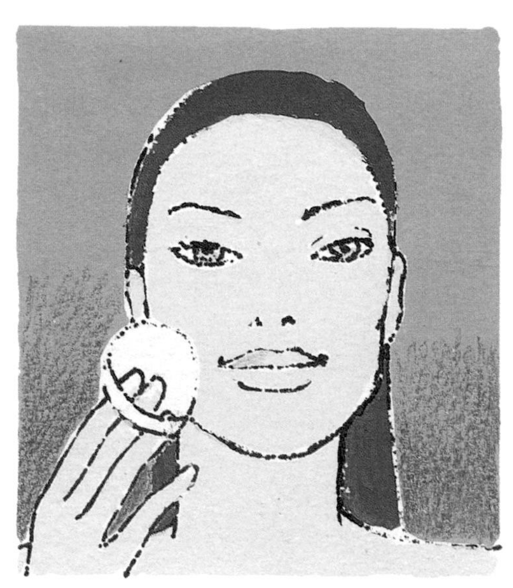

3. Set the base by applying a little translucent loose face powder. Use a puff, not a brush, to press rather than dab the powder into the skin and it will look smoother. More mature make-up users should be careful to use powder sparingly, avoiding areas of the face that are particularly lined.

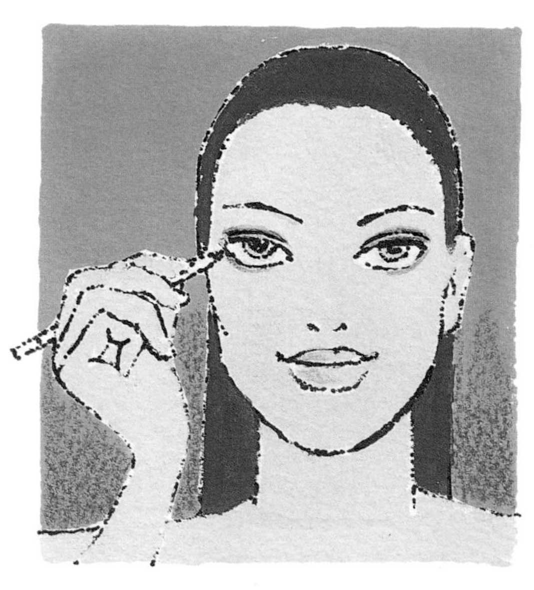

4. Once you've found the eyeshadow shade that works best bear in mind that eyeshadow applied with a foam applicator will appear stronger than that applied with a brush. Always blend out your eyeshadow with a blender brush for more professional results. Most make-up users wear eye colours to enhance and enlarge their eyes, so when applying eyeliner, remember to apply it only to the outer third of the eye (otherwise the eye may actually look smaller).

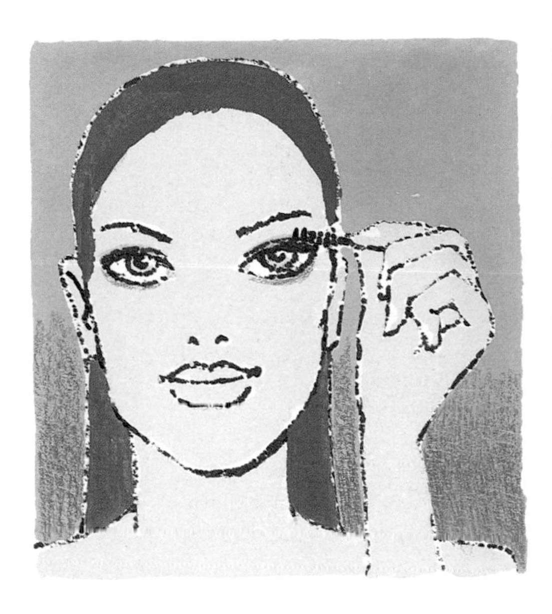

5. Mascara can be used to lengthen or thicken the look of the lashes. Before applying it, be sure to wipe any excess off the wand. By combing through the lashes after every coat of mascara, the lashes will appear more abundant. If you use more than two coats of mascara, the lashes tend to look clogged. After applying mascara, don't forget the brows: set them by combing through a brow gel, then define with an eyebrow make-up.

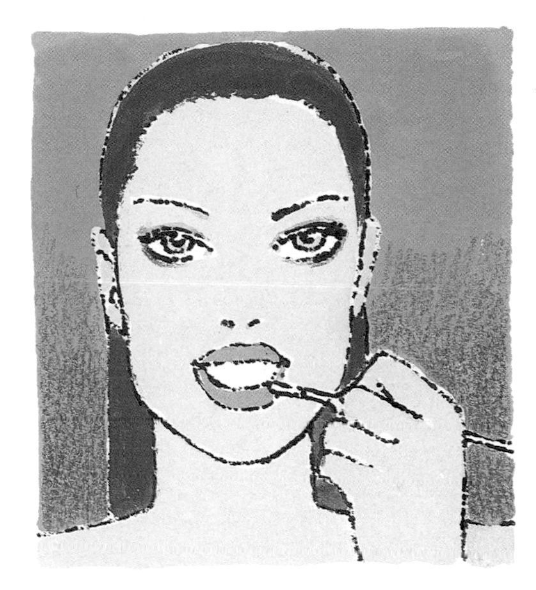

6. Use a lip liner to keep lipstick in place and stop the colour "bleeding". Sharpen your lip pencil regularly to ensure a finer line and practice lining your lips by starting at the centre of the cupid's bow and working out to the corners of the lips in short strokes.

For a longer lasting lipstick, apply with a brush. After applying, blot with one layer of tissue, apply a little loose powder over the tissue, remove carefully, apply a second coat of lipstick and blot lightly.

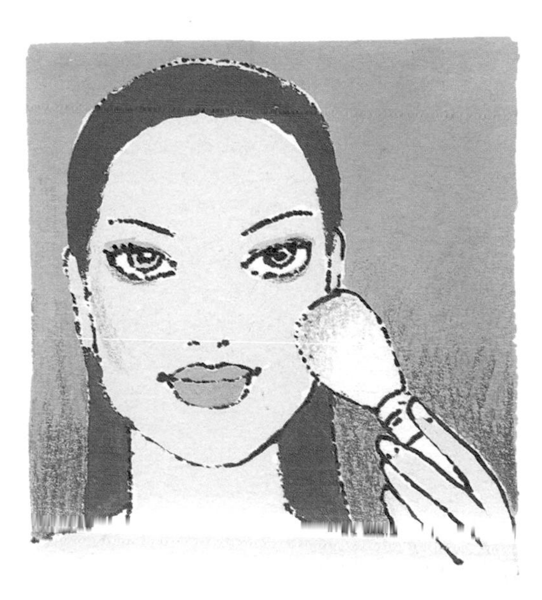

7. Blusher should complement your look and provide a balance between the strength of your make-up and lip make-up. To avoid the "dolly cheek" look, blusher should always be applied at the end of your make-up routine. Apply blusher with a large-headed blusher brush to the apple (the fattest part) of the cheek and then sweep the colour up towards the temples. To ensure your blush looks natural, use your powder puff to blend away the edges of the colour.

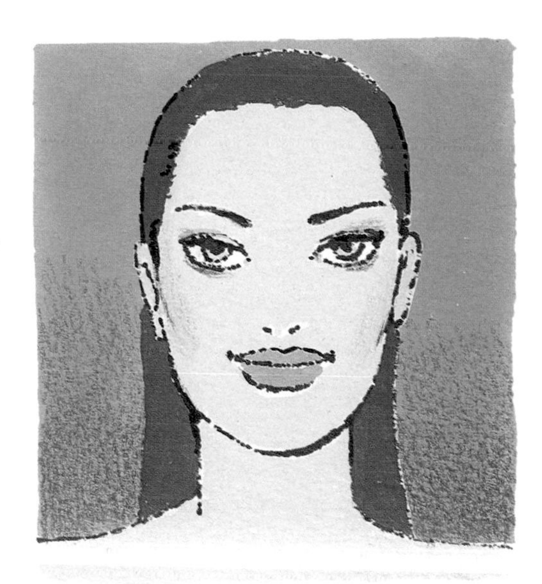

8. Take a large clean blusher brush or a fan-shaped finishing brush to dust off any excess powder or any flecks of eyeshadow that might have fallen onto your cheek. Now you're ready to go!

- More interest in using more unusual natural extracts where they can be proven to benefit the performance of the product.
- More products developed specifically for the "mature" make-up wearer.
- Make-up that works like a skincare product, moisturising and conditioning the skin.
- Higher SPFs in make-up (and not just in the usual foundations).
- Make-up with greater durability.
- Dual or triple action products such as Complete Colour, Colourings' three-in-one stick for eyes, cheeks and lips.

AND NOW FOR SOMETHING COMPLETELY DIFFERENT...

Men and make-up have a longstanding relationship. In Ancient Egypt, both men and women painted their nails, the colour of the paint signifying their place in the social order. Red was for the Pharaohs, the men at the top of the social pyramid. And both sexes mixed ground beetle shells and malachite to make glittery eye shadows. Tutankhamen's tomb contained jars of skin cream, lip colour and rouge that were still usable more than three thousand years after their formulation.

Charles Baudelaire, 19th century French poet, advised the use of black eyeliner: "It makes our look deeper and more particular, converting the eye into a window open to infinity."

Roman centurions painted their faces and lightened their hair with preparations picked up on the easternmost fringes of the empire, while their commanders went into battle with matching lip gloss and nail varnish, their careful manicures a token of their sophistication and social superiority.

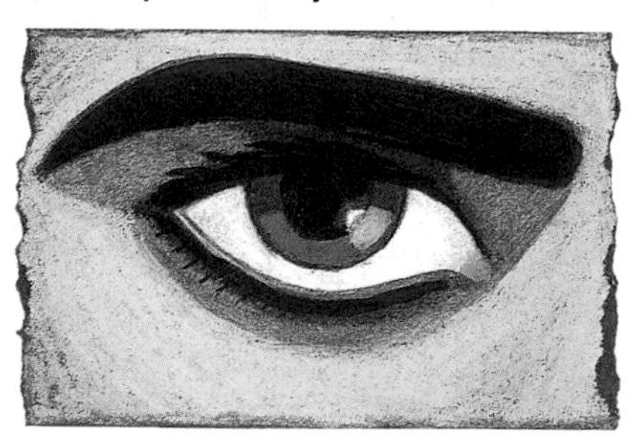

From Elizabeth I to Louis XVI, the courts of Europe were full of men painted, varnished and periwigged often to ludicrous degrees. When the 19th century spread its pall of sobriety across England, make-up on men became a sign of social deviation that proved irresistible to would-be dandies. Much the same situation prevailed during this century when any whisper of paint on a male face was used as proof by conservatives that the fall of the Western empire was just around the corner.

The 1960s introduced a different kind of self-consciousness. Men or, more truthfully, boys were encouraged to move on from using hippy body paint and the woad of Woodstock to tasteful embellishments created specifically for them by the likes of Mary Quant. But encouragement wasn't enough. Though the more outrageous pop stars like Mick Jagger and Jimi Hendrix had no qualms about a kohl-rimmed eye or a glossed lip, the man in the street tended to resist the blandishments of style leaders. David Bowie probably did more for men in make-up than anyone since King Tut, but the paint he sported had a blatant theatricality that limited its appeal to the mainstream man.

And yet it's precisely that mainstream that is now being drawn to cosmetics. More than 10 per cent of men polled in a 1993 UK survey felt that it is as important for a man to tend to his looks as it is for a woman. In a world in which everyone judges a book by its cover, anything that enhances the appearance is bound to appeal. As the skin-care market for men has grown alongside the fitness boom and more and more men opt for a little "surgical refreshment", it makes perfect sense that cosmetics should eventually get a look in.

But cosmetics for the modern man mean a subtle application of products that women use every day: foundation, concealer stick, powder, clear lip gloss and bronzers for a healthy glow. As yet, there have been no new cosmetic ranges developed with men in mind so anyone choosing to use women's product lines should bear these points in mind:

- Given the oiliness of men's skins, it's best to opt for oil-free foundations. Colour-free foundation offers an even skin tone with no change of hue. And make sure the skin is well-shaved before application.
- A little translucent powder helps dull the sheen of oily skin.
- Concealer sticks are an excellent way to redress morning-after ravages without going for a fully cosmeticised look.
- Lip balms offer lips moisture and protection without giveaway colour.
- Though clear mascara can't be seen, it goes a long way towards giving the eye a brighter, bolder appearance.

THIN LIPS, BIG LIPS & EYEBROWS

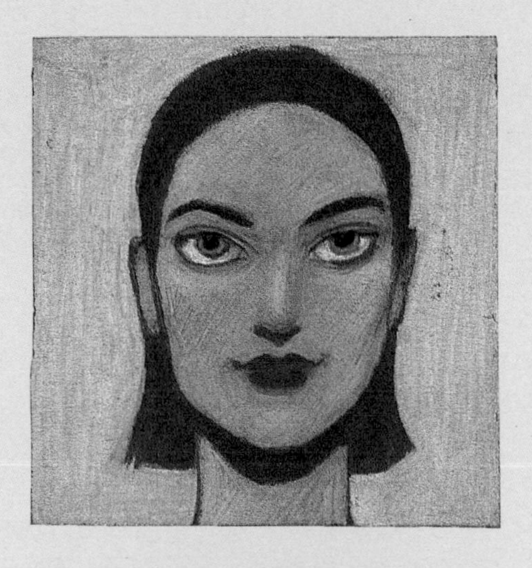

1. Dark, intense shades of lipstick will make thin or narrow lips seem even narrower.

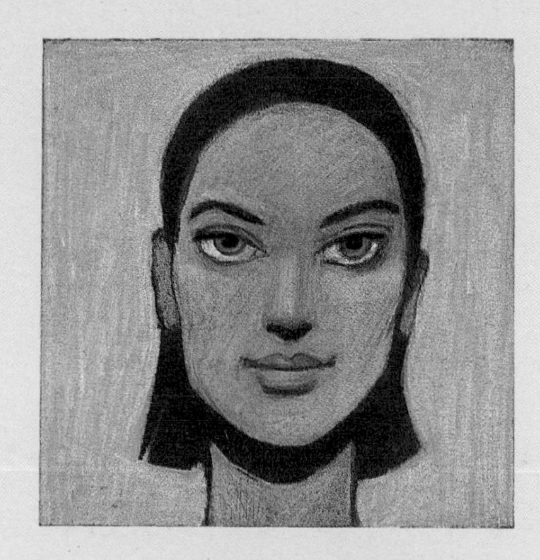

2. But by applying a paler shade of lipstick, narrow lips will appear more generous.

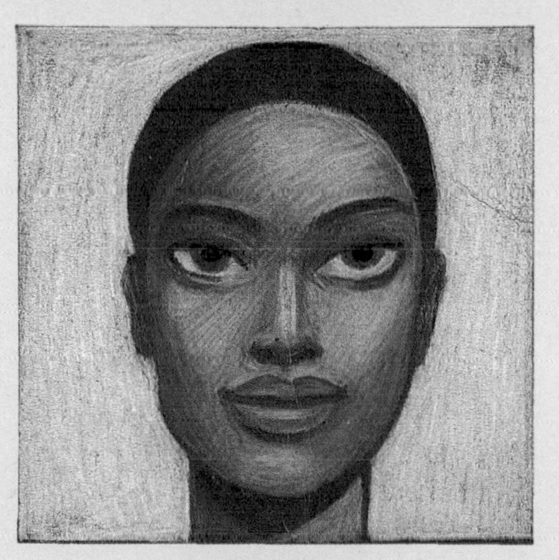

3. Wearing a pale lipstick will make full lips appear larger.

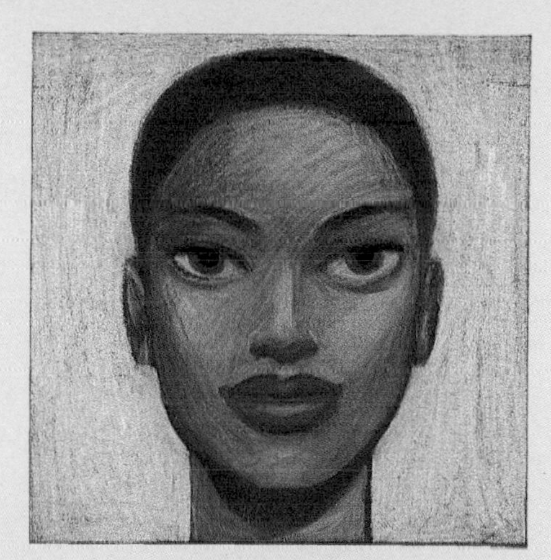

4. To minimise full lips, simply apply a darker, more intense shade of lip colour.

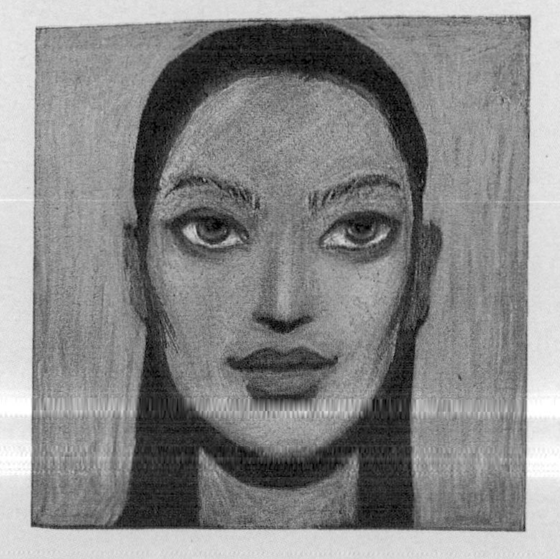

5. Undefined eyebrows add little to the overall effect of the face.

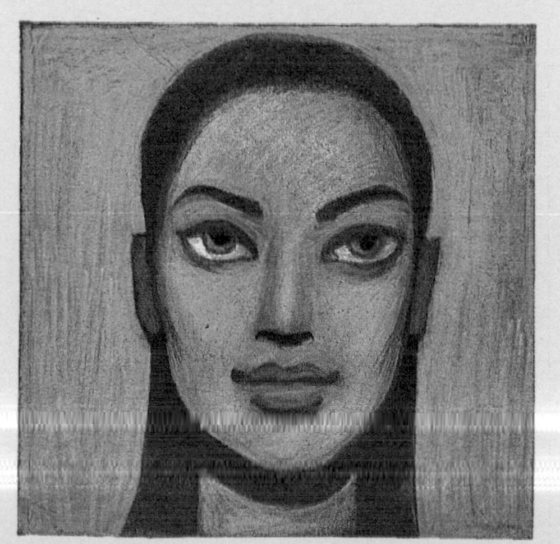

6. By making-up the brows, the entire eye area appears to have more definition. Defined eyebrows seem to form a "frame" for the face.

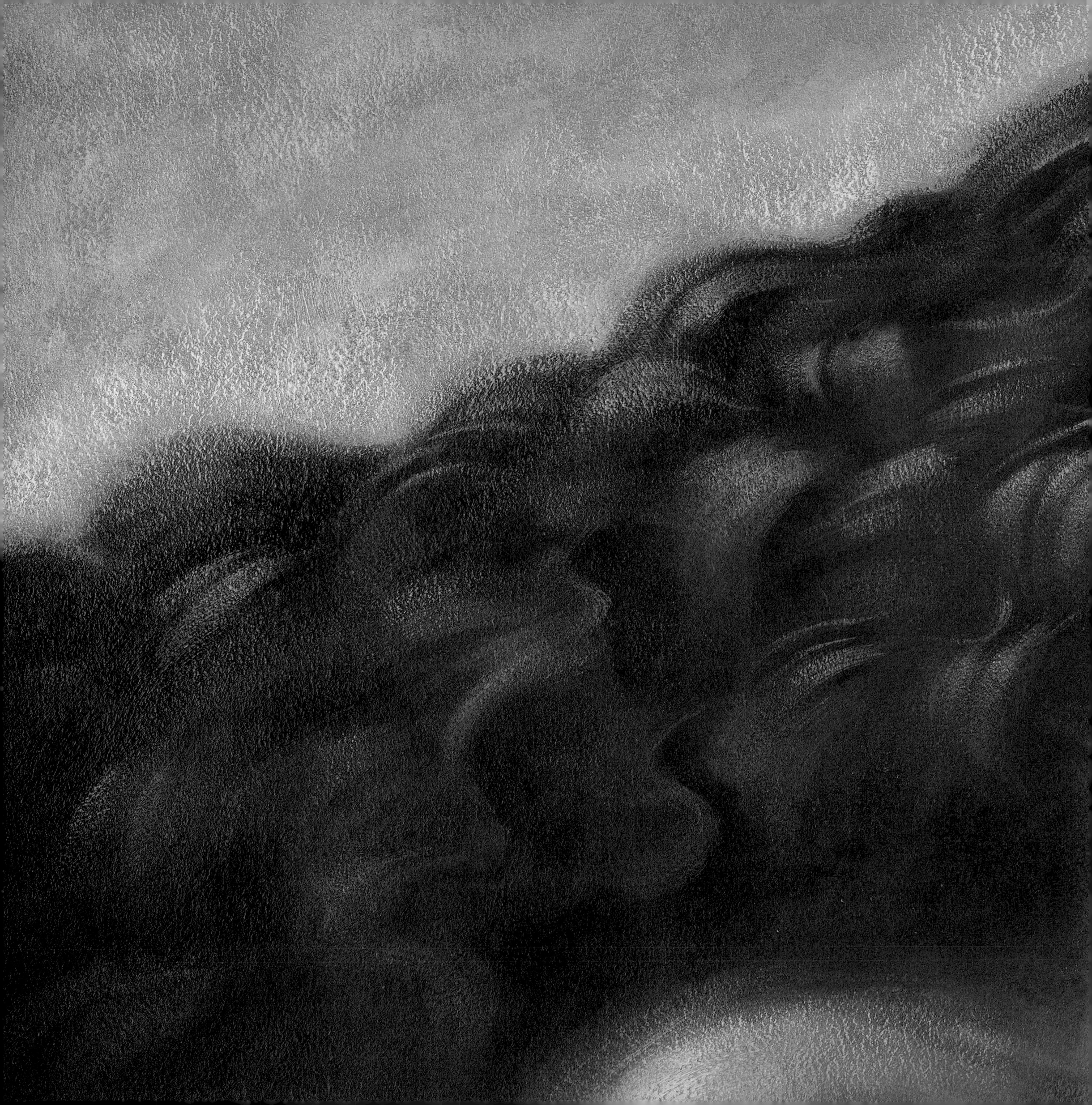

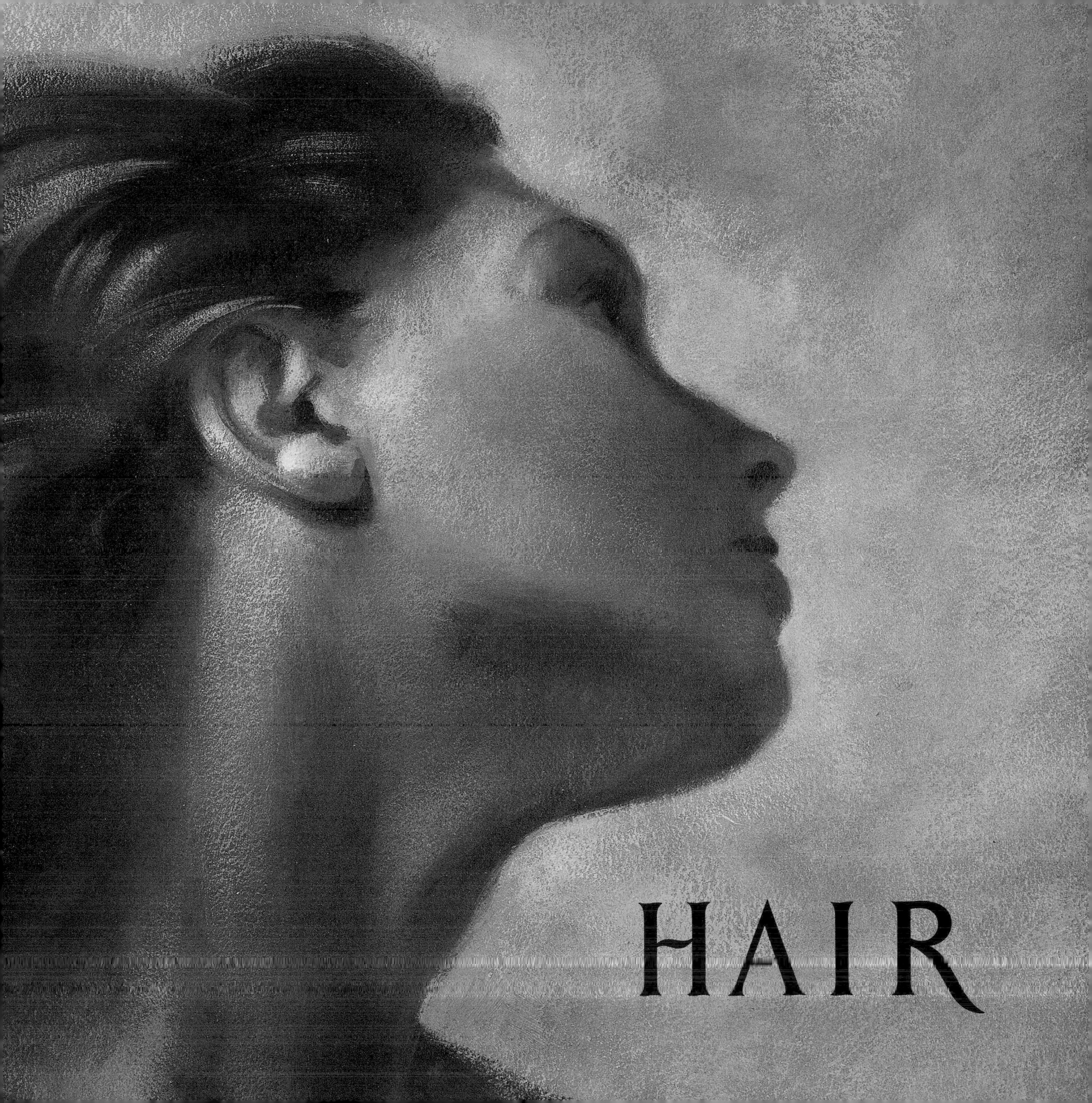
HAIR

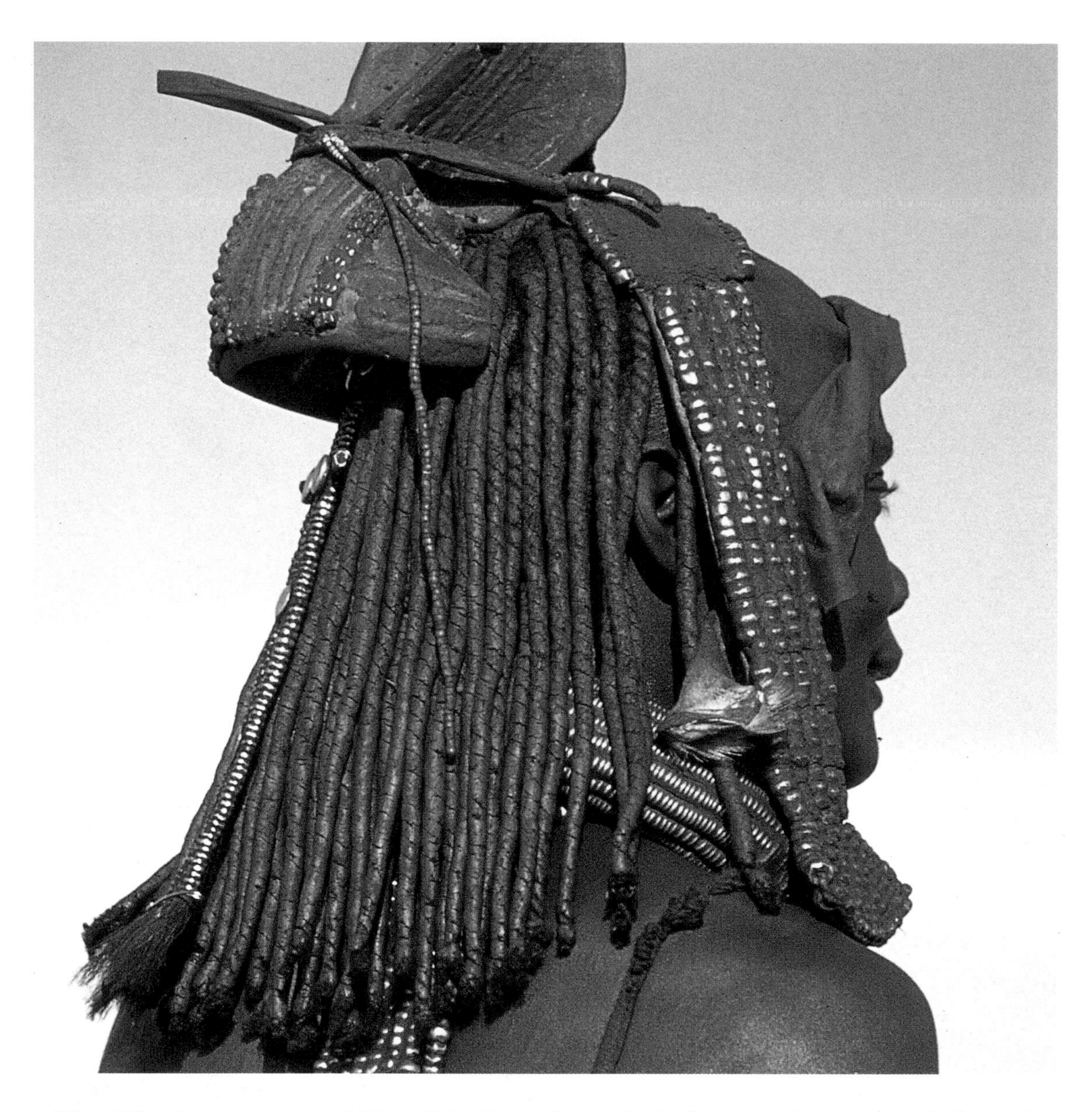

The Himba women of Namibia lengthen their hair with twists of sheep's wool, then set it in place with a mixture of mud, fat and ochre.

hair

Throughout history hair has been one of the easiest ways to signal social, religious, even political allegiances. Whether long, short, braided, loose, coloured, au naturel or not there at all, hair sends a signal - and rightly or wrongly, people make judgements about us based on those signals.

But we can constantly manipulate the information our hair sends out. It gives us an amazing variety of choices. If blondes aren't having more fun, they can always choose to become redheads or raven-tressed. By changing our hair at will, we can transform how other people "read" us. You don't have to be Madonna to appreciate hair's transformational powers.

> ***Your hair is your identity badge. As well as declaring who you are, it says how you belong. Wherever you live, whatever you do, it's one of the first things strangers notice.***

RITUAL HAIR

While in the Western world we tend to be intensely private about the body, we're quite happy to go public with our hair care by heading off to the hairdressers. The haircut is, in fact, a collective activity for many cultures. Native American groups like the Sioux are terrified of cutting their hair and all do so at the same appointed time, just like social butterflies in London or Manhattan who coordinate visits to smart salons so they can catch up on news.

The Maasai warriors of East Africa have a similar, social, view of hair care. They spend hours together, plaiting their hair and swapping tips on how to beautify it. So do the Moran, the warriors of the Samburu tribe of Northwest Kenya. They can spend up to 12 hours a day collectively braiding their long locks and applying yellow ochre for colour. Unsurprisingly, the Moran set enormous value on their hair. Imagine how you'd feel going to the hairdresser's for a crewcut; that's nothing compared to the way a Moran would feel. The warriors never trim their hair, but they must shave it right off when someone dies. It is an act of ultimate sacrifice, demonstrating kinship with and honour to the dead in an act that strips the warriors, temporarily, of their prized personal beauty.

MAGIC, SEX AND SYMBOLISM

Hair has always been a major component of primal magic. It's easy to see why. Like the earth, it can be harvested and it will grow again. And it seems to have a life of its own - it continues to grow after we are dead.

Hair has always been used as a fundamental representation of the power of the whole human organism. "Kaiser" and "Tsar" both mean "long haired". Headhunters in Borneo and Indians on the American Plains took scalps not as trophies but to enhance their shields with the powers of their victims. In societies where sorcery is practised, people take care to hide their hair clippings so that witch doctors can't put curses on them. Along with tail of newt and eye of toad, hair has always been a sorcerer's standby in all sorts of folkloric potions.

Hair also stands for virility. The idea that hair is the visible symbol of a man's hidden penis has been around since Delilah unmanned Samson with a short back and sides. Hair grows faster when we are young and strong, and slowly, or not at all when we are old. Its growth is also mysteriously stimulated by sexual activity.

A good diet will show in your hair. High protein foods are important, as are dairy products, fresh fruit, salads and vegetables.

It was once believed that comets shooting through the night sky were tendrils of the Great Mother's hair, the last the ancient world would see of her before she abandoned it to its destiny. Perhaps that forsaken feeling helps explain why abundant female tresses have on occasion inspired male distrust and fear. Or perhaps it's simply a deep-seated and abiding male fear of female sexuality.

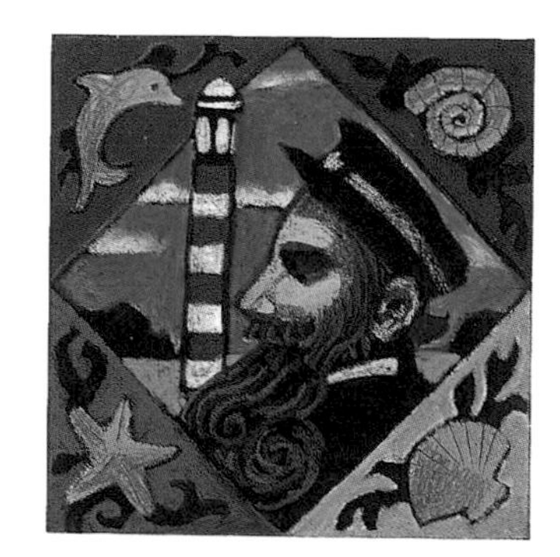

Hair growth is stimulated by sexual activity or the expectation of it. One case study involved a lighthouse keeper whose beard growth was recorded; growth peaked just before he went home on leave and was at its lowest after he had returned to work.

In myth, a woman with masses of hair was seen as positively terrifying. India's Tantric sages warned that unbinding a woman's hair would unleash catastrophe. Medieval Christians believed witches unbraided their hair to brew up tempests. Scottish girls from seafaring families still honour that conviction, leaving their hair alone on the nights when their brothers set out to sea. Even today, the quaintly folkloric tradition of the maypole dance refers to the mythical properties and the power of plaiting and unplaiting hair. And when the wild animals hunted by the Inuit Indians of the frozen North grow scarce, the bravest magic man in the tribe must carry out a ritual which represents an effort to appease the Mother of the Sea Beasts by combing out her hair. Only then will the animals caught in it be released and the hunters freed to take up the chase once more.

Fear of another kind motivated the early Christian church. It was believed that bats, the devil's own messengers, would become ensnared in it, which is why women had to wear hats to church. The tradition persists even though we now know that bats have precise natural radar and better places to nest than churchgoers' hairdos!

So much for fear. But the powers that were attributed to female hair were undoubtedly sexual, and sex is indeed an awesome force. The fear of female hair endures in some societies. Strict Muslim women may not show their hair and must cover it with a Hijib so that men won't be seduced. Some Hassidic Orthodox Jewish brides must shave their hair and don wigs, for fear that their natural hair could work spells on their husbands. Without it, they are less able to lure their husbands into sex for anything other than procreative purposes.

Other croppings have an even more sinister subtext. During World War Two, concentration camp inmates were shorn to signify that they had been robbed of everything, even their individuality. After the war, those who had collaborated with the German invaders of France were shorn to symbolise their shame.

But as well as the issue of punishment through shattering someone's vanity and looks, hair is an obvious target for purification when the body and mind are considered to be defiled. Because it is essentially an excretion from the body, it can be seen as contaminated. So women accused of witchcraft during the Middle Ages were "purified" by shearing before they were burned. Cropping their own hair didn't save them from the stake. A woman who cut her own hair short was seen as odd, which tended to mean she was also a witch. At least, that was the reasoning used against Joan of Arc. Then, a self-shorn head could mean antisocial individuality. Today, it can stand for antisocial instincts of quite another colour. The shaven heads of neo-Nazi skinheads betoken a pack mentality of the worst kind.

HAIR AS PROTEST

In our century, the removal of hair on face or head has often been the first step towards a declaration of conformity. In the military, a shearing on induction is the great leveller. So there was no simpler way for young men to protest against their governments' military and defence programmes in the 1960s and 1970s than to grow their hair. And long hair quickly became a badge of distaste for establishment mores of all kinds. In the black community, the Afro, sported to iconic effect by 1960s' activist Angela Davis, signified an awakened political consciousness. The poster for the smash-hit musical "Hair" became the emblem of the style.

In some mammals, such as whales and elephants, hair is restricted to scattered bristles. A rhinoceros's horn is actually a dense tuft of fused hair.

HAIR'S GOT SOUL

So that's hair's serious side: a pointer to where we stand on society, religion, politics and the status quo, as well as a symbol of sexuality and virility. But what about hair as a simple thing of beauty? Hair's got soul. A lock of hair is a traditional token of love. A medieval knight would ride to battle with a lock of his lady's hair, anonymously given because milady would often be married to another long before the knight returned from his adventure. Or the knight might even take a snip of pubic hair.

If it's soulful, hair can also be doleful. In some societies where hair is usually worn long, it is shorn to indicate grief and vice versa - if hair is usually kept short, it is allowed to grow excessively long. In Imperial Japan, when a woman's husband died, she would cut off her hair and put it in a pilgrim's bag. Her husband's ghost could thus take something of her with him to the next world. By sacrificing a part of the body, cutting the hair stands for a symbolic sacrifice of the whole body.

In the Western world, we too make a connection between hair and trauma. Though we tend not to scar our bodies, as some tribes do, to mark passing phases in our lives we may react by cutting our hair. A recent example would be the severe bobbed style adopted by Princess Caroline of Monaco after the death of her husband. And hair itself reacts physically to trauma, by falling out, or by turning white or grey overnight in times of great stress or grief.

HAIR WHAT

But what is actually at the root of all this magic and mystery? A hair follicle is a cavity in the skin surrounded by clumps of cells called papillae. Gorged with blood from the capillaries that feed them, papillae are stimulated to produce hair cells, which harden or keratinise, die and become the hair shaft. The hair is then pushed out through the follicle like toothpaste through a tube.

Everyone is born with a finite number of hair follicles which remains static. An average count would reveal between 90,000 and 150,000 hairs per head. It's the follicle that determines the shape and size of the shaft. The larger the follicle, the thicker the hair. The natural oiliness or dryness of hair is also determined by the follicle. Attached to it are sebaceous gland sacs which pump out sebum, the hair's lubricating oil.

The hair fibre core, or cortex, is made up of two components. The larger is the paracortex, which is relatively tough. The other is the orthocortex which is less resilient. The relative amounts of orthocortex to paracortex vary in human hair according to racial type. Negroid hair has the highest relative level of orthocortex. Mongoloid hair has the least and is therefore the toughest. Caucasian hair is somewhere in between. The different cells in the orthocortex and the paracortex are thought to contribute to curl in hair fibres, hence the curl in Negroid hair and the straightness of Mongoloid hair.

We actually have fine downy hair, called vellous hair, everywhere on our bodies, except on the lips, soles of the feet and palms of the hands. Eyelashes, eyebrows and nostril hairs are classed as terminal hair. They are coarser to protect the sensitive eyes and nose from irritation, bacteria and germs. Pubic hair is also terminal hair. It is generally long, possibly because its purpose is to prevent chafing of sensitive skin areas, though it is also useful to have longer hair to allow sweat a route through to the air. Sweat serves to cool the body and does so marvellously.

But it is the hair on our heads that unsurprisingly gets most attention. In good condition, this hair is so flexible and strong - stronger even than copper wire - that you can suspend an egg from one strand.

Hair has three layers: the cuticle, the outer layer made up of overlapping scales; the cortex of cells, which provides stretch, strength and the colouring pigment; and the medulla, the inner core of round cells which gives

Rastafarians are proud of the sheer mass and size of their dreadlocks, which they regard as high-tension cables to heaven in the same way that medieval church builders regarded soaring steeples as heading straight up to God. Rastas call their coiled hair Dreads because they aim to inspire fear with them.

TEN STEPS TO CLEAN HEALTHY HAIR

1. Begin with a pre-wash to condition the hair or to moisturise or stimulate the scalp. If your scalp is dry, massage Joboja Oil or Aromatherapy Scalp Oil thoroughly into the scalp and leave for 20-30 minutes. Rinse.

2. When washing, lean forwards over bath or basin to stimulate circulation in the scalp. Never wash hair while taking a bath - water can be dirty and teeming with undesirable elements!

3. Use only one capful of shampoo and spread it between the palms of your hands.

4. Massage shampoo gently into the scalp using the pads of your fingertips. DO NOT use the length of your hair as a pad and do not massage shampoo into hair growing below chin length. If you wash your hair frequently most shampoos are effective enough to warrant only one shampoo per wash.

5. Rinse hair thoroughly - any residue will leave hair dull and sticky, attracting dirt.

6. Blot dry on a towel. Do not rub, pull or wring as this can make wet hair lose much of its resilience and elasticity.

7. Condition the hair - especially the ends. For long hair use a tablespoon of conditioner, for short hair, a teaspoon. Use a wide-toothed comb to ease the conditioner through the hair gently.

8. Rinse again - a general rule is to rinse for twice as long as you think you should. Wrap a towel around the head.

9. Comb gently. Wet hair is fragile. Section the hair and comb from the ends working up to the roots.

10. Dry naturally if possible. If using a hair dryer - blow the air down the shafts of the hair and stop drying when it is still a little damp.

hair its thickness. The medulla was once thought to be the life shaft of the hair. In the past, split ends were singed to keep life in, which is nonsense. Hair is, of course, quite dead to begin with!

Human hair has one of the most prolific growth rates in the body, particularly between the ages of 11 and 30. It can grow up to half an inch a month. This growth is a cyclic activity, the active or anogen phase alternating with a resting period known as the telogen phase. The anogen phase can last up to three years. Its duration determines the terminal length of hair fibres Between the anogen and telogen phases there is a short transitional stage, the catogen phase, in which newly formed hair moves towards the scalp surface.

HAIR WHY

Hair protects the brain from the heat and ultraviolet rays of the sun and helps to insulate the skull against cold and pressure. It also acts as a sensor. Beneath each follicle is a small muscle, the arrector pili muscle, which contracts with fear or cold. So hair standing on end is a kind of early warning system.

CARING FOR THE HAIR

It may be technically dead but that doesn't stop hair responding not only to our state of mind but also to our general health and the care we take of it. It has long been recognised in India that the health of the hair depends upon the fertility of the ground from which it springs. So the scalp is regularly anointed with oils. Hair unguents include almond, jasmine, clove, rose, orange, henna, even mustard. Scalp care, cleansing with shampoo, massage, and a regular workout with a clean hairbrush to remove dead skin particles and dirt, work wonders for the hair.

It wasn't always so. In the Middle Ages, washing hair wasn't a popular option. All that was needed for "clean hair" was pest control. By the 18th century, women had taken to carrying antiseptic fluid in their cleavages to kill the bugs that dropped from their hair. The regular application of soap and water to the hair was regarded as a health hazard, even by doctors, up to the 19th century.

SHAMPOO - WHAT'S IN A WORD?

In 19th century England, "shampoo" signified the kind of massage you got in a Turkish bath. Derived from the Hindu word champo "to knead", it came into currency at the same time as a vogue for all things Indian swept England. By the end of the 1870s, fashionable English hairdressers had refined the term to mean massaging and washing the scalp with a combination of soap, water and soda. Each salon had its own closely-guarded variant on this basic recipe.

But shampoo as we know it needs a detergent to remove the scalp's natural oil from the hair shaft - it is the oil that causes dirt to stick - and soap wasn't a really effective cleanser because it left its own scum on the shaft. Ancient Egyptians used citrus juice, the citric acid effectively cutting the oil.

The first *real* detergent-based shampoo was developed in Germany in the 1890s, though it was Massachusetts fireman John Breck who made it the household product it is today. Obsessed with heading off his own baldness, Breck spent his life developing hair and scalp products. He opened his first scalp treatment centre in Springfield, New England in 1908. By the end of the 1930s, he had a hugely successful nationwide business.

One detergent used in The Body Shop shampoos is sodium laureth sulphate, a mild and effective cleanser derived from coconut oil, rather than a petro-chemical oil.

CLEAN HAIR WAYS

There is a school of thought which says that you should never wash your hair because its natural oils will keep it moisturised and clean. In fact, the desirability of clean hair is a suprisingly recent development in the Western world.

It was only at the beginning of this century that regular washing of the hair caught on, made necessary by the clinging fumes and effluvia of big city life. Modern plumbing, particularly the shower, has made it easy for people to wash their hair every day. Though this is undoubtedly an improvement on brushing with bran, it is not necessarily a good thing. The scalp can be over-stimulated. Holding out for two days can lead to glossier hair in some cases.

FIRST THE PRE-WASH

Everyone can benefit from a pre-wash conditioning. Whatever your hair type, begin your hair care once or twice a week with a pre-wash, if you have time. Some pre-washes can help to moisturise or stimulate the scalp. Pre-wash conditioners smooth the cuticle and add emollients - like most conditioners they are designed for the hair itself, not really the scalp.

FACTS AND TIPS

STRIPPING Rather than too frequent washing causing the scalp's oil glands to work overtime, it is believed that washing with shampoos that are too harsh can strip the hair of natural oils and force the scalp to overcompensate.

EXTRA OILY Water and oil don't mix, so next time you wash your hair, apply diluted shampoo to dry hair and start working up a little lather. Once you've worked the shampoo in, wet and wash as usual.

ALL CHANGE Hair condition may benefit from alternating shampoos - choose a few of your favourite ones. If you alternate a conditioning shampoo with a non-conditioning shampoo, you may overcome the effects of build-up. Hair can also benefit from the application of different ingredients.

HOW OFTEN? Shampoo as often as necessary to keep hair looking good and your scalp feeling comfortable. The frequency may range from daily to weekly, depending on oiliness, hair style, scalp condition, physical activities and the environment you live in.

MYTHS AND FACTS

The more lather there is, the more effective the shampoo and the cleaner the hair.

WRONG One common mistake is to equate the amount of lather with the shampoo's potential to clean. Lathering agents are often added to shampoos, but

Here's a backhanded compliment to the social desirability of clean hair: the Fakirs of India signal their renunciation of this earth by keeping their hair long, matted and teeming with lice (not an easy thing - lice actually prefer squeaky clean hair!).

FACTS AND TIPS

TIP: DRY HAIR TREAT Soak the scalp with warm olive oil and wrap your hair in a hot towel for 20 minutes. Rinse with cold water, then shampoo.

TIP: OILY HAIR TREAT Dilute your shampoo; pour one capful into a cup, add warm water and egg yolk; stir thoroughly. Use one lather.

TIP: DON'T TAKE YOUR HAIR FOR GRANTED If your hair is dull due to damage to the cuticle layer from excessive dryness, overzealous use of heat-stylers, improper use of bleaching, waving, straightening or colouring, you will have to allow new hair to grow for permanent shine and gloss to return. But in the meantime use a gentle shampoo and conditioner to make it more manageable and steer clear of harsh treatments.

TIP: GO GENTLE Hair sometimes becomes limp and dull from a build-up of mousses, gels, hairsprays, shampoos and conditioners. If your hair is suffering, shampoo it for two weeks with a gentle, non-conditioning shampoo to remove build-up and bring back bounce and gloss.

TIP: IN THE SWIM Daily exposure to chlorine and salt water has a drying effect on hair that can lead to various problems - breakage, tangling, dull appearance. Make sure you use a mild shampoo and rinse out well after every swim. Apply a conditioner to counteract dryness, add gloss and make combing easier. Wrap hair in a towel and gently pat dry. Comb with a blunt-toothed comb. Leave to dry naturally if possible.

FACT: THE FINAL SOLUTION Split ends are the proof of a severly damaged cuticle. The only solution is to have them chopped off. Nothing mends split ends.

TIP: ANIMAL MAGIC Take a tip from the vet - vitamin B supplements improve the coats of animals and can work wonders for human hair.

more foam doesn't mean cleaner hair. Some more natural shampoos, like Henna Shampoo, don't lather up excessively but that doesn't mean they're not doing their job.

The more shampoo you use, the cleaner your hair will be.

WRONG Just one dollop of shampoo, about the size of a ten pence piece, slightly diluted and smeared between the palms of your hands is usually sufficient for shoulder length, frequently washed hair. Vary according to length, time between each wash, and whether your hair is dry or oily.

Conditioner helps repair split ends.

WRONG Conditioner may help to smooth down the cuticle and make hair seem in better condition but ultimately nothing will "repair" a split end, the only solution is cutting.

It is good always to use the same shampoo and conditioner.

WRONG Always using the same shampoo and conditioner means a residue can build up on the hair shaft, leaving hair limp and dull looking.

Not rinsing out conditioner properly is good.

WRONG Not giving the hair a thorough final rinse will undo all the good you have done by washing it. So unless it is specifically stated to the contrary on the bottle, rinse out all conditioner, otherwise your hair will be lank and your scalp prone to oiliness.

The longer you leave the conditioner on, the more effective it will be.

WRONG Conditioners usually only coat the hair - they do not penetrate the hair shaft. They are therefore as effective after only one minute, as after ten minutes. Oil or panthenol-based deep conditioning treatments do penetrate the hair shaft and should be left on longer.

Dry hair is damaged by too frequent washing.

WRONG Dry hair is generally only damaged if the shampoo used is too harsh, stripping the hair of all its natural oils. Hair is much more likely to be damaged if it is left too long between washes, clogging the follicles of the scalp with dirt and dead skin cells, blocking the flow of sebum (the scalp's natural oil) and making the hair dry and brittle. Apart from permanent hair styling and bleaching, damage is most likely if hair is combed harshly when wet with no conditioner.

For centuries the American Indians have used jojoba oil to care for their skin and hair. Its superb conditioning qualities leave hair soft and silky.

GARDEN SOLUTION

You can even look beyond the kitchen into the garden hedgerow, where you might find soapwort growing wild as a weed. It was once used in the textile mills in the North of England to clean cloth, and fabric conservationists still use it to clean silks and tapestries.

SHAMPOO ALTERNATIVES

Never wash hair in washing up liquid. Its effectiveness in stripping grease from dirty pots is not what is needed for the gentle removal of dirt from your hair. If you run out of shampoo, there are other things from the kitchen that will do the job as effectively - and far less harmfully.

TREAT FOR LIMP HAIR

Give shine to hair with flat beer. Try diluting one cup of flat beer with three cups of water to put spring back into flat hair. Be sure to rinse thoroughly if you don't want to smell like the local pub!

GO TO WORK ON AN EGG

For dry hair, separate an egg yolk and white. Whisk each separately, then fold together, massage into hair and leave for five minutes. Rinse with warm - not hot - water. If you use hot water you may end up with lumps of cooked egg in your hair! For the more adventurous, a paste made of mashed bananas applied to damp hair makes a rich pre-wash treatment. Leave it on for 15 minutes then shampoo out.

FRESH AND CLEAN

For a quick fresh-smelling hair cleanser and scalp astringent, cut a lime into thin slices and rub thoroughly over scalp. Lime or lemon juice and vinegar mixed together and diluted make a shiny final rinse. Leave the citrus juice on and sit in the sun for a while to help lighten blonde hair.

CONDITIONING

The fact that conditioners exist at all is testament to the effectiveness of modern shampoos. Before World War Two, shampoos didn't strip hair of dirt the way modern versions do, so a vinegar or lemon rinse was all that was necessary to give hair shine.

Conditioners are made up of emollient ingredients that help to smooth erratic cuticles and soften the hair leaving it tangle free. Despite the promises, conditioners can't mend split ends. What they can do is coat the hair shaft, cut down on static and ease tangling, and smooth down the scale-like cuticles so they lie in one direction, thus making the hair look shiny. They can also offer protection against the sun and other environmental threats.

HOW TO USE A CONDITIONER:

DO blot hair dry after shampooing for most effective application of conditioner.

DO start at the roots for general conditioning and gently work through with the fingers or a comb.

DO use a conditioner primarily for the ends of the hair, not necessarily for the scalp. Long, normal hair will benefit from a conditioner just on the ends. It's more economical too.

DO rinse conditioner out thoroughly.

DO condition scalp as well as hair. A massage with slightly warmed olive oil is simple and effective.

Home conditioning hints:

- **egg yolk or beer add body after shampooing**
- **1 tbsp vinegar in a pint of warm water helps combat tangles**
- **malt vinegar is especially good for dry or treated hair**

BANANA

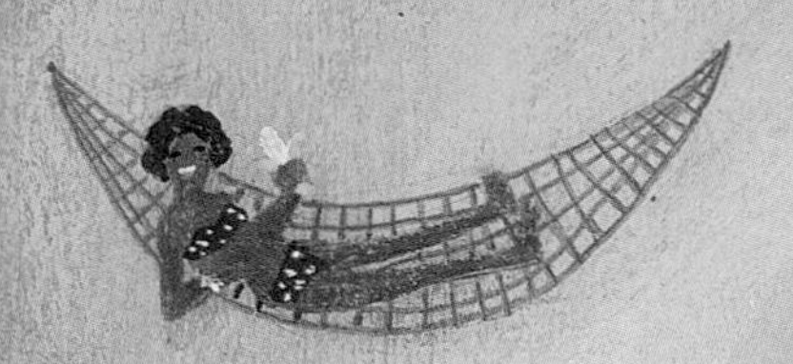

Bananas are rich in carbohydrates, potassium and vitamins A, B and C. They're also a natural relaxant because they contain tryptophan, a sleep-inducing amino acid that can have antidepressant qualities.

The Body Shop uses up to 250,000 bananas a year for our banana products.

Bananas are ideal for use in hair products because of their lubricating properties.

The English saw their first banana in April 1633 when shopkeeper Thomas Johnson mounted a large display in his shop window in Snow Hill, London. These fruit were just off the boat from Bermuda.

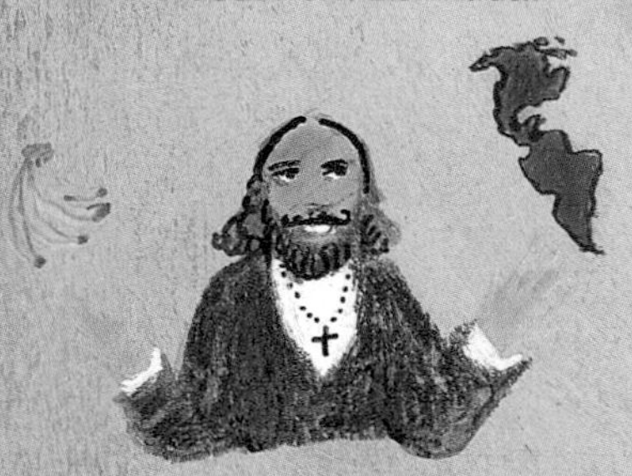

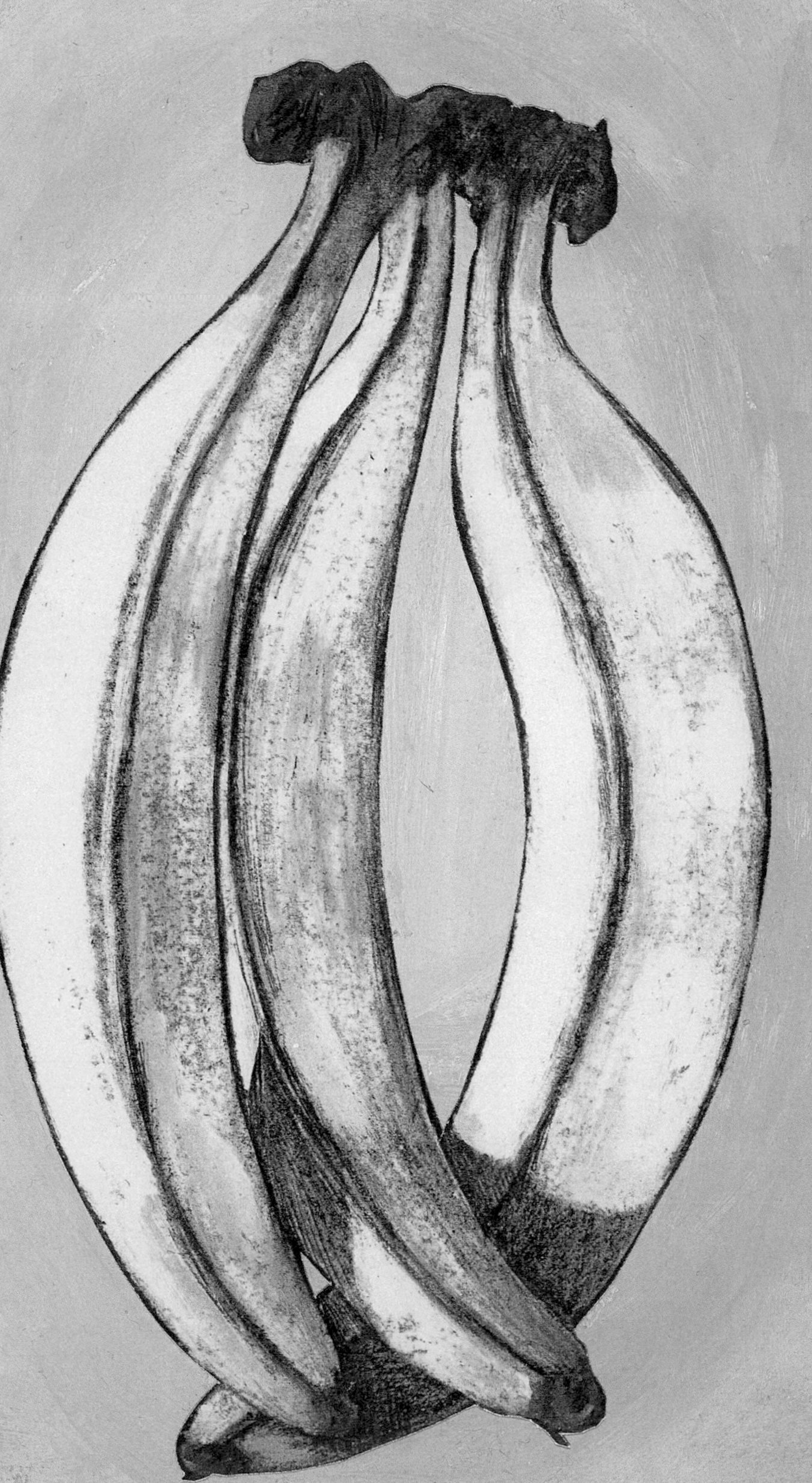

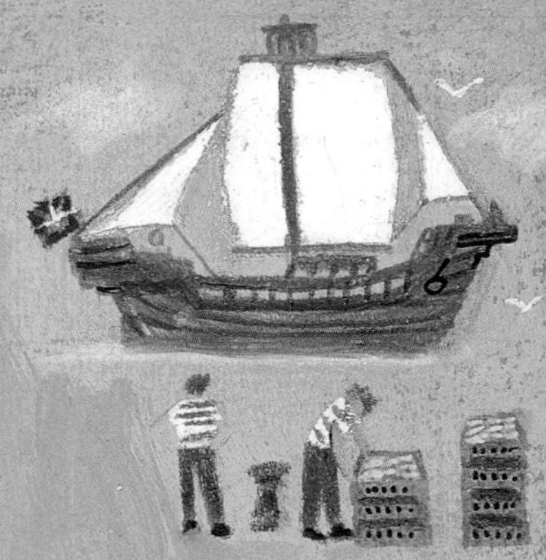

The world's favourite smell is banana, according to a 1988 study undertaken by the University of California.

The banana was introduced to the Americas by a Spanish missionary in 1516.

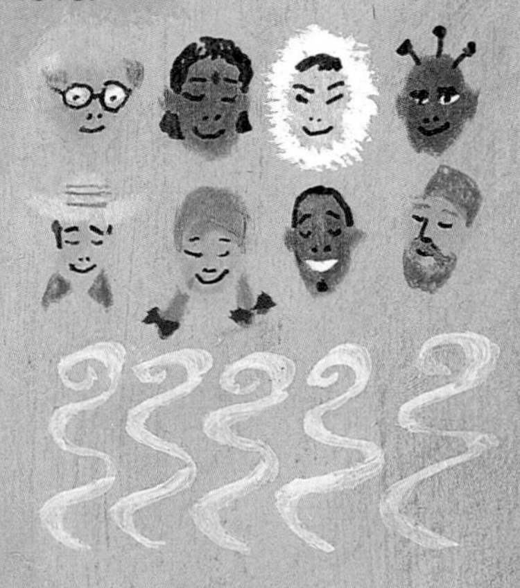

The Taiwano Indians treat scalp problems with heated extract of banana.

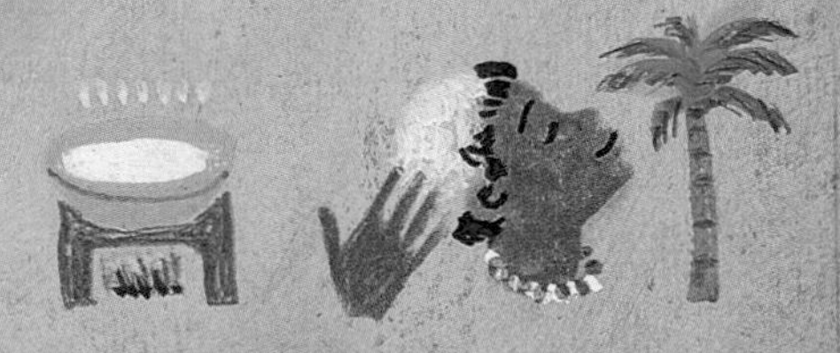

HAIR UNDER ATTACK

BLEACHING

Bleaching destroys the hair's colour pigments and usually damages the cuticle, leaving hair dry, dull, porous and prone to tangles.

COLOURING

Permanent colours generally lift the cuticle and bleach the natural colour so the new shade can penetrate the hair shaft. The colour is formed by the ingredients reacting together in the hair and fixing to the hair structure. This can leave hair dry and dull. Semi-permanent colours generally only penetrate slightly into the hair shaft and will wash out in 6 to 12 washes, sometimes longer. Temporary colours last for one shampoo unless the hair is very porous. They generally coat the hair shaft and do not penetrate the hair.

PERMING

Hair is wrapped around curlers and a lotion is applied. This penetrates the hair shaft and breaks the bonds in the hair that give it shape and strength. The hair adopts the new shape set by the curlers and is fixed into curls using a fixing lotion which causes new bonds to form in the hair. Perming damages the cuticle and cortex and can make the hair dry and prone to breaking.

RELAXING

Relaxing the hair is virtually the same as perming except hair is changed from curly to straight and the process can be even more damaging as stronger solutions are used. The cuticle has again been assaulted and the hair can become very dry and dull.

GENERAL ABUSE

Curling tongs, styling brushes and hair dryers can all break the hair. They are also notorious for burning it, dehydrating it and encouraging split ends. Elastic bands damage hair by ripping off the cuticle - always use material-covered bands. The sun will also dry and bleach the hair - keep it covered or protected, just as you would your skin.

A Mexican tip - wet the hair with aloe vera, allow to dry, rinse out at night. Adds lustre and manageability to the hair and acts as a partial sunscreen.

HAIR STYLING

People in the past may have been reluctant to keep their hair clean, but otherwise they had no qualms about fussing over it. Burnt bear claws made hair ornaments for primitive man and woman. They also used swallow droppings as a Neanderthal hair gel to keep hair out of their eyes.

THE PERM

One of the earliest permanent waving methods dates from the time of Louis XIV. It was known as "Frisure Infernale", or "Hell's own curls". Tresses were pulled over clay rollers then cooked for three hours in the oven. Thankfully, the technique was only used on wigs and not on people.

It wasn't until 1906 that the first perms were produced on a human head. Strands of hair that had been soaked in borax were rolled on metal curlers and enclosed in a heater brought to 150°F.

The process took a whole day and the heater was removed with a nutcracker, sometimes taking shanks of hair with it. Society women bragged of their burns.

Modern perming methods use a chemical called ammonium thioglycollate or one of its derivatives, to prise open the sulphur bonds which give hair natural stability and strength. Hair is wound around rollers and then neutralised to enable most of bonds to reform in the new position. Never perm hair more often than once every three months and avoid perming entirely if your hair is already damaged or weakened.

Wild hair styling peaked - literally - in 18th century France. The bigger the wig, the greater one's social status. The pillars of hair worn by both men and women were called Macaronis (hence Yankee Doodle Dandy's aspirational headgear). They were so high and heavy that they caused occasionally fatal abscessing on the temples.

BE KIND TO YOUR HAIR

We are our hair's worst enemy. Even the "magic face-lift" of pulling hair up in a pony tail can heighten the hair line, and eventually lead to partial hair loss. Straightening can lead to hot comb alopecia, or hair loss. And traditional practices, such as wrapping scarves tightly around the head as in Libya, twisting Sikh hair into a ball on the scalp or the tight braiding practised in the Sudan, can also lead to marginal alopecia.

We torture our hair with backcombing, twist it and pull it and yet expect it to look fine when we let it down. Why should it always behave as we want?

Tahitian women traditionally washed their black hair daily with sandalwood-scented coconut oil to leave it soft and glossy.

FOR THE BEST STYLING OF ALL:

DO blot dry your hair.

DON'T towel strenuously, as this can cause snags and loss of elasticity.

DO let your hair dry naturally. Avoid dryers whenever possible.

DO use a conditioner as defence against overstyling.

The first real hair stylists were the Ancient Assyrians whose cutting, curling, crimping and colouring 3,500 years ago would have been the envy of any modern hairdresser.

BRUSHING AND COMBING

Brushing helps to massage the scalp, loosen flaky skin and spread natural oils down the hair, which help protect it. Go for brushes set in rubber or with flexible bristles and wait until your hair is dry before brushing it.

Combing is not as damaging because it puts less pressure on the hairs. Choose a wide, round-toothed comb to remove tangles and help prevent the frizzies in curly hair. Do not comb wet hair more than is essential as it is very susceptible to damage. Don't tug tangles; comb out the ends and work upwards.

HAIR SHINES

Coconut oil, wheatgerm oil and avocado oil all help the hair retain water which keeps it looking healthy. These oils also smooth the hair shaft so that its scale-like structure lies flat, which has the effect of making dark hair shiny. The Body Shop Coconut Oil Hair Shine works in the same way, by adding shine and condition.

STYLERS

Styling products are not just limited to styling, they can protect the hair from the heat and the environment - and they're fun to experiment with. Gels, mousses, lotions and sprays all contain some form of film-forming polymers to create a thin, clear film on each hair strand. Curl, uncurl, mould, or add volume and shape to your hair - the choice is yours.

MOUSSES

Ideal for thin, limp or fine hair, mousses add control and volume to all hair styles. Some mousses also contain conditioners and sunscreens. Work through damp hair, then style with a brush and dryer, or scrunch dry to add volume. Also good as a conditioner between shampoos.

GELS

Gels can shape hair firmly and give extra hold, body and shine. Choose from traditional gel form or a lighter gel spray which gives firm control without stickiness. On damp, freshly washed hair, gels give volume and control. On dry hair, gels create a slick, wet appearance that holds hair in place. Apply gel on wet or dry hair and spread evenly. Shape with fingers, a brush and/or a dryer.

HAIR SPRAY

Originally formulated in the 1950s, hair sprays are used after the hair is dry and styled to provide a final layer of control. Today's hair sprays control styling by both protecting the hair from moisture and holding hair together. And pump-activated mechanisms are an effective replacement for ozone-damaging aerosols.

SETTING LOTIONS

These provide control and body when you're setting your hair with rollers or hot rollers. They're usually used for soft, waved natural hair styles.

DRYERS

Hair dryers speed up the drying process and help to style - but use on a low setting and protect hair with a styling product first. The same goes for curling tongs, hot irons and heated rollers.

FINGER-DRYING

Don't overlook your fingers as a styling tool. Run them through your hair, scrunch and fluff hair up. Finger dry after towelling and eliminate the need for some blow-drying and setting.

HAIR COLOURS

Note: it is very important that you ALWAYS CARRY OUT A STRAND TEST before you apply any Herbal Hair Colour.

HAIR COLOUR	**STRAWBERRY TO DARK BLONDE**	**LIGHT BROWN**	**MID-BROWN**	**DARK BROWN**	**BLACK**	**REDHEAD**	**GREY** (less than 30 per cent sprinkling of grey)
BLONDE HERBAL HAIR COLOUR	After 10 minutes. Golden/ honey tones.	After 30 minutes Golden/bronze highlights.	Unsuitable.	Unsuitable.	Unsuitable.	Unsuitable.	Unsuitable.
EXTRA RED HERBAL HAIR COLOUR	Unsuitable.	Unsuitable.	15 minutes to 5 hours. Bright auburn sheen.	15 minutes to 5 hours. Deep auburn hue.	1-5 hours. Imparts subtle red lights.	15 minutes to 5 hours. Brings out red lights.	Unsuitable.
RICH RED BROWN HERBAL HAIR COLOUR	Unsuitable.	Unsuitable.	15 minutes to 5 hours. Auburn/ chestnut colour.	15 minutes to 5 hours. Deep chestnut lights.	Unsuitable.	15 minutes to 5 hours. Brings out auburn lights.	1 hour. Will give bright auburn lights.
BROWN HERBAL HAIR COLOUR	Unsuitable.	Unsuitable.	15 minutes to 3 hours. Rich, dark brown colour.	15 minutes to 3 hours. Deep walnut tone.	Unsuitable.	Unsuitable.	1 hour. Helps to blend in grey
BLACK HERBAL HAIR COLOUR	Unsuitable.	Unsuitable.	Unsuitable.	15 minutes to 1 hour. Raven black hair.	15 minutes to 1 hour. Enhances black hair and adds shine.	Unsuitable.	Unsuitable.
	Note: Blonde Herbal Hair Colour is unsuitable for hair that is sun-bleached, highlighted/ bleached, colour treated or permed.	**Note:** Blonde Herbal Hair Colour is unsuitable for hair that is sun-bleached, highlighted/ bleached, colour treated or permed.	**Note:** if you have colour treated, permed hair you must do a strand test when using Brown, Extra Red and Rich Red Brown Herbal Hair Colours.	**Note:** if you have colour treated, permed hair you must do a strand test when using Brown, Extra Red and Rich Red Brown Herbal Hair Colours.	**Note:** All other Herbal Hair Colours may add shine to the hair, but will impart little colour, except on grey strands.		**Note:** If you have a sprinkling or less than 30 per cent grey on mid- to dark-brown hair you must do a strand test when using Rich Red Brown and Brown Herbal Hair Colour.

HAIR COLOUR

For as long as people have been styling their hair, they've been colouring it. Caesar reported seeing Saxons with hair dyed blue with woad. Peculiar nuggets of folk wisdom have attached themselves to hair colour over the centuries. Did you know, for instance, that blondes, brunettes and redheads are supposed to smell different? Certainly, different hair colours carry all sorts of stereotypes, which are now completely scrambled because so many people no longer sport the hair colour they were born with.

White hair is usually thicker than coloured hair so people who go grey at a young age often have an enviable head of hair.

Lead combs were the rage in the 17th century because they turned wet hair a fashionable shade of black - as well as inducing lead poisoning and kidney failure.

In 1950, 7 per cent of American women dyed their hair. Today, that number is more like 75 per cent. That's why hair colour has not been a required physical feature on passports since 1969.

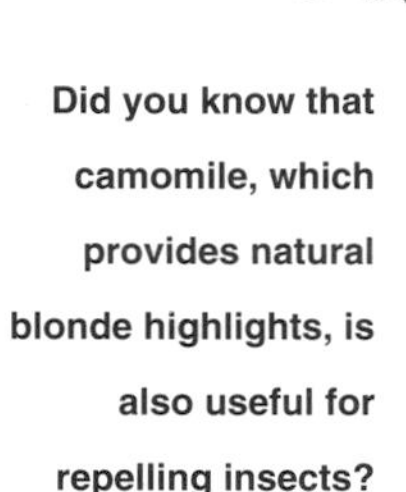

RED HAIR

Because red hair has never been common, it has always had many strange associations. Red is the colour of Mars, so redheads are supposed to be fiery. Until the Middle Ages, they were also viewed as innately treacherous because it was thought Judas was a redhead.

Did you know that camomile, which provides natural blonde highlights, is also useful for repelling insects?

Copper was judged to be the metal of Venus, so 16th century Venetian women tried all sorts of tricks to turn their hair into Titian red-gold curls. They suffered sunstroke from sitting out during the hottest part of the day with their hair drenched in caustic soda. Then, with Elizabeth I, red hair became the shade of royalty in England. Women who wanted to look like her applied saffron and sulphur powder to their hair. The result? Headaches, nausea and nosebleeds, along with a reddish tinge.

BLONDE HAIR

Blonde hair has had a rollercoaster ride over the millennia. In Ancient Greece, it was the shade of heroes like Achilles and Paris. The Romans favoured dark hair until Caesar's armies returned home with Gallic captives they'd taken as slaves. Their blonde tresses started a new trend with brunette Roman matrons who started experimenting with hair lighteners. After these potions had made their hair fall out, they made wigs from the hair of the captured Germans.

Contrast our own century during which blonde hair has suggested dumbness due, no doubt, to the tireless efforts of Hollywood to promote strings of feather-brained platinum-haired sexpots. Appropriately, it's show business that has redressed the balance with Madonna, whose multimillion dollar business patently belies any connotations stirred up by her defiantly artificial hair colour.

Blondes generally have the largest number of follicles and usually have the finest hair. Redheads can appear to have the most abundant hair because their hair follicles are often larger and each strand is therefore thicker.

CHEMICAL HAIR DYES

The first chemical hair dye was patented by Monnet et Cie in Paris in 1883 and was based on a new chemical, paraphenylenediamine, which was used for dying textiles. Addressing safety concerns that were already evident, French chemist Eugene Schueller founded the French Harmless Hair Dye Company in 1909.

But how safe are chemical hair dyes? Links between certain hair dyes and cancer were first suggested in the 1960s. In 1975, a series of tests was conducted on common commercial products to see which, if any, might be cancer-inducing. Two showed up as mutagens - cigarette tar smoke and a permanent hair dye. Further tests revealed that 89 per cent of chemical hair dyes could cause mutation. These conclusions suggested that the products should be further investigated. And yet after rigorous testing, American statisticians announced in 1978 that the chances of dying as a result of using readily available hair dyes were 1 in 160,000,000, though the risks for beauticians in regular contact with the dyes were believed to be ten times greater.

In any event, chemical hair dyes are more likely to

cause allergic reactions than any other cosmetic preparations so that ought to be incentive enough to try herbal alternatives. The symptoms of hair dye allergy can be terrifying. The head may swell as large as a football and the tongue so large as to cause asphyxiation. Because of this, permanent hair dyes should be patch-tested 24 hours before use.

Colourless henna powder (henna with the dye removed) coats the hair shaft without colouring it - that is why it is used for adding body to hair.

And even without conclusive proof of links between hair dye and mutagens, some doctors feel mothers-to-be are wise not to dye their hair chemically when they are pregnant, because harmful agents might leach into the body and harm the foetus.

HOW CHEMICAL HAIR DYES WORK

Permanent hair colours are aniline dyes which react in the hair to give it the desired colour. The pigment lodges in the cortex of the hair which initially looks healthy and shiny. However, repeated applications of dye can swell the cortex and damage the cuticles so that the hair looks dull. And hair can also become brittle and fragile.

HENNA - A HERBAL ALTERNATIVE

In recent years, henna has been extensively tested due to hair dye scares, and has come out with a clean bill of health. It comes from the dried leaves of the *Lawsonia inermis* plant, whose shoots and leaves are crushed and made into a paste with water. This paste has been used to tint hair, hands and feet, as well as breasts and navels, for thousands of years without adverse or allergic reactions. Henna has associations other than decorative - Berber woman in Morocco dye their hands and feet to ward off the earth devil.

When you use henna, check that it is pure. Any product which promises a complete colour change in 10-15 minutes may be a compound with aniline dye or metallic salts to speed things up. Many processes using natural ingredients can take far longer to work. Equally, any smooth viscous liquid that pours beautifully from a bottle is unlikely to have much to do with pure henna, which is messy to use and smells earthy.

DO carry out a strand test first and check the colour after the minimum time given in the instructions.

DO wrap the Herbal Hair Colour in a plastic cap or cling film to help develop the colour.

DO remember, the shorter the time, the brighter the colour.

MIX IT UP

- For darker tones, mix approximately 200ml of strong coffee with a packet of red henna and paint the paste over your hair. This will dull the red tones and give a darker hue.
- Henna can sometimes have a slightly drying effect, so if you have dry hair add one whole beaten egg to the cooled mixture before adding the coffee.
- If your henna tone is too red, you can apply a Brown Herbal Hair Colour over it. Alternatively you can give your hair an olive oil treatment: rub olive oil into the hair, use a hair dryer for five minutes, then wash the oil out. Repeat until the hair loses its reddish colour.
- Lemon juice will accelerate the dyeing process. Red wine gives a richer red colour to hair.

SPECIAL HAIR NEEDS

AFRO-CARIBBEAN HAIR

Conditioning is especially important for Afro-Caribbean hair. Beautiful braiding takes its toll on the hair, as do chemical straighteners, though these are thankfully going out of fashion. Because of the tight curly structure of Afro-Caribbean hair, it picks up the sun's rays at several different angles and absorbs light which makes it an effective block to the damaging effects of UVA rays. But this also means it can look dull if not conditioned sufficiently.

Afro-Caribbean hair is invariably dry. Its curled structure allows moisture to escape from the hair shaft so that it becomes difficult for sebum to travel down and

Middle Eastern women have traditionally used henna to condition their hair, after which a paste of crushed indigo leaf and water is applied for a blue-black sheen. Different hennas yield different tones: henna from Iran gives a deep red colour, Egyptian and Moroccan henna an orangey hue.

HOW TO USE HERBAL HAIR COLOUR

YOU WILL NEED
• plastic gloves
• a henna brush
• a bowl
• an old towel (henna stains)
• approx. 200ml hot water
• an old wooden spoon
• optional - a henna cap
or clingfilm

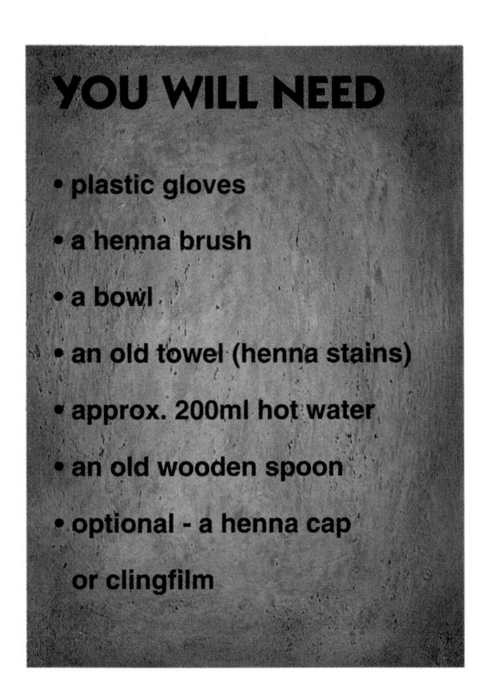

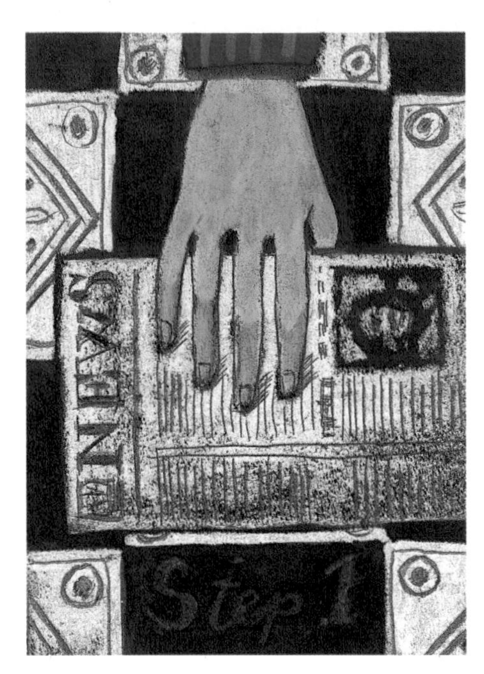

1. Henna is messy! Cover the floor with newspapers, wear plastic gloves.

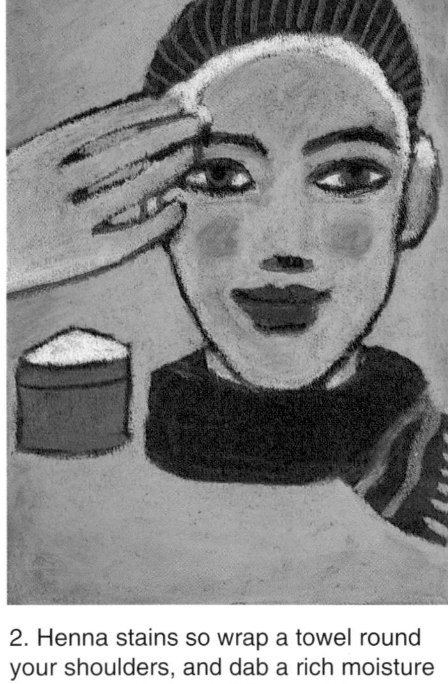

2. Henna stains so wrap a towel round your shoulders, and dab a rich moisture cream round your hairline and ears.

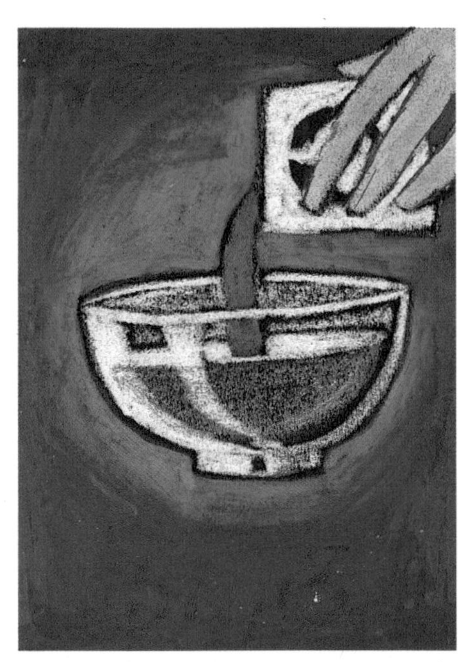

3. Mix the whole packet with 200-250ml boiling water until it is pourable. Leave to cool for 1-2 minutes. If hair is shoulder length or longer, you will need at least two packets and double the water.

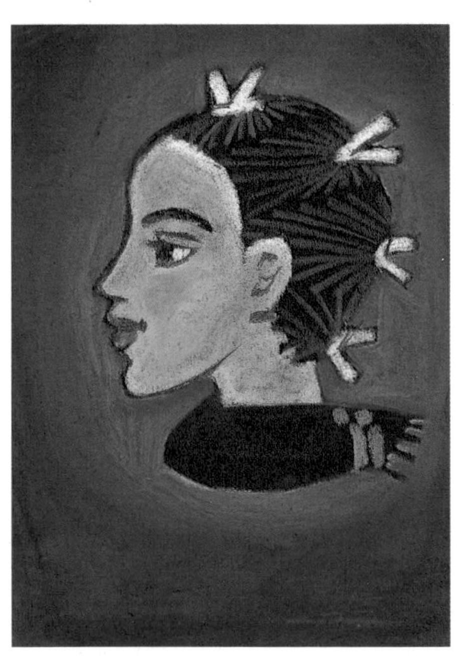

4. Section the hair - using grips if it's long - so that the hair at the nape of the neck is exposed.

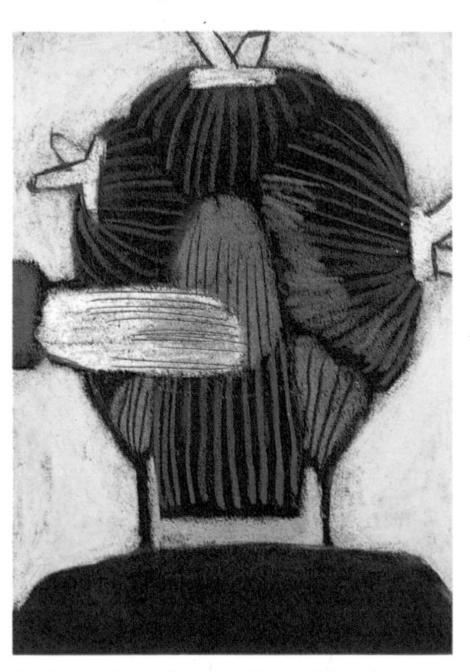

5. Apply the mixture either with a brush or gloved fingertips to small sections of the hair, starting at the roots and massaging down the length of the hair.

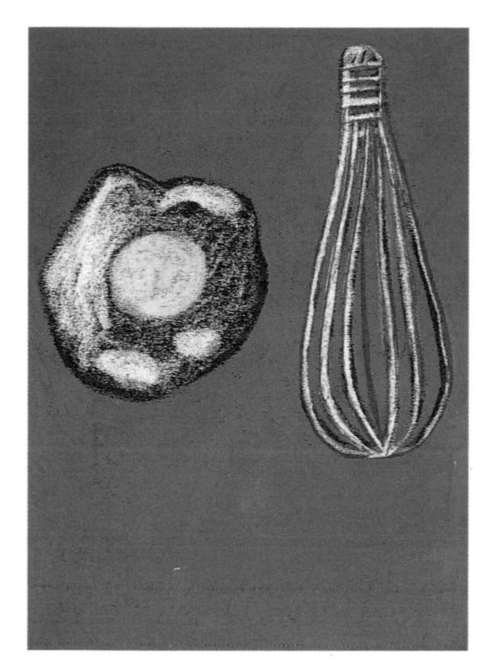

6. If the mixture is too watery, add one boaton raw egg to the cooled mixture which can help it stick.

7. Twist each strand to ensure all hair is evenly coated.

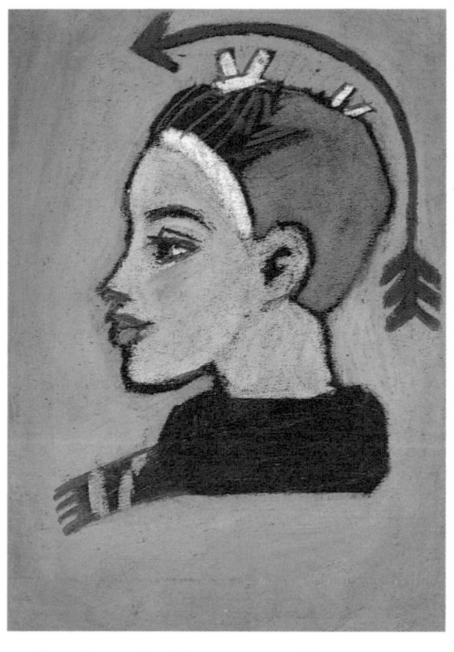

8. Continue in this way, working towards the front of the head until all the hair is coated.

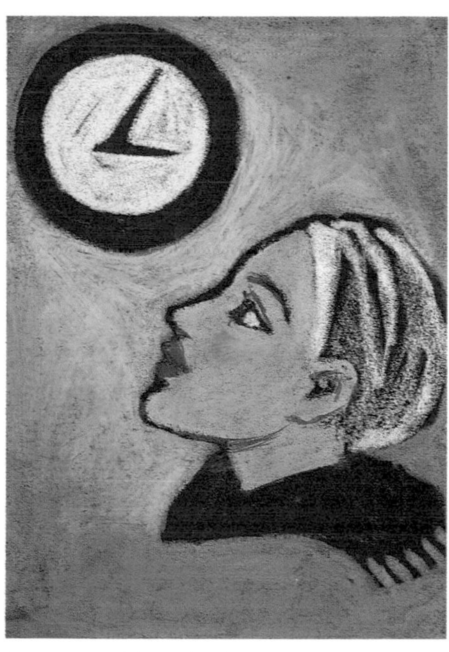

9. Cover with a plastic cap and leave to develop (for timing, see back of packet). Remember - the longer you leave it, the deeper the colour. The shorter the time, the brighter the result.

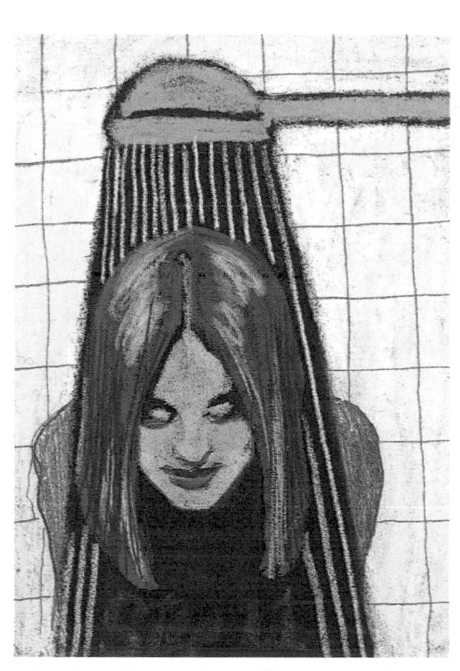

10. Rinse thoroughly with warm water

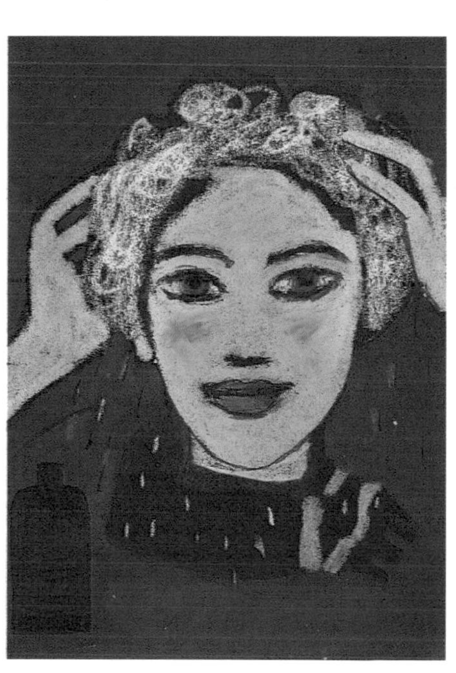

11. Shampoo and condition as normal.

HAIR-CARE GUIDE

	DRY	OILY	NORMAL	MIXED (Oily roots, dry ends)	DANDRUFF
CAUSES	Usually coarse and can have fewer follicles or less active oil glands. Hair gets drier with age as the production of sebum slows. Most dry conditions are due to self-inflicted damage including perms, blow-drying, harsh shampoos, overexposure to the sun and even insufficient washing and grooming.	Common with fine hair because of more numerous follicles pumping out sebum. Hormonal imbalances, especially in teenagers, also speed up oil production. Poor diet, stress, overhandling and cold weather all contribute to greasy and oily hair.	Fortunate genetics, healthy diet and sensible precautions	As hair grows long, its condition often changes, with ends becoming dry and brittle. Harmful treatments, sun damage and rough handling exacerbate the mixed condition.	Possible causes: 1. Metabolic imbalance within body. 2. *Pityrosporum ovale*, a yeast normally present in less than 50 per cent of total micro-organisms on scalp appears on more than 70 per cent of dandruff scalps 3. Excess oil on scalp. 4. Vitamin deficiency, particularly A and B6 (pyridoxine).
SYMPTOMS	Dull, coarse, brittle and easily damaged. Scalp can be tight and flaky.	Lank, dull and stringy; holds style poorly. Unless frequently washed, will trap sebum, sweat, cigarette and food odours.	Glossy throughout; fine hair may be static	Hair needs frequent washing which seems to make the ends worse.	Everybody sheds dead skin cells from the scalp, normally in tiny clusters. In dandruff, the outer cells stick together to form large visible flakes.
REMEDIES	Wash regularly - dry, dirty hair is fragile. Before washing, massage the scalp with oil to prevent the build-up of dead skin cells. Use a conditioner after every wash. Avoid heated stylers or dryers - use mousse or gel instead. Protect the hair in the sun.	Nature remedies this condition because hair becomes drier with age. Until then, wash frequently avoiding harsh shampoos. Avoid rich, fatty foods; expose the hair to fresh air at least half an hour a day. Use a conditioner as protection on the ends of long hair.	Maintain this happy state of affairs by washing every 2 to 3 days. Use conditioner to protect the ends; avoid perms.	Apply shampoo only to scalp (alternate one for oily with one for normal). Use a conditioner as for dry hair, especially on ends. Remove with diluted lemon or vinegar rinse. Rinse with fresh water. Alternately, use pre-wash treatment.	Use an anti-dandruff shampoo regularly till scalp is clear, then twice weekly to help keep dandruff at bay. Products not especially designed for use with dandruff can irritate scalp - use them only on hair, not scalp. This applies to conditioners and stylers too.
OCCASIONAL PRE-CONDITIONER	Aromatherapy Scalp Oil, Banana Hair Putty, Jojoba Oil, Henna Wax	White Grape Skin Tonic	Aromatherapy Scalp Oil, Banana Hair Putty, Henna Wax	Banana Hair Putty	Aromatherapy Reviving Scalp Oil, Sweet Almond Oil
SHAMPOO	Coconut Oil, Camomile, Jojoba, Henna Cream	Frequent Wash Grapefruit, Ice Blue	Camomile, Seaweed & Birch, Banana, Tangerine Beer, Shampoo and Conditioner in One	Camomile, Seaweed & Birch, Coconut Oil, Ice Blue, Ginger Anti-dandruff	Ginger Anti-dandruff
CONDITIONER	Banana, Brazil Nut Oil, Protein Cream Rinse	Light Conditioner	Banana, Light Conditioner	Brazil Nut Conditioner, Banana	Brazil Nut, Light Conditioner
STYLER	Coconut Oil Hair Shine, Slick, Aloe Gel	Aloe Hair Gel, Hair Gel	Aloe Hair Gel, Slick, Hair Gel, Coconut Oil Hair Shine	Coconut Oil Hair Shine, Slick, Aloe Hair Gel, Hair Gel	

lubricate the hair. This makes the hair more brittle than Caucasian, Asian or Oriental hair. But it does not follow that the scalp is also dry. The most common mistake is to apply lots of oils to dry hair on a greasy scalp which only serves to block the follicles. Treat such greasy skin before washing by separating the hair into sections and dabbing with cotton wool soaked in a gentle freshener along the partings. This will lift excess oil and tone the skin. Shampoo gently, kneading the scalp as you wash the hair. Use shampoo sparingly and leave it on the hair for a few minutes. Apply conditioner to the hair, and not necessarily the scalp.

Here's one procedure for braided hair. Using the shower attachment, wash hair between the braids. Massage Henna Wax into the braids, wrap the head in hot towels or shower cap and sit in a steamy bath. After 15-30 minutes shampoo out and condition as usual.

When colouring grey hair, don't try to return to the shades of your youth - much better to go for a tone between three and five shades lighter

GREY HAIR

Grey hair is not actually grey at all - it's white. But as the white hairs grow in among your darker coloured strands, they create an illusion of greying. The first "grey" hair usually appears around the age of 30 (though it can be much earlier), and, for many women and even more men, this foretaste of receding youth is enough to send them rushing to the dye bottle. Around 80 per cent of all women who dye their hair are doing it to hide the grey. The fact is that grey hair looks distinguished on any other head but your own.

For smokers at least, one way to slow the process is to give up cigarettes, which appear to accelerate greying. But by the age of 50, some 50 per cent of the hairs on any Caucasian scalp will be grey. The temples usually grey first, caused by a reduction in the activity of melanocytes, which give the hair pigment and which are usually age-dependent. The greying process happens later to Afro-Caribbean hair.

Grey hair can be covered up with vegetable dyes and herbal rinses - or it can be enjoyed. Grey hair is associated with grace and charm in India.

SPECIAL SCALP NEEDS

CHILDREN

Young children usually have oil-free scalps as they don't produce as much sebum as adults. Baby shampoos are gently formulated to cleanse dirt, but will not remove oils from the scalp. For that reason baby shampoos are not suitable as mild family shampoos.

BABIES

Babies often develop a scalp condition called cradle cap. It looks like patches of scaly skin, usually on the crown of the head. One recommendation for this is to use an oil to moisturise and soften the dry scales. Sweet almond oil has long been a firm favourite.

OILY SCALPS

Very oily scalps can benefit from parting the hair and dabbing a cotton pad containing skin freshener along the scalp. Do this between washes to absorb excess oil.

DANDRUFF

A normal scalp has between 24 and 40 layers of dead cells which are constantly moving up to the surface where they are shed. The cycle for each layer takes 28 days. Although we tend to describe flaking scalp as dandruff, true dandruff is skin cells flaking 20 to 30 layers deep, thus exposing the cells before they have hardened and are ready to shed, making the skin feel tender and itchy. The most likely physical cause is a fungal infection, coupled with accelerated hormonal reaction which pushes out the new cells without giving the old cells a chance to shed.

It is almost universally agreed that dandruff is stress related. Scalp massage is helpful because it aids circulation and relieves tension whilst easing headaches and constriction of the scalp. Parting the hair and dabbing the scalp with a scalp oil or rosemary oil between washes also helps to loosen

Brazil Nut Conditioner is made with the richest, purest Brazil nut oil in the world. The oil is sourced by the Kayapo Indians in the Amazon rainforest. It is believed The Body Shop is the first cosmetics company to use Brazil nut oil in hair care products.

dead skin particles and moisturise the scalp.

Dandruff is one of those problems most people think they suffer from - 10 per cent of all shampoos sold in Europe are anti-dandruff. But what we think is dandruff is often just residual shampoo that has not been removed while washing the hair.

To treat dandruff: beat 2 egg yolks into 115ml warm water, massage into scalp, leave 10 mins and rinse. Rinse again with 2 tsps vinegar in 225ml cool water.

DO rinse your hair for twice as long as you think necessary to remove all loose debris.

DON'T wash your hair in the bath. Floating bits of dead skin and soap scurf are likely to lodge in your hair!

The scalp peels after sunbathing, just like the rest of the body. After a holiday, expect to have to brush and wash more skin particles from your hair than usual. Better still, wear a hat while you are in the sun.

For real dandruff, try invigorating shampoos containing natural ingredients such as ginger and birch bark extract to treat the scalp. Infusions of nettle and rosemary can also cleanse and stimulate the scalp.

Dandruff isn't a modern problem. The Chicksaw Indians of North America traditionally used a solution of wood and twigs from the willow tree to stop scurf in their long hair. Today the Hopi Indians of Arizona prefer to bathe their hair in an infusion made from the leaves of the Rocky Mountain juniper.

FLAKY SCALPS

Flaky scalps are often mistaken for dandruff. They can be caused by dry skin, just like dry skin on any other part of the body. Especially dry and flaky scalps will benefit from a hot oil treatment before washing the hair. You may find you need a treatment more often in the winter. Excellent oils to use are jojoba oil and sweet almond oil. Just as beneficial is the accompanying massage (see Massage chapter).

HOT OIL TREATMENT FOR DRY SCALPS

- Warm the oil by standing the bottle in hot water for a few minutes. This makes it easier to apply.
- Place a small amout of oil in the palm of one hand and with the fingertips of the other, massage it gently into scalp.
- Leave on for at least 10 minutes; wash normally.

SUN, SEA AND SAUNAS

The sun is one of the hair's worst enemies. Wearing a hat in hot climates not only helps protect from sunstroke, it prevents hair from scorching and weakening. Where a hat isn't practical - in the sea for example - the hair should still be covered with a protective cream, lotion or gel. Styling gels can offer minimal protection since they coat the hair. And remember, sun-parched hair always benefits from conditioning after every shampoo.

Salt and chlorinated waters also exact a toll. Between them, the sun, the sea and chlorine can drive harmful chemicals and minerals right into the hair shaft. Dyed or treated hair is specially vulnerable so you must make sure you rinse it thoroughly after swimming. The effects of a summer in the sun stay with us for the next six months because of damage to the cells that are pushing out new hairs.

Don't be lulled into believing dark hair can cope better with the sun. Quite the contrary. Dark hair absorbs more harmful UVA rays and therefore is even more prone to damage than fair hair. But as we've seen, black Afro-Caribbean hair is sun resistant.

Hair doesn't like saunas - the temperature is just too hot. Wrap a cool damp towel around your head and change it as it heats up.

HAIR LOSS...

It is quite normal to lose between 50 and 150 hairs a day. For your hair to show as thinning, you would have to lose between 40 to 50 per cent from one area. That can happen if capillaries are constricted, if the papilla is damaged or if it is genetically programmed to stop producing hair. Then the follicle will not produce replacement hair.

Alopecia areata is a condition that causes hair loss either in patches or a diffused fall all over the scalp. It affects one in a hundred women, of whom a fifth will lose all their body hair, though in most cases it grows back.

...AND WOMEN

Nearly 60 per cent of women suffer some form of hair loss during their lives. Many develop thinning hair as they grow older. It may resemble that of male baldness with a receding hairline, but most often there is a diffuse thinning across the top of the scalp, which is slower than in men. Then, towards the back of the crown an oval-shaped bald patch may appear. Women practically never go totally bald because they don't produce the same level of androgen hormones as men.

Don't wear your ponytail, rollers, barrettes or combs too tight - this causes traction which can lead to temporary hair loss.

Exact causes of female baldness can be hard to trace: factors ranging from head injuries, emotional problems, stress and diet to menopause and especially changing hormone levels during pregnancy have been linked to hair loss. However, mistreatment through indiscriminate colouring or heating can cause more than breakage and lead to permanent hair loss.

Concern is growing because an increasing number of women are beginning to lose their hair. Some researchers argue that women are producing more androgen hormones. The normal ratio of hormones in women is eight parts oestrogen (female hormone) to one part androgen. This balance affects skin texture and hair resilience. If the balance is disturbed, some trichologists believe that regrowth of hair is affected. That is why hormone replacement therapy can help arrest hair loss in women.

Heredity plays a role in both male and female hair loss. Clever hair styling is the most practical way to conceal female pattern alopecia. If you have fine or thinning hair, wash it weekly with shampoo and use a daily regime of warm water rinsing and gentle massage to help rid the scalp and hair of excess dirt. This is designed to prevent fine, thinning hair from looking lank very quickly, without actually washing it every day. Use body builders, protein conditioners and mousse products. These will not make the hair grow any better, but the existing hair will seem thicker.

...AND PREGNANCY

Many women are distressed by hair loss after the birth of a baby. This is particularly noticeable as the hair is so lush during pregnancy - there is little hair loss at all over the nine months' gestation. After the birth, substantial hair loss is quite usual. It is essential to look after your hair and scalp well during pregnancy to stand it in good stead for when normal growth resumes after delivery. Don't worry - your hair will grow back, though it may take six months to make up the loss.

...STRESS AND DIET

But this may not be the case with hair lost during a crash diet. These can be low in essential proteins and vitamins so the body loses its stores of raw materials which are necessary for growth and repair. The body then channels its resources into keeping more essential functions going and has fewer resources for starting new hair growth. The solution is to stop the diet and balance your intake of food.

Likewise, over work and stress can cause permanent hair loss. The incidence of stress-related baldness in women is increasing, possibly because women in high-stress positions produce a high quantity of male hormones. As with all stress-induced symptoms, relaxation techniques do help and regular scalp massages can minimise the effects of stress.

Long illnesses and major surgery are frequently accompanied by hair loss which should stop when the medical problem is corrected.

...AND MENOPAUSE

The menopause is most commonly accompanied by hair loss, particularly in women who have a quick menopause. As a woman gets older, her body grows more slowly and the cells do not reproduce as quickly. This slowing down process affects the growth of the hair which falls out faster than it can be replaced and so begins to look sparse. Hormone treatments administered to alleviate other menopausal problems can minimise hair loss, but it is generally inevitable that some hair-thinning will take place in women between the ages of 45 and 55. At the same time however, coarser body hair may develop.

Hair has traditionally held healthy magic for young mothers around the world. Irish women once believed that their hair, which had grown so abundantly in pregnancy, must therefore possess special powers. So they pulled skeins of it from their heads and wove it into amulets for their babies.

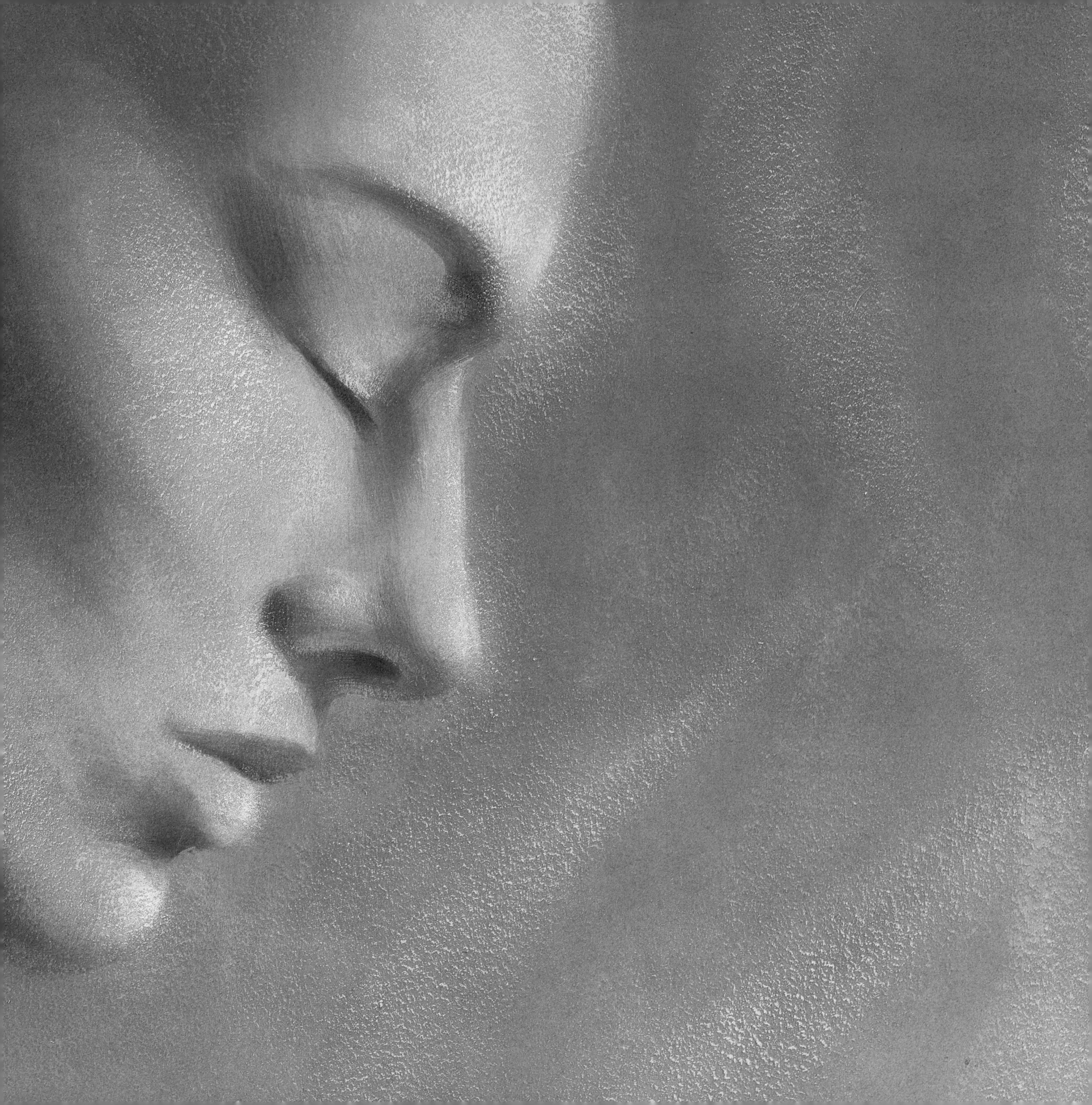

SMELL

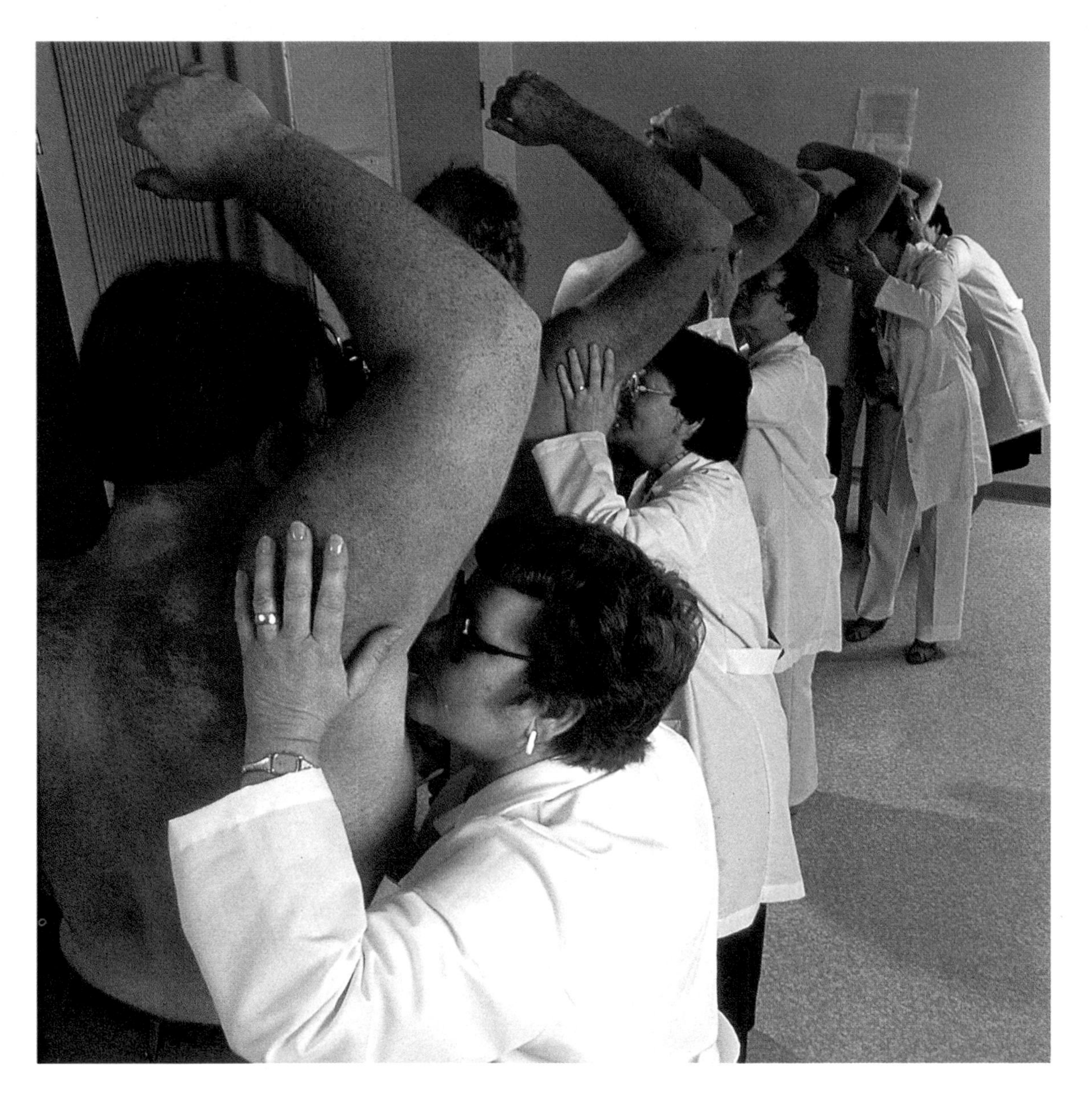

Though the fresh scent of our bodies is one of the most alluring smells known to man or woman, this laboratory in Ohio, USA goes on looking for new ways to disguise the heady odour of humanity.

smell

It's as though we are swimming in a rich soup of smells from birth until our final breath. The sense of smell is the last sense to leave a dying person.

Perfume's power is primitive and primary. Smell was the first ever sense, and guided single-celled organisms through the earliest sea billions of years ago. From these smell receptors the first brain evolved - the smell brain, known to scientists as the limbic system. In animals, the limbic system remains the most highly developed part of the brain. One of the things that makes humans different from other animals is that we have come to ignore the limbic system in favour of the cerebral cortex or "thinking cap". This is where rational thought originates.

Descartes wrote: I think therefore I am *(Cogito ergo sum)*, but I smell therefore I am *(Olfacio ergo sum)* would have been more appropriate, as all brainpower is descended from our sense of smell.

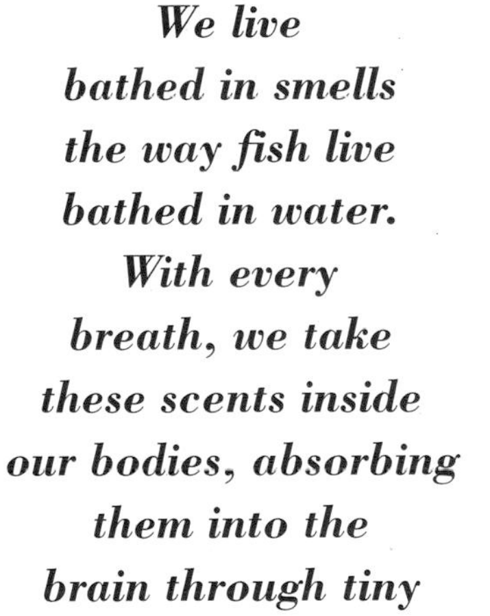

THE EMOTIONAL BRAIN

We respond to odours emotionally rather than intellectually. Smell receptors high in the nostrils are directly linked to the limbic system, which is responsible for a great range of emotions: fear, rage, aggression, nostalgia and pleasure, as well as regulating reproductive cycles and sex drive. Some of the olfactory nerves that transmit smell signals pass through the limbic system, so certain smells or fragrances stimulate intense memories and recreate experiences. The associations they provide us with may, or may not, be pleasant. Smells can warn, frighten or arouse us. Console us too.

What we call gut feelings are reactions produced by the limbic system. When you are ruled by the heart rather than the head, you are being ruled by the limbic system rather than the rational thinking cap above it.

Ruled by the abstract, rational brain as we are, we tend to downgrade the importance of the more sensual senses like taste, touch and smell. Sight and hearing, our preferred means of gaining information, work by analysing waves that bounce off ears and eyes. Scents, however, have to react chemically with chemicals inside our bodies for us to smell them. So smell is a more intimate sense.

Certainly, smell has the most direct access to the brain. Unlike the other senses, there are no stopping points along the olfactory nerve pathways. A smell signal speeds without interruption to the area of the brain that is most strongly connected to the subconscious. Scent receptors are also the only brain nerve cells that repair and reproduce themselves, possibly because

Smell is less acute in humans than in most animals, which is just as well because, were we to have the senses of a cat, many of us might choose to wear gas masks! The male silkworm can detect a female of the species five miles away by her smell. Horses are said to smell water a mile off.

reaching out into the environment makes them vulnerable to pollution. Scientists are studying this ability in order to help research into brain damage.

HOW WE SMELL

THE MECHANICS

Much remains opaque about the hows and whys of smell, but recent research such as that done by Warwick University's Olfaction Research Group is beginning to illuminate the probabilities.

Scent molecules are drawn into the nose where they dissolve in the mucous membrane on two tiny patches of tissue, one in the upper half and one in the roof of each nostril. When your nose is plugged up with a cold, these areas are blocked, so you can't smell. In humans, the sensory patches form a total area of three-quarters of a square inch. Compare this with hunting dogs, which have a minimum of ten square inches, sharks with 24 square feet, or rabbits, with an area that equals the skin surface area of their entire body. Black people have bigger scent receptor patches than white, though no conclusive research has been done to show whether this gives them a better sense of smell.

Tiny hairs protrude from the nerve cells at the end of the fibres that pack the sensory patches. These are rich in many different receptor proteins. The leading theory is that different proteins will bind only with the molecules of certain odours, setting off a chain reaction of chemical changes, and then electrical changes, that the brain registers as a particular smell.

It's a bit like an incredibly complex jigsaw puzzle. Think of receptor proteins as having specific shapes so that only matching pieces of the smell puzzle can attach to them. When all the dewberry-shaped protein receptors are fully occupied, for example, there is nothing in the nose for dewberry molecules to fit into and we cannot smell them, however many are pumped into the nostrils. This is why we often lose the ability to smell a fragrance on ourselves soon after we apply it. After a while, scent molecules are probably metabolised by the body. We can then smell them again because the jigsaw-like receptors are once more free.

Some odours have a much greater effect on us than others. There is a universal attraction to musk smells for example. A vast proportion of commercial fragrances contain one of the group of musky/sandalwood/urinous/amber notes. Our preference for these could be because we were aware of them in our mother's womb (humans secrete musky molecules) or it might be the result of a special type of receptor site which gives a stronger imprint than others, leading to an innate preference for this type of odour. Perhaps there are primary scents, like primary colours, waiting to be discovered Science is still at the crawling state where the sense of smell is concerned.

THE REJECTED SENSE

Animals use their limbic systems to gain intricately detailed information about the world and to evaluate it in ways we cannot even dream of. We consider the limbic system, emotion and the sense of smell as inferior compared to "intellectual" thought processes. And we are prejudiced in favour of the senses that are most easily expressed by the rational structure of language: sight and sound.

For other cultures, like the Dogon of Mali, smell is the ruling sense, integral to language. They classify words according to their aroma: good words smell sweet, bad ones rotten, and they talk about hearing a smell.

A good sense of smell is important to doctors when making a diagnosis. Many diseases have their own particular smell: yellow fever smells like a butcher's shop, typhoid fever like freshly baked bread, plague like apples and measles like freshly plucked feathers.

Are we losing out by repressing the importance of the sense of smell? Psychiatrist Oliver Sachs published a case history of a young man whose sense of smell became incredibly fertile after habitual use of mind-altering drugs. One night he dreamt he was a dog and afterwards, for three weeks "all other sensations...paled before smell". He entered the clinic, sniffed, and "in that sniff recognised, before seeing them, the twenty patients who were there. Each one had his own olfactory physiognomy, a smell face, far more vivid and evocative, more redolent, than any sight face." During this time he had felt no need of his human cognitive abilities. They

HOW OUR SENSE OF SMELL WORKS

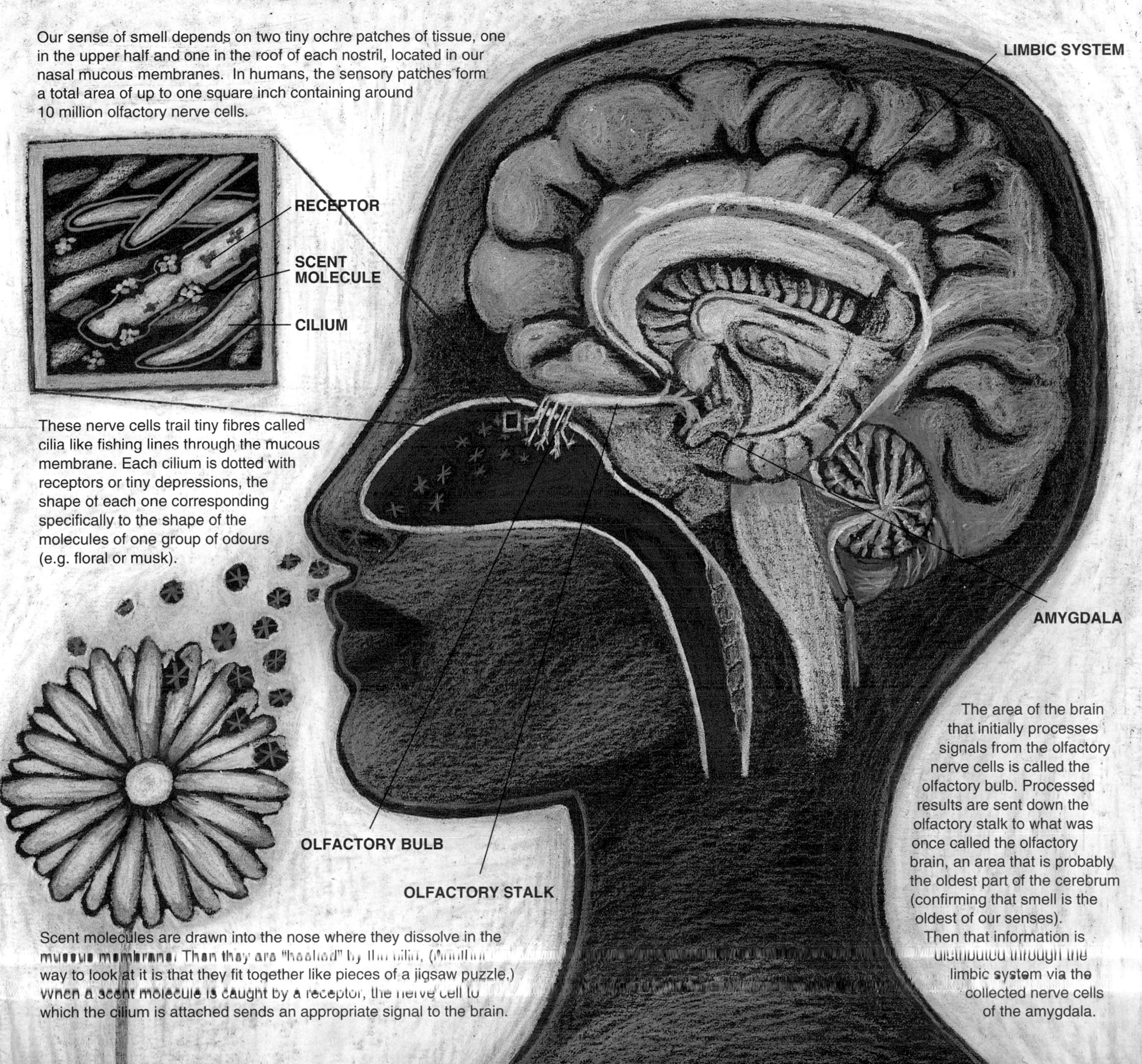

were superfluous once he had tapped into his smell brain. He said afterwards, "I see now what we give up in being civilised and human".

This experience gives a glimpse of the unmined riches that lie waiting in the limbic system, if only we could raise our smell consciousness and unleash its possibilities. At present, we are sensually starved when it comes to scent. But, as computers take over more and more of the cognitive functions of the human brain, perhaps we will adapt. Freed to focus more on the potential of the smell brain we could be guided to new perceptions by the deep and as yet alien scent-maps that underlie our very visual world.

The odour of sweat can be altered by body weight, alcohol and spicy food. Vegetarians smell different from meat eaters and smokers from non-smokers.

Literary scent stories: Kipling wrote that "smells are surer than sounds to make your heart-strings crack". When travelling away from home, Goethe would carry his lover's bodice so that her fragrance was with him always. Somerset Maugham asked why H.G. Wells was so successful with women, as he didn't look the part! A mistress of Wells' replied that he smelt of honey.

FRAGRANT ID CARDS

Perfume has helped us to kill, to make love, to worship our gods and to survive. One of scent's most basic functions is to warn all animals of danger. Substances that are poisonous to us often smell noxious, while the smell of an enemy lying in wait is still a beacon to the members of hunter-gatherer societies like the Kalahari bushmen and Australian Aborigines.

One of the first uses of applied, rather than natural, scent was as a disguise. Hunters would smear their bodies with the scent from a fresh kill to mask their own odour and help them get nearer to other prey undetected. In shaman-centred tribal societies, the practice often came to be highly symbolic of the hunter's identification with the animal he hunted and his profound respect for it. Smearing himself with its blood or fat was a way of magically taking on its character, its wisdom and its particular prowesses.

In numerous cultures it's a woman's scent which proscribes her from certain activities. The smell of menstrual blood is, almost universally, a powerful taboo. Some African tribes forbid a woman to hunt, explaining that it's because the animals would detect the smell of her menstrual blood or maternal milk, and flee. The Kwoma of Papua New Guinea ban sexual contact with women before a battle because it is believed that the erotic aroma of female sexual fluids would adhere to the warriors' skins so that when the enemies' spears smelt it, they would be overcome by an insatiable urge to penetrate their bodies.

Because of its roots in the emotional centre, scent is a fundamental way of identifying a loved one. Babies identify their mothers at first solely by smell and are able to do so within hours of birth. Adults often find the smell of an absent loved one just as comforting, but are ashamed of admitting it (the girlfriend's T-shirt on the teddy bear syndrome). In New Guinea, one tribe's method of saying goodbye involved putting a hand in the other's armpit, then stroking the scented hand all over themselves to remind them of the other's odour.

DIFF'RENT STROKES FOR DIFF'RENT FOLKS

Havelock Ellis, writing in 1910, noted that every race has its own odour overtones. Australids, he said, were almost phosphoric; Central African women had a slight nut smell; while native Carib Indians reeked of the kennel. The Inuit were apparently fishy, which is not surprising, because diet plays a large part in tingeing the natural body odour.

The smells you like or dislike are strongly influenced by your culture. Europeans eat a lot of milk and cheese, which Asians detect as a foul, rancid butter smell. The Japanese diet is mainly vegetables, fish and rice, which leaves only a neutral smell.

It's the hairier races, those of Caucasian and African origin, who also have the most apocrine glands, which produce the sweat that makes the natural human smell. Our modern phobia about this smell might lead us to worry about it. Apocrine glands are so sparse in Koreans that half of the population has none at all. Similarly, most Japanese have little or no armpit odour. Perhaps this odourlessness explains the subtlety of their approach to smell. Commercial modern fragrances are rarely purchased by them for scenting their bodies - they are considered far too strong. Instead, they are put on display as objects of conspicuous consumption.

Traditionally, saints carried a fragrant ID. They wafted the "odour of sanctity", a sign of their closeness to God. Saint Trevere smelt of roses, lilies and incense; Saint

Cafetan of oranges; Saint Catherine of violets; Saint Theresa of Avila of jasmine and irises, and Saint Lydwine of cinnamon bark. The scent of Saint Benedicta, mingled with that of the angels, the Virgin Mary and Christ Himself, composed a perfume known as "The Bouquet of the Lake" which could be appreciated hovering above a lake from a great distance. By contrast, the stench of the sinner enabled Saint Philip to recognise immediately those souls destined for Hell.

In Europe, until the 18th century, there was thought to be a mysterious connection between the womb and the sense of smell. Doctors treated the pox (syphilis) with inhalations of burning cinnabar, whereas amenorrhoea (lack of periods) was treated with fumigation of old shoes. The treatments made a valid connection. In recent experiments when male sweat was smeared regularly on the upper lip of women who weren't menstruating, it triggered off a resumption of periods. (Sweat must certainly have been present in old shoes.) We now know, too, that the menstrual synchronicity between women who live or work together is due to scent signals emitted by their sweat.

In the Trobriand Islands, they put a spell in you, not on you. The spell enters the body in the form of an aroma, smell being the active ingredient in love magic.

SEX AND SMELL

THE SEXUAL SEA

Richard Burton's pet name for Elizabeth Taylor was apparently Ocean. The sea has always been a symbol of the womb - that inner Atlantic of salty fluids where the embryo floats - and of woman. But it's the smell of the sea, and of fresh fish, that has also been used to describe the sexual smell of a woman in many cultures. Mermaids, whose myth is universally one of luring men into lust, are fishy below the waist - and not just in order to swim. Could it be that men make love to women solely because their fishy smell reminds them of their primordial home in the ocean? Sex would thus be a way of returning not to the human womb but to the womb of the world the ocean.

Victorians were terribly afraid of the sexual power of smell. In no circumstances were perfumes to be put directly on to the skin itself. Instead, a fashion for scented hankies, mittens and slippers grew. Only the much diluted eau de toilettes were acceptable on bare skin - preferably "innocent" smells like rose, plantain, bean or strawberry waters.

But even a flower could be flagrant. The Victorians were concerned that the expression of enjoyment on the face of a woman smelling a flower, and on the face of a woman making love, were alarmingly similar. According to some experts of the time, this shady relationship between female and flower could end in orgasm.

MUSK, LUST AND DISGUST

Until the 18th century, musk was the most fashionable fragrance. Then came the Victorians with their unshakeable conviction that musk reeked of debauchery. In Edmond de Goncourt's novel *Cherie*, the heroine somehow manages to procure some musk, which she inhales furtively in bed like a forbidden drug. The resulting intoxication leads to an illicit orgasm. Divine retribution decrees that she die a virgin without ever having known the real smell of a man which, in fact, is incredibly close to the fragrance of musk. Musk is a key factor of the male fragrance ID card. While it is heavily aphrodisiac to both sexes, women secrete a much smaller amount of "musk", about a third as much as men.

The musk used in fragrance comes from the penile sheath of a small deer found in China and the Himalayas. One of the most expensive perfume ingredients, it is worth much more than its weight in gold. Unfortunately, although the pod can be extracted without harming the animal, the deer is nearly always killed in order to get at the musk. However, the synthetic version smells every bit as sensuous as the real thing - in fact, chemically speaking, it is the same as the real thing.

Why are the penis scrapings from a remote deer so provocative to men and women alike? The answer lies under our arms. We have two types of sweat gland in our bodies, eccrine glands, which occur all over, and apocrine glands, which are concentrated under the

Smell is important subliminally to us in accepting, even falling in love with, a person. The word for kiss and smell is the same in many languages. Social kissing or nose-rubbing is a form of greeting used all over the world. It sprang from a desire to catch a whiff of someone to see how they were, where they came from and what they were like. Dogs use the same approach.

SANDALWOOD

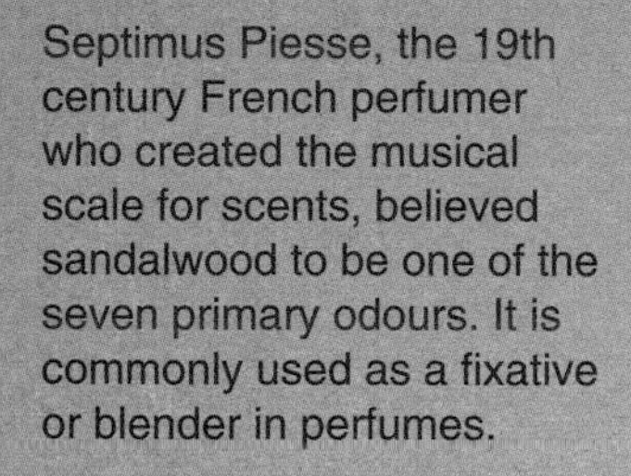

Septimus Piesse, the 19th century French perfumer who created the musical scale for scents, believed sandalwood to be one of the seven primary odours. It is commonly used as a fixative or blender in perfumes.

Sandalwood is one of the oldest known perfume materials - 4,000 years ago, it was the general panacea of Ancient India, where it was also used to build temples.

Legend has it that Solomon used sandalwood for the pillars of his temple to perfume the devotions of worshippers.

The Egyptians used sandalwood in scent and incense as a relaxant. Sandalwood oil is steam-distilled from the roots and inner wood of *Santalum album*, an evergreen tree native to India and Indonesia. The tree itself can grow to 30 feet high, with oval, furry leaves and blood red flowers.

Famous for its rejuvenescent powers, sandalwood was also used in oil form as an external disinfectant and to calm inflammations of the skin.

Sandalwood's deodorising properties work well in this fragranced body powder.

Combine:
2 oz cornstarch
1 oz powdered sandalwood
1 oz powdered blue malva
(or rose or vetivert) sifted through a fine sieve.

arms, in the pubic area, round the anus and nipples. Apocrine glands don't function until puberty, a clue to their main role, which is not to sweat but to release sexual body signals through smell. It's at puberty that the apocrine glands begin to advertise your sexual ID This is why in experiments, volunteers were unable to tell the sex of a pre-pubescent child, while they could discriminate between the smells of an adult man and a woman.

SMELLS LIKE SEX APPEAL

Scent messages produced by one sex for the purpose of being detected by another are called pheromones. They can carry messages about our emotional state but, above all, they convey information about sexual attractiveness and availability. Their chief aim is to enhance a mood that will lead to mating. It's well known that animals and insects are highly responsive to them. Much research is still being done in the area of human pheromones, but the general consensus seems to be that we do respond to them. American research into sensory disorders suggests that about a quarter of people with smell disorders found their sex drive diminished. Sometimes a pheromone smell is detected subliminally - you react to a scent molecule, but you are not aware that you can smell it.

The scent exuded from the apocrine glands is a mixture of pheromones and other body chemicals, which in the right, carefully modulated doses, smell appealing, even exciting. Should their concentration step over a threshold, however, we perceive them as unpleasant, even repulsive. Fatty acids from the apocrine glands develop into the aroma of the great unwashed if left too long. When fresh, they give off a light, creamy scent that most people find delicious.

The main human pheromone is androstenone which, with the related steroid, androstenol, is what gives humans their muskiness. It drives the libido in both sexes. It's because these musky steroids are a major part of sexual attraction in humans that we find perfumes which contain musk or ambergris (which originally came from whales but is now made synthetically) so sexy.

The highest concentration of androstenone is produced in the genital area. Its output is directly linked to the amount of testosterone in the body; production in women more or less ceases at the menopause. Androstenone is also present in saliva, which could be the one reason why we find kissing so arousing.

A MASS OF CONTRADICTIONS

When puzzling over the narrow threshold between attraction and repulsion we should remember that the limbic system is the emotional core as well as the smell centre of the brain. Could the mysterious connection between lust and disgust be an echo of the strong connection between the emotions of love and hate? Could it be a relic of a time when we were open to the appeal of a broader range of smells than we are now? Europeans and Americans are definitely less tolerant of natural human smells than they were before the mid-18th century. Until then, the fondness for musk led to children's excrement being included in tiny amounts in fragrances. (A child's excrement was thought to be purer than an adult's.)

Certainly, it's a signal that lust and disgust are more closely connected than they seem, and that pleasure and repulsion are not opposites, but different points on a sliding scale. Our sensual responses are not bland black and white, but richer hues that blend a rainbow of possibilities.

THE WORLD DEODORISED

The beginning of this chapter suggested we live in a soup of smells. But in the last two centuries, this soup has lost much of its flavour. In the 18th century, with the rise of the cult of the individual came the notion of individual space. We were no longer a common mass linked by our common smell; we were each different and following a different destiny. Cities became deodorised as they became disinfected. Musk, a major component of the smell of human scent and a human sexual attractant, became taboo. The less we smelt, the less we were bound together. Excrement, as well as human scent, became a source of horror and outrage. The idea of dropping a minute ball of a child's faeces into a

A hundred million years ago, dinosaurs became extinct and flowers appeared on the planet. These new plants put on a tremendous sexual display, visual and odiferous, all over the earth. According to one of the more poetic extinction theories, dinosaurs didn't like the smell of flowers and avoided eating them. Gradually, as flowers proliferated, dinosaurs died away. Hence the scent of flowers may have helped rid the planet of its longest-lasting inhabitants.

Rosewater contains the alcohol form of phenylethylamine (PEA), credited by some scientists as being instrumental in creating feelings akin to post-coital bliss. Chocolate is also a source of PEA; is that why we use the combination of roses and chocolates to win hearts?

perfume to heighten its pheromonal echo would have brought a rictus of revulsion to Victorian features. The less you smelt, the more acceptable you were.

This situation has lasted until today. We are still obsessed with deodorising ourselves and our world. "The extensive use of deodorants and the suppression of odour in public places results in a land of olfactory blandness and sameness that would be difficult to duplicate anywhere else in the world" wrote E. T. Hall of Western society. "This blandness deprives us of richness and variety in our life." Perhaps we have gone in for overkill. The fresh scent of our bodies is, after all, one of the most alluring odours known to man and woman. Perhaps we should take a leaf out of Napoleon's book. He once said to Josephine, "Je reviens en trois jours. Ne te laves pas." ("I'll be back in three days. Don't wash.")

Not all cultures feel as we do about the naturally fragrant body. Among the Suya of Brazil, everything - animals, plants, people - is classified according to its smell: bland, pungent, rotten or strong smelling. Strong-smelling people are identified with jaguars, their fetish animal, and rule society. They are said to be the most powerful people.

Androstenone, the main human pheromone, has also been called "the male essential oil". In one study, it was sprayed in three different concentrations on seats in a dentist's waiting room. Many women chose seats with a high concentration - did it remind them of men? Men, on the other hand, got uneasy and chose seats with a low concentration similar to levels secreted by women.

CREATIVE SMELL

FLOWER POWER

A flower is the sex organ of a plant - many, curiously, echo the shape of animal sex organs. The scent is the plant's equivalent of a pheromone: aimed at attracting. Almost all perfumes contain flower oils and women usurp the sexual attraction of blossoms whenever they wear a fragrance. But why should women - and men - wrap themselves in sexual aromas of plants in order to attract each other? The theory used to be that as sophisticated, civilised beings, we had come to reject the musky/urinous/sweaty body odours that we emit, but that we still need a scented come-on to make ourselves alluring. We washed off the nasty sweat smells and chose the sweet and innocent breath of flowers as our representatives instead.

The theory is changing. Flowers exude their scent in order to attract, not each other, but animals. The aim is for their pollen to be picked up, as the animal or insect sticks its nose into the flower, and transferred to another plant, fertilising it. Many ingredients of scented flowers copy insect pheromones for this reason, and are not arousing to humans. Others though, contain the same steroids as animal attractants. The male sex hormone testosterone and the related androstenone have been found in pine, for example.

Jasmine is known as the most erotic of all flowers, a narcotic blend of warmth and coolness, of flower and flesh. The animal note comes from an ingredient called indole, also present in large quantities in tuberose, that other heavy, heady flower. It's a question of proportion once again. In the right dose, indole is an incredibly sexy smell. Too much and you can get a headache, which isn't surprising when you consider that indole is also one of the more disgusting odour notes in human and animal faeces. It's also found in smaller doses in many other perfume plants: neroli, hyacinth, jonquil, orange blossom.

The theory that sweet flowers mask musky body odours is giving way to a more intriguing idea. It seems we wear perfume not to disguise our smell but to enhance it, to elaborate on it with natural human creativity, and to spread its net wider. The base notes of modern perfumes are often in the musk/amber/sandalwood range, akin to human pheromones. The mid-notes may be jasmine, tuberose, orange blossom or other flowers with indole. The top notes are often citrusy (also containing a touch of indole) or rose - essence of post-coital bliss. We may choose a light, flowery scent with a delicate appeal like apple blossom when we want only to hint at attraction, and a stronger, more suggestive scent like patchouli when we want to deepen our sexual aura. Yes, we unwittingly use scent in a sophisticated way, a way that often works to enhance its primitive bonding power.

The scent of flowers and fruits, then, is often related to our own secretions of sexual attraction. But there is a further unexpected connection to be made between scents used in seemingly different ways. The musky smells that can lead to sexual rapture are of the same chemical family as the balsamic smells which are used to evoke religious rapture. Is there, then, one fundamental, primary aroma of euphoria?

SYNESTHESIA

Hindus say that the different senses once formed one great original sense which combined them all. In the womb, it's thought that we experience all senses as one: we see touch, hear smells, feel light with our bodies in a phenomenon known as synesthesia.

While Western culture classifies and separates sensory experience, other cultures often perceive senses as fused together. This gives them a perspective that we miss. The Kwoma of Papua New Guinea picture the world as primarily one of sounds/smells. Their language has a single word for to hear and to smell, a connection also made in many African languages.

This would make sense to perfumers, who correlate fragrance with music. The 19th century perfumer, Piesse, was the first to classify fragrance by notes corresponding to particular musical notes. These notes form accords like musical chords, and perfumers speak of composing a fragrance, as though it were a piece of music. Piesse speculated that perfume composers should practically be able to "play" their composition on the piano as well as formulating it into a perfume. Modern advertisers use visual imagery to sell fragrance. Would it not make more sense to play on this innate human connection between the olfactory and the audial and use sounds to sell scent? By reawakening our sense of smell and reuniting it with our other senses, we can open ourselves to experiencing the world in new and richer ways.

The ancients sprinkled scents on the burning carcasses of animal sacrifices to mask the smell. "Perfume" comes from* per fumus, *Latin for "through the smoke".

DIVINE PERFUME

We prize perfume as a luxury; other societies prize it as a divine bridge between our world and the spiritual worlds. Perfume has always been central to magic and religions everywhere. In Ancient Egypt, as in many other antique cultures, it was initially forbidden for any but sacred and royal use.

The smoke of incense, of burning woods, resins and spices are the most ancient scents. The word perfume comes from the Latin *per* (through) and *fumes* (smoke). The Ancient Greek words for scent and offering to the gods were the same. Burning incense was offered to the gods because it was pure and invisible, moving with ease into their invisible world. It was thought the gods nourished themselves only on this most exquisite substance. The Huichol of South America still believe this, and burn their incense, copal, night and day, as food for the gods.

Frankincense, myrrh and sandalwood, all recognised as sexual scents, are the three scents most widely used in religious ceremonies all over the Far East, the Middle East and in Europe. The resins used for incense in South America are of the same family. Why have so many religions chosen this one group of essential oils as elements of worship? The odour of sandalwood and the human pheromone, androstenone, have proved very similar in tests, just as the chemical components of myrrh are strikingly similar to testosterone. These religious resins, while they may smell ascetic, contain alcohols very similar to human pheromones and hormones. Could this mean that the odour of incense, reminiscent of human sex attractants, activates the repressed limbic system and so harnesses some of the emotional exhilaration we associate with sex to feelings of spiritual uplift?

Perhaps the scent of the sublime in religious ritual and the sublime in sexuality are essentially the same. The power of smell to evoke religious rapture or sexual rapture is the same power. Once again, scent transforms us. Scent is, in this respect, the essence of magic.

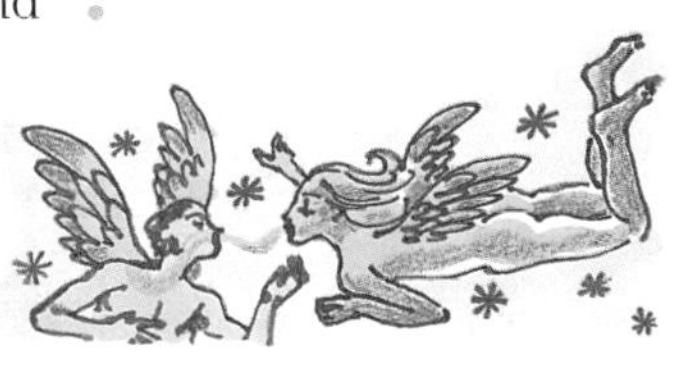

Saint Benedicta's fragrance grew particularly powerful during her religious ecstasies. At those times, her odour was said to transmit God's love to the people around her.

MAGIC SMELLS

It's very Western to use perfume as a means to get words through to God. More radical is the notion that scent itself can be prayer. For the Maya-Tzotzil of Chiapas in Mexico, the burning of copal is a prayer for health, unaccompanied by the baggage of words. In Papua New Guinea, spells work in a similar way. As spells are spoken, they are thought to infuse into odiferous substances. The magic of the spell is contained in the aroma as much as the words.

FRAGRANCE WHEEL

Every fragrance can be classified by a geneaology based on dominant notes. For women's fragrances, there are about 15 such notes, including spicy, floral, oriental and combinations such as floriental. Aldehydes are simply dominant synthetic notes (the most famous belong to Chanel no. 5).

A simple way to come to grips with the concept is to think of fragrance notes as musical notes. A perfume is like a piece of music, notes blended to create a harmonious whole.The top note is the first impression you get when you sniff a fragrance, the base note is what you'll smell on your skin all day. To show the whole idea at work, we've given you breakdowns of The Body Shop's best-selling fragrances, Dewberry and White Musk (which uses aldehydes in place of the natural musk that is cruelly extracted from the musk deer).

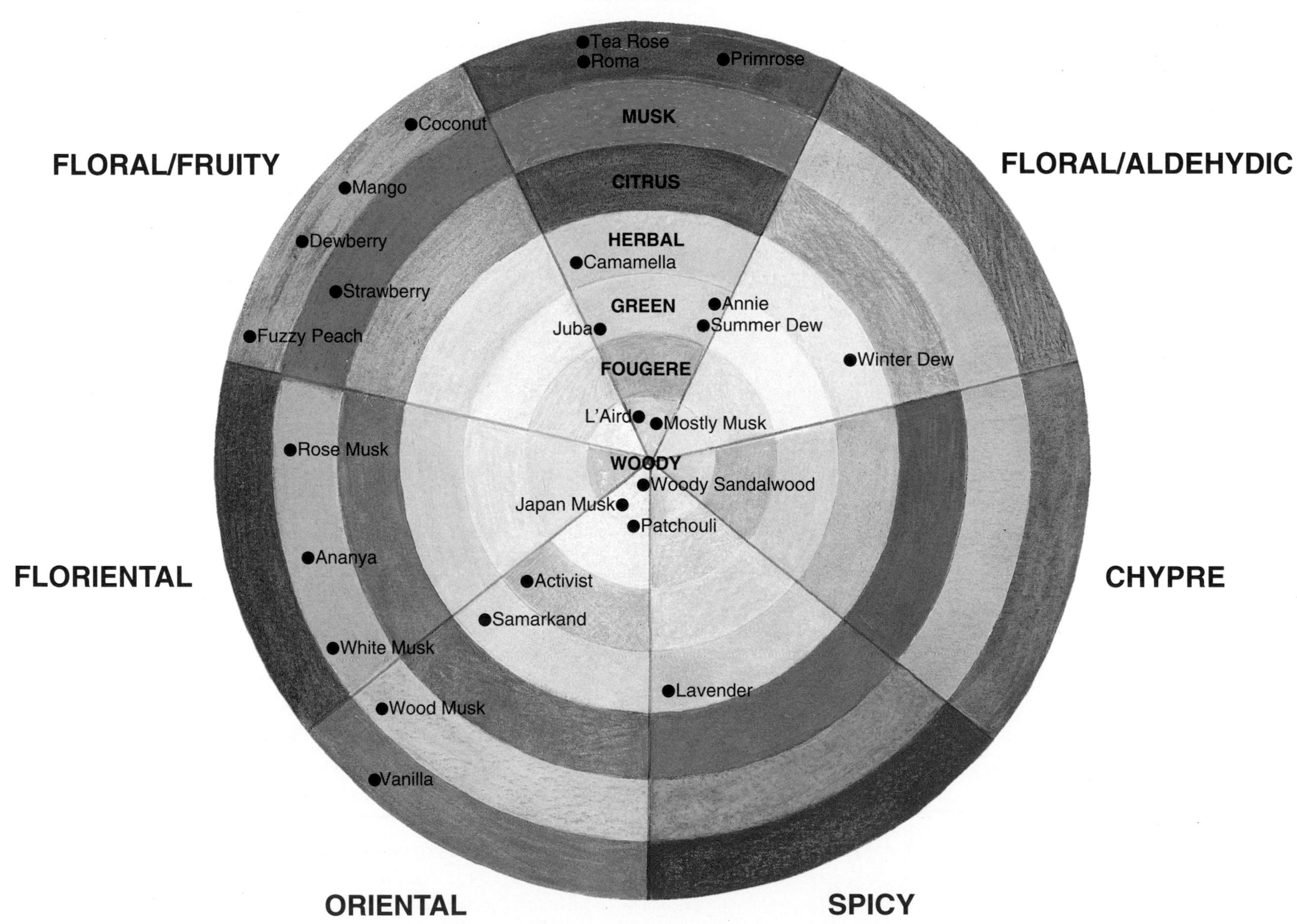

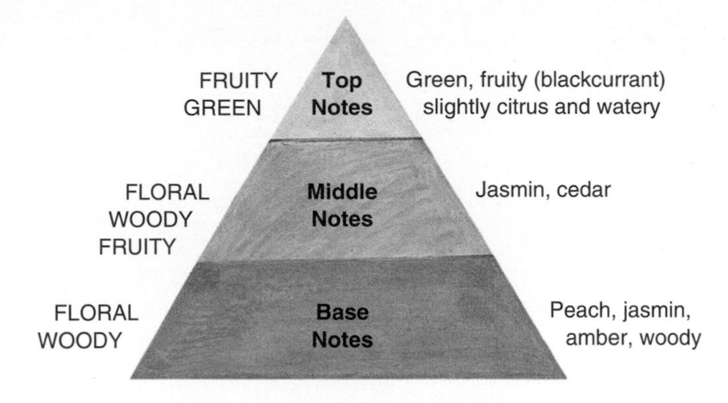

DEWBERRY
An original fruity complex with woody ambery undertones.

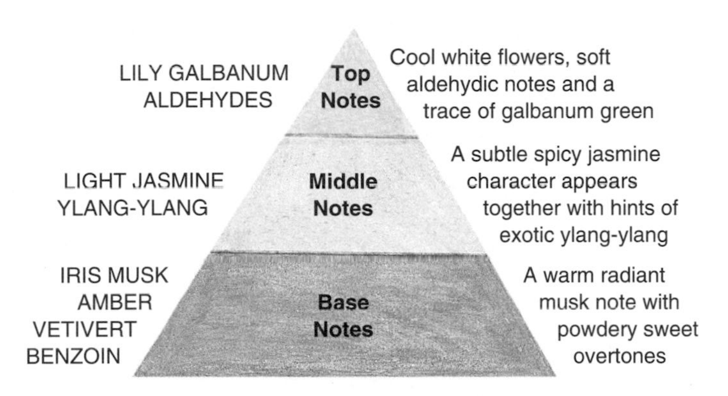

White Musk
The classical musk note enhanced with floral, powdery and sweet woody character.

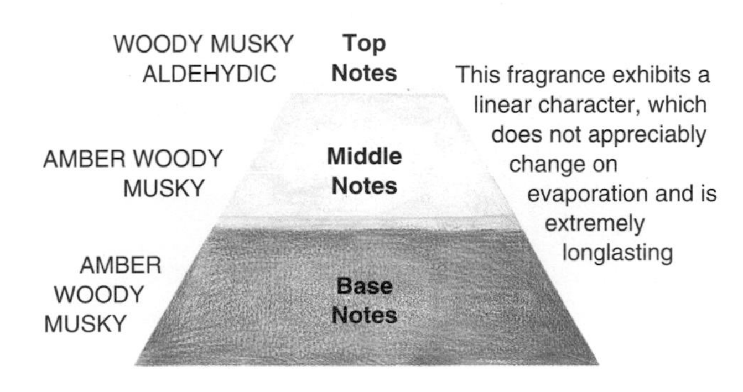

Mostly Musk
An original combination - musk is enhanced with sandalwood, and other precious wood notes, and enriched with amber tones.

The link between scent and magic is potent. The aim of magic is to transform things, for example to make someone who is indifferent to you love you. Scent has the power to transform because it has a non-rational, emotional effect on the brain.

Scent is also used worldwide in rituals of passage such as birth, coming of age, marriage and death. In the Opaque myth of how men lost their immortality, death came because they smelt its stench. It is smell which finally signifies that death, not sleep, is here. And it's by scenting the corpse and burning perfumes over it that cultures like the Ancient Egyptians masked the unbearable reality of death as they masked its stink, and symbolised the transcendence of the soul in the scented smoke that rose from their fires.

This, like scent's role in magic, is connected with its mysterious nature. Unlike visual objects it is not concrete or definite. It crosses boundaries between the concrete objects it emanates from and the invisible that it moves towards. It can transcend physical barriers, permeating the air, passing under doors. All of these are important symbols in rites of passage. It escapes, it cannot be held or contained. Perfume is powerful magic.

Egyptian priests inhaled smouldering incense as a mind-altering sacred drug so they could reach a higher plateau of consciousness that allowed them to communicate with the gods more easily. Prayers were always accompanied by the burning of perfumes, because it was thought that scented smoke created pathways to heaven on which the prayers could travel, and would sweeten earthly pleas on arrival. The Catholic ritual of burning a candle as you pray is a reminder of this.

THE MAKING OF A FRAGRANCE

Creating a perfume has often been compared to preparing haute cuisine, or better still, to composing a piece of music. Balance in music is achieved by the careful harmonisation of instruments. In perfume, the "nose" or perfumer also seeks to balance a fragrance by careful harmony of different "notes". The top note of a perfume is the first impression you have of it. The middle note comes into play after you have been wearing the perfume long enough for it to dry on your skin and for the different essences to "expand". The bottom or "base" note is the final lingering scent. One or more of these perfume notes may occur in the same scent. A perfume may have a floral top note, for example, and dry down to a woody base note. The main perfume families are the greens (citrusy and sharp), the florals, the orientals, the woody and leather notes, the synthetic aldehides (which can be floral, woody or oriental) and the chypre notes.

HOW TO USE SCENT CREATIVELY

What you need to know about using scent is simple: wear what gives you pleasure and nothing else. Don't let scent snobs cajole you into believing a perfume that costs five times as much is somehow better than the one that you instinctively feel is right for you. A breakdown in cost of the average perfume reveals that only 7.6 per cent is spent on the ingredients. Packaging and advertising take up over 25 per cent of costs with most perfumes, and the shop where it is sold cleans up a hefty 40 to 60 per cent profit. Selling perfume in this way is about selling an image as much, if not more, as it is about selling a smell. Remember that only you see the bottle, which, all too often, is the expensive part. Others only detect the smell. Don't let marketing pull the wool over your eyes. Choose your fragrance for the way it smells on you.

Afro-Caribbean skin can be particularly sensitive to fragrance in cosmetic products - the best advice is to use the simplest fragrance-free products.

DIY essential oil: fill a glass jar with sweet scented herbs or flowers, such as lavender; cover with the most odourless vegetable oil you have, and stopper the jar securely. Leave it in a warm place for a fortnight or so, then strain off the oil, which should be delicately scented.

WHICH SCENT SUITS?

So how can you find the right perfume? Start by thinking about you. There's no reason why you can't have different perfumes for every occasion, as no single scent will ever suit all your moods.

When choosing a scent, bear in mind the climate in which it is to be worn. Cool showery weather will bring out scent and strengthen it, whereas strong, dry heat will make it more difficult to smell. Fragrance is intensified in warm, humid countries - so choose a lighter scent and apply more frequently.

A perfume will not smell the same on everyone - equally one scent will even vary at different times on the same person. So don't just pick up a bottle and sniff the contents - always try out a perfume on your own skin. Your skin colour and type affect a perfume's performance. Acidity and oiliness are key factors: the oilier the skin, the richer and longer-lasting the fragrance will be. Diet is also important: spices and garlic can emerge through the skin hours after a meal and affect the skin's chemistry for days. And be aware that other products you use (shampoo, hair spray) leave their own fragrance too, which can affect your perfume.

Don't try too many scents at once - unless you have a trained nose, you will soon become confused. Stick to three or four at a time, testing them on parts of the skin that are as far away as possible from each other. And remember, wait for 20 minutes after applying a scent to allow it to develop and enable the true nature of the fragrance to come through. This is the scent which lingers.

Fragrances conjure up powerful memories and emotions since smell is the most evocative of all the senses. The scent you wear will identify you as clearly as the way you look. The Body Shop's perfume oils are based on natural essences derived from flower extracts, aromatic resins, balsams and synthetic fragrances - but no alcohol and no animal extracts. The Body Shop's perfume oils are concentrated so you only need a small amount.

MAKING THE MOST OF YOUR SCENT

Whether expensive or reasonably priced, there are a very few simple practicalities you need to know about fragrance.

DO store it in a cupboard or at least away from direct sunlight and radiators. Heat and light change the smell.

DO store the bottles in the fridge, if you have a large supply. They will keep at least four time longer than they would outside, though different fragrances deteriorate at different rates.

DO remember it's best to buy fragrance in small amounts to ensure it will stay fresh.

DO test a fragrance on your own skin. A perfume that smells good on someone else may not smell good on you. It depends on the exact nature of the acid mantle that naturally covers everyone's skin.

DON'T bother with the old advice about dabbing fragrance where the pulse points are. Research has shown that this has a negligible effect on its dispersion into the atmosphere. Instead, why not follow Coco Chanel's advice and put perfume wherever you want to be kissed?

DON'T wear fragrance while sunbathing - it can stain skin when affected by strong sunlight. And many essences are photo-sensitising and can cause a rash.

DON'T spray it on pearls.

And DON'T limit yourself to chaste dabs at the neck for big evenings out. Fragrance is one of the loveliest pleasures of life. Why deny yourself?

SYNTHETICS VS. NATURALS

Synthetics are often regarded as the poor relations of natural substances and have the reputation of being cheaper and poorer in quality than the real thing. Neither of these ideas is true. Some synthetics now cost more than natural substances and some are, in fact, better than the natural products.

There are a number of reasons for this. Firstly, no two harvests of flowers are ever the same, so maintaining quality is very difficult with natural substances, especially when environmental wild cards such as acid rain conspire actively to alter once familiar fragrances. Synthetics, on the other hand, can always be produced to the same quality level.

Also, some natural scents are notoriously disappointing once extracted.

Lilac and hyacinth rarely smell as good as they do in the garden. Artful use of synthetics can actually give a truer rendering of the perfume.

Natural ingredients are also limited in supply and, in the case of animal scents, may involve animal exploitation. Musk is a perfect example. It is extracted from the male of the species *Moschus moschiferus*, a small deer (the largest weigh no more than 22 pounds) that lives in the rhododendron and birch groves of Central Asia. The male of this species carries a small sac in the front of his abdomen that secretes a fluid something like a tomcat's spray. These secretions can be collected from the deer, but it is easier and cheaper for hunters simply to kill the animal and extract the scent pod. As an alternative to this brutal practice, The Body Shop's White Musk perfume uses a synthetic version of musk. It is so popular it ranks as our number one best-selling fragrance.

SCENTING YOUR SURROUNDINGS

Most of us enjoy scenting ourselves, but what about scenting the environment around us? The smell of a room has a huge effect on mood.

- Use pot-pourri to "lift" a room, particularly the bathroom; and keep a little bundle of patchouli roots in your underwear drawer or with stationery. Dab a handkerchief with your favourite fragrance and place in your wardrobe or drawers.
- Perfumed wooden balls can be rolled into nooks of the linen cupboard as was the custom in previous centuries to scent pillows and sheets very subtly.
- If you don't like the proprietary scent of most fabric conditioners, buy a non-perfumed one instead and scatter a few drops of your favourite essential oil into the dispenser in the machine along with it.
- An aroma pot is one of the most ancient ways of scenting a room. A few drops of special scented oils for burning or aromatherapy oils are placed in the bowl-shaped top, and a small candle lit underneath. The heat will waft the fragrance into the air (there's more on this in the Aromatherapy chapter).
- Add a few drops to a dish of water and place on a warm radiator to add fragrance to your home.
- Dab a little perfume oil on a light bulb, which will diffuse the scent around the room as it heats up.
- Create your own aromatic notepaper: impregnate a tissue or other absorbent paper with a few drops of perfume oil. Cut the paper into several pieces and place it at regular intervals in a box of notepaper. Keep the box closed for at least 24 hours.
- Turn an ordinary candle into a fragrant one: light the wick and wait until a small amount of wax has melted, then add a few drops of perfume oil to the melted wax. A few minutes later the room will be filled with fragrance.
- Sprinkle two clean dry towels with your favourite scent, pop them in the clothes dryer for a few minutes, retrieve and give yourself a vigorous rubdown.

The Chinese believed that jasmine could clear an oppressive atmosphere and favoured its use in the bedroom at night. In India, the wedding bed is often decorated with jasmine.

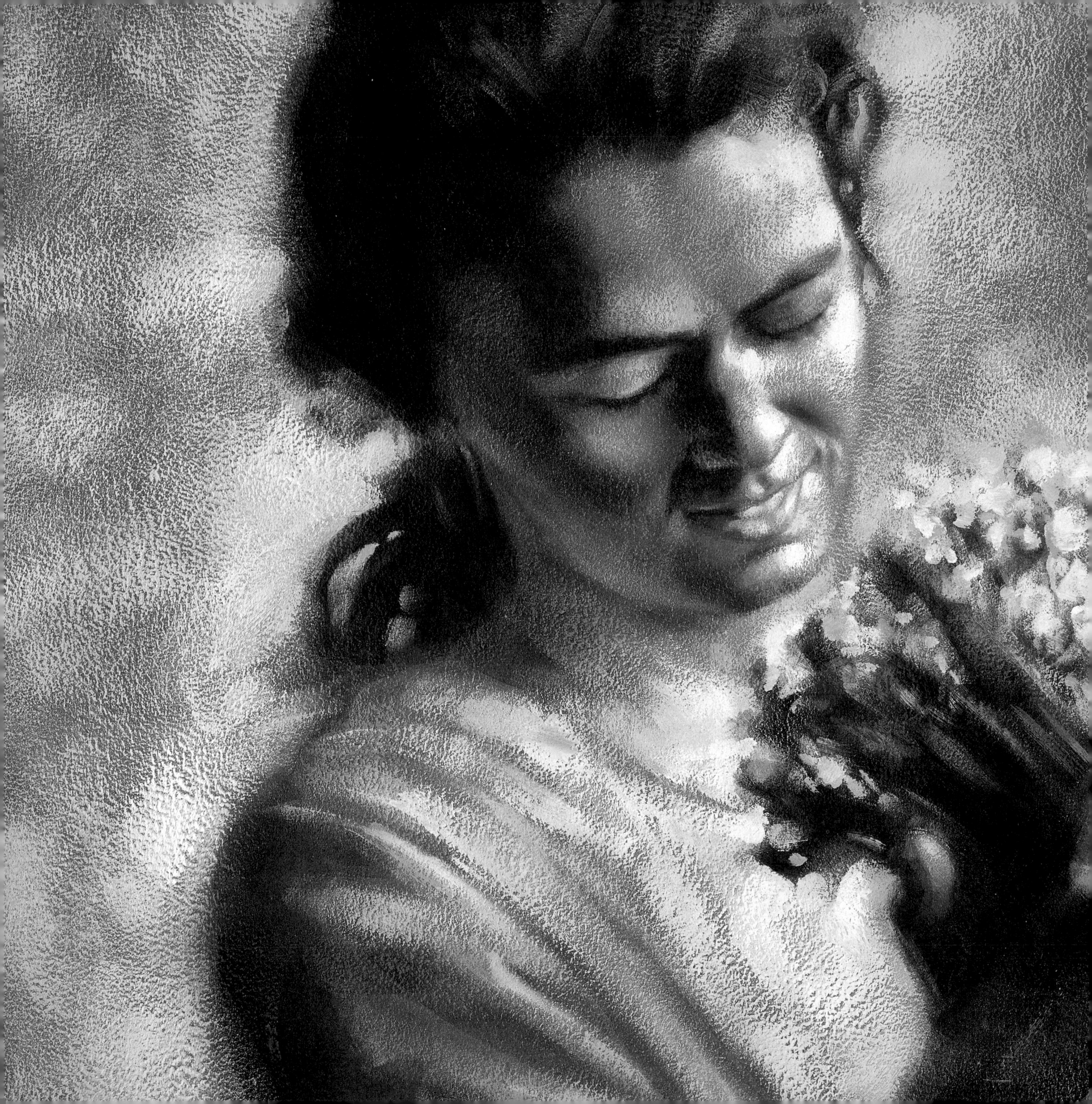

AROMATHERAPY

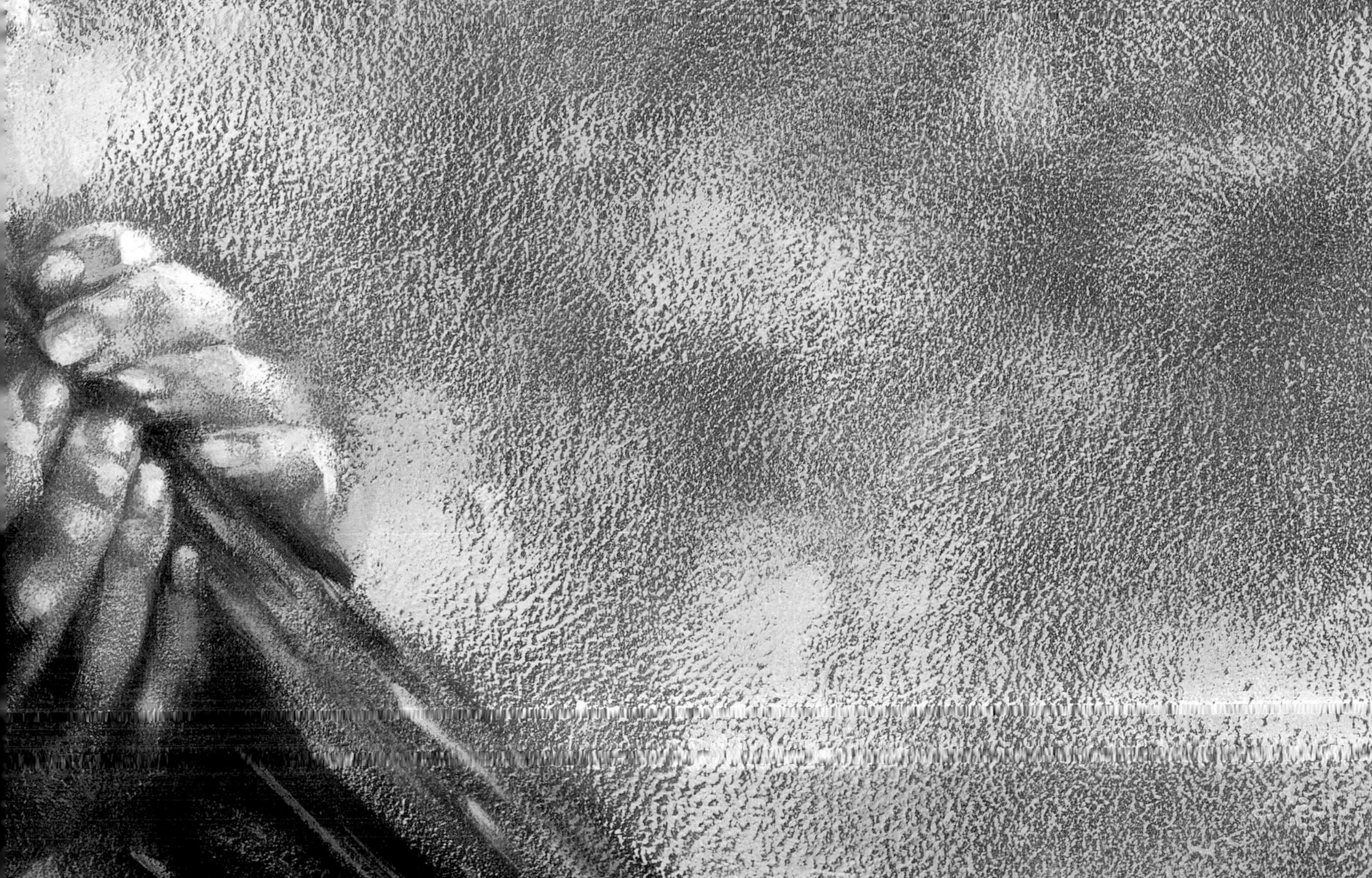

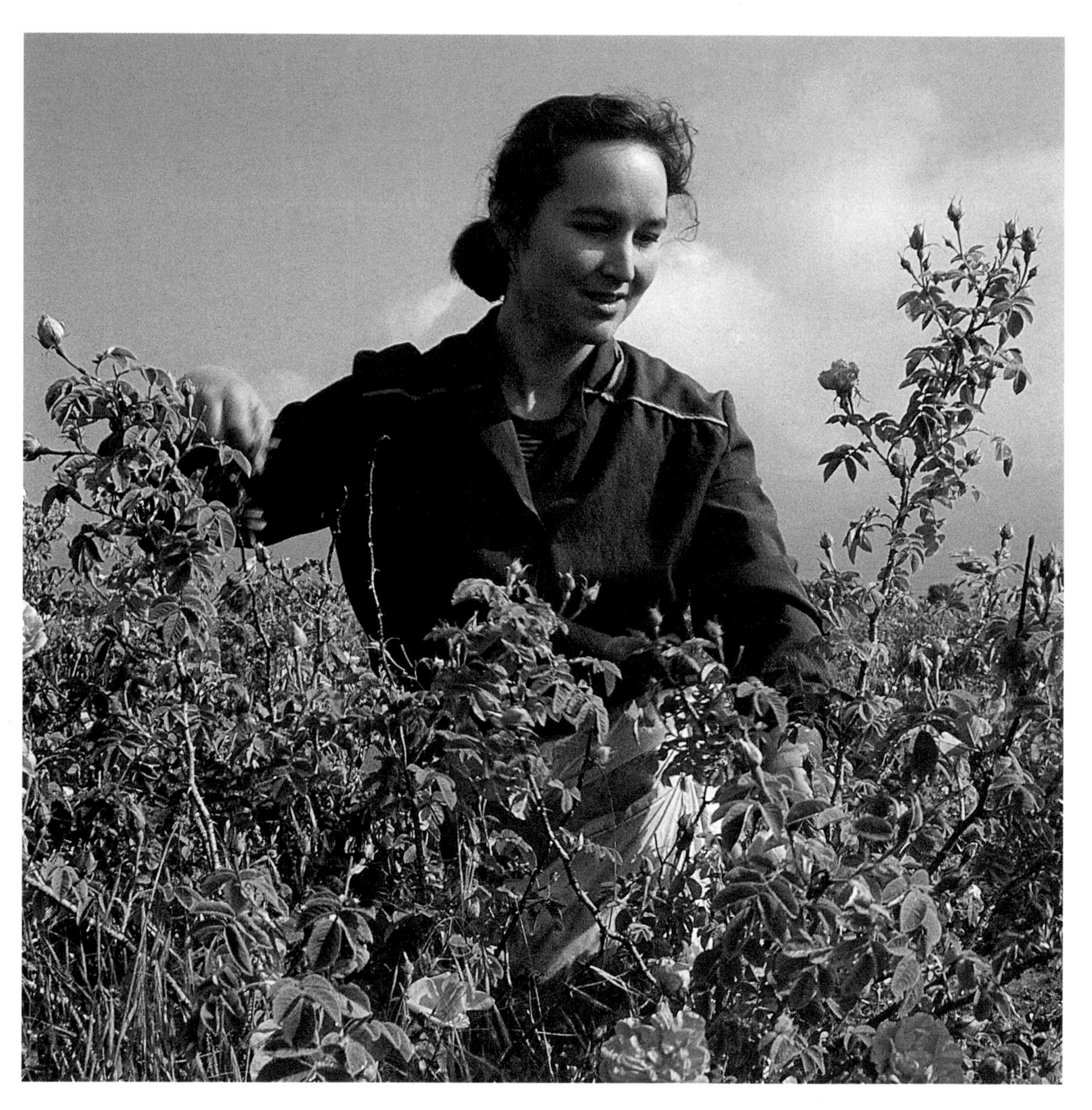

Bulgaria brought attar, the essential oil of roses, to Europe from the East, and even today Bulgarian roses are the most prized in the world. The oil they produce has been used for centuries to revitalise all types of skin.

aromatherapy

Even if we can't possibly determine at what point in pre-history we first looked beyond plants as food and began to use them for medicine, perfume and magic, we can still be reasonably certain that aromatherapy, the practice of using essential oils extracted from aromatic plants to enhance health and appearance, dates from the dawn of human time. Legend provides support for this theory: supposedly, every aromatic plant that has ever existed grew in the Garden of Eden. For the Ancient Egyptians, the first living thing was a voluptuously scented flower: the lotus. As it ripened, its petals unfurled to reveal the Supreme God hidden within. The lotus was sacred to the Ancient Egyptian, as it is to Buddhists and Hindus today.

There is something primal and instinctive about the principles of aromatherapy. You have only to look at the ways that other animals make use of the fragrant pharmacy that grows all over the planet. Dogs seek out particular grasses when they are sick; and birds are now known carefully to choose specific aromatherapeutic plants to build their nests. Each chosen plant has different anti-bacterial or insecticide properties. When woven together, they keep a broad range of pests and diseases away.

Aromatherapy uses essential oils, the soul of the plant. They are its volatile, aromatic part, perceived by us as fragrance. But fragrance is only the beginning. Our sense of smell is just one route by which the powers of essential oils affect us.

Essential oils are not truly oils - the name itself is actually a bit of a misnomer - and will evaporate if placed on blotting paper, leaving only a faint mark. They are completely different from true fatty oils like almond oil, avocado oil or soyabean oil, which can all be used as "carrier" or "base" oils and which do not have aromatherapeutic effects.

Different essential oils come from different parts of a plant: the flowers, as in camomile; the leaves, as in thyme; the roots, as in vetiver; the bark, as in cinnamon; or the wood, as in sandalwood. They can also be extracted from grasses (such as lemongrass) or fruits. A few plants yield different essential oils from more than one of their components. The bitter orange tree, for instance, provides orange from the fruit skin, petitgrain from the leaves, and neroli from the exquisite smelling orange blossom.

Essential oils are a highly complex harmony of many different components. Most have about 100 ingredients. Eucalyptus has 250; rose oil, 3,000. Science uses a technique called gas chromatography to identify the different chemicals present in an essential oil, but it's proving to be far from foolproof. Twenty years ago, scientists thought jasmine had 100 ingredients, now they know it has 150, and the figure is still climbing. Essential oils offer us constituents and compounds of a range and usefulness that the best chemicals in the world can scarcely match.

Scientists have succeeded in isolating some of the key ingredients of essential oils, and can make synthetic copies of these in the laboratory. These copies are used in food, cosmetics and the drug business. In the USA, for example, 25 per cent of all prescriptions dispensed in pharmacies contain an active ingredient synthesised from a plant original. These synthetic copies of "active ingredients" have revolutionised medicine. But, sometimes they are too brutal, causing side-effects or allergic reactions. Occasionally they prove not only to be less safe, but also less effective than the original essential oil. For example, essential oil of oregano is 26 times more powerful as an antiseptic than phenol (the active ingredient in many household cleaners). Yet the active ingredient of oregano is phenol, and it makes up 20 per cent of the essential oil.

The Russians sent their astronauts into space with phials of essential oils to remind them of earth and to overcome the emotional deprivation of scentless space.

What seems to be happening is that essential oils are proving to be an excellent example of the principle of synergy. Two things work synergistically when their action together is more than the sum of their individual actions. The ingredients of essential oils, many of which are still mysterious to science, heal in harmony. This explains why synthetic equivalents - which are never complete, but only what scientists deduce as the active ingredients - do not always have the same effects. In addition, though oils are effective on their own, they often work synergistically with other oils. For example, camomile's anti-inflammatory properties are more than doubled when blended with lavender in the right proportions.

AROMATHERAPY AND THE HEALING POWER OF PLANTS

One of the great modern aromatherapists, Marguerite Maury, called essential oils "the purest form of living energy that we can insert into man". They are also frequently referred to as the soul of the plant. They are its volatile, aromatic part, perceived by us as fragrance.

Hot Compress for Blemished Skin: add 2 drops juniper berry oil and 2 drops lavender oil to bowl of warm water. Soak wash cloth, wring out and cover face. Repeat.

But fragrance is only the beginning. Our sense of smell is just one route by which the powers of essential oils potently affect our brain and our endocrine system.

Our great-grandmothers knew how to heal with plants and every country had its own pharmacopoeia of plant lore. The healing power of these plants is often contained in their minute quantities of essential oil. However, aromatherapy - the use of the pure distilled essential oils - was largely lost as an art for hundreds of years. Then, at the beginning of this century, a French chemist, René Maurice Gattefosse, was experimenting in his laboratory when a small explosion burnt his hand. He instinctively plunged it in to the nearest bowl of liquid which happened to be pure lavender essential oil. The burns healed more quickly than usual and there was no scarring. This aroused his interest and he pioneered research into essential oils. It was Gattefosse who coined the term aromatherapy.

Aromatherapy means therapy using the aromatic, volatile part of plants, but not always through the sense of smell or aroma. In fact, the most usual way for aromatherapists to administer the oils in this country is by a massage. In France, where every aromatherapist has to be a medical doctor by law, most aromatherapy prescriptions are to be taken internally; this would be extremely inadvisable without expert medical guidance.

At any rate, many aromatherapists now believe that swallowing essential oils is one of the least effective ways of taking them, as the chemistry in the stomach can alter them. In massage, or when in a bath, the oils are easily and quickly assimilated through the skin, and inhaled at the same time. Experiments have "tagged" essential oils with radioactive isotopes which can be detected by a geiger counter. They are rubbed onto a patch of skin. Later, when the geiger counter is moved over the body, the isotopes, and hence the oils, show up in the liver, kidneys, lungs, and all over the body.

One of the benefits of aromatherapy oils over conventional drugs for healing, is that while they are usually slower acting than drugs they rarely have side effects, though epileptics and women in the first three months of pregnancy are cautioned against the use of some oils. For this reason, research is focusing on essential oils as the medicines of the future. Unlike many synthetic drugs, they are not, as far as we know, stored in the body. They are quickly excreted in the urine, faeces, and through sweat and the breath. Different oils escape by different routes. Sandalwood and juniper can clearly be smelt in the urine; geranium will scent your perspiration.

Powerful stuff: scientists have killed the typhoid bacillus with cinnamon oil in 12 minutes, clove oil in 25 minutes, and geranium oil in less than 50 minutes.

THE PROPERTIES OF ESSENTIAL OILS

Essential oils are antiseptics and disinfectants. Until the Second World War, the most effective oils such as thyme, lemon, clove and camomile were used to sterilise instruments and fumigate hospital wards. What a healthy contrast it must have made to the pungent synthetics we use now!

As naturally derived antibiotics, essential oils do more than simply kill bacteria and viruses, they also stimulate the body's immune system to fight the infection; exactly the opposite of synthetic antibiotics, which weaken the immune system as they work. The frequent use of antibiotics for minor ills is often described by aromatherapists as using a sledgehammer to hit a pin. While antibiotics are obviously necessary and remarkable in their place, the gentler, immune system boosting action of essential oils can be a better choice where antibiotics would be overkill.

Different oils have a huge variety of different effects. Peppermint, for example, prevents flatulence when taken as a tisane and its antifungal properties make it an effective treatment for the feet.

About 300 oils, at present, are well known for their healing powers, but it is highly likely that there are many more waiting to be discovered in areas like the Amazon. The Amazonian rainforest and the people who inhabit it and are knowledgeable of the huge natural pharmacy of plants within it are incredibly valuable resources. Their shortsighted and cruel destruction could deny all of us the key to cures for many diseases.

AN ANCIENT SCIENCE

The Ancient Egyptians possessed a wealth of knowledge about the power of plants and their oils. Egyptian priests used many aromatic substances in embalming. The Greek author, Herodotus, explained the process. First, the brain was drawn out with infinite care through the nose with fine hooks, and the skull stuffed with aromatherapeutic herbs and oils. Next, the abdomen was slit open, the viscera removed and the cavity packed with myrrh, galbanum and other resins and spices like cinnamon, clove and nutmeg rich in antiseptic and antibiotic essential oils. The viscera were then washed in palm wine mingled with aromatic oils and stored in canopied jars. The body was soaked in natron (sodium carbonate solution) for 70 days and then washed and wrapped in mummy-bandages that had been steeped in essential oils such as cedar and cinnamon.

The oils proved to be mightily effective preservatives: bits of Egyptian mummy intestine examined under the microscope have proved to be intact after thousands of years, which unwittingly vindicates the modern usage of essential oils as preservatives in many "natural" cosmetics, and as "youth preservers" in formulations aimed at living skin.

CLASSICAL GAS

Ancient Egypt's priests made great use of aromatics for releasing the powers of the subconscious during ecstatic religious trances. One of the most famous euphoric perfumes was kyphi, described as having anything from 16 to 60 ingredients. Originally sacred to the gods and burnt only in temples, kyphi eventually became a major Egyptian export. It contained myrrh, incense, broom and calamus, now known to be a potent narcotic that would indeed be able to "allay anxieties and brighten dreams" as Plutarch claims.

The Egyptians had a holistic attitude to life. For them, perfume and medicine were one and the same thing. Aromatic substances such as those used in embalming

As far back as Ancient Athens, physicians have used aromatic smoke to keep infection at bay. Aromatic fumigations were used to try and halt the Plague, but don't seem to have had much effect. In the 19th century, 120 juniper wood stakes lit all at the same time in the street of Bois-le-Roi in France, apparently kept an epidemic at bay.

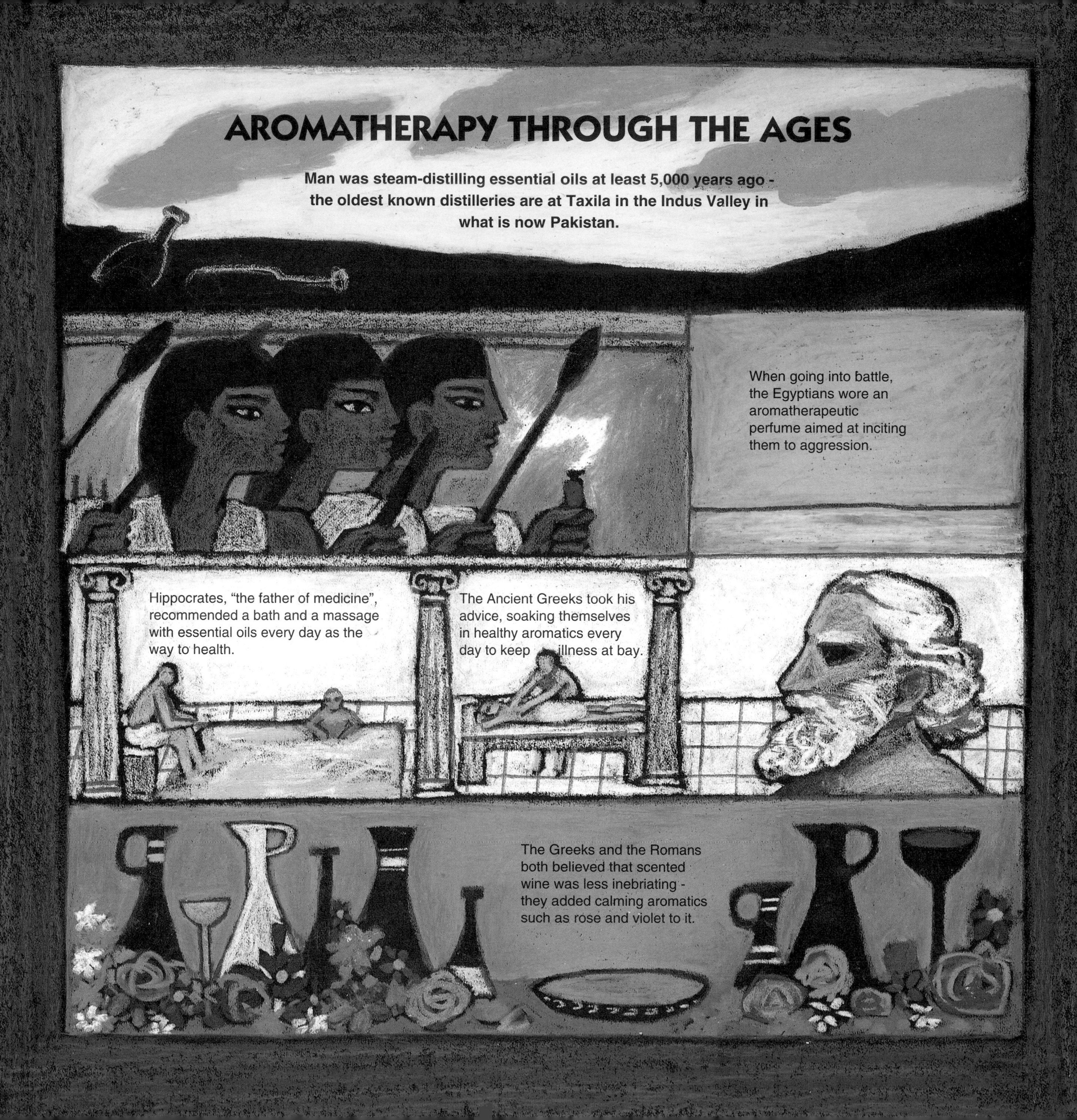
AROMATHERAPY THROUGH THE AGES
Man was steam-distilling essential oils at least 5,000 years ago - the oldest known distilleries are at Taxila in the Indus Valley in what is now Pakistan.
When going into battle, the Egyptians wore an aromatherapeutic perfume aimed at inciting them to aggression.
Hippocrates, "the father of medicine", recommended a bath and a massage with essential oils every day as the way to health.
The Ancient Greeks took his advice, soaking themselves in healthy aromatics every day to keep illness at bay.
The Greeks and the Romans both believed that scented wine was less inebriating - they added calming aromatics such as rose and violet to it.

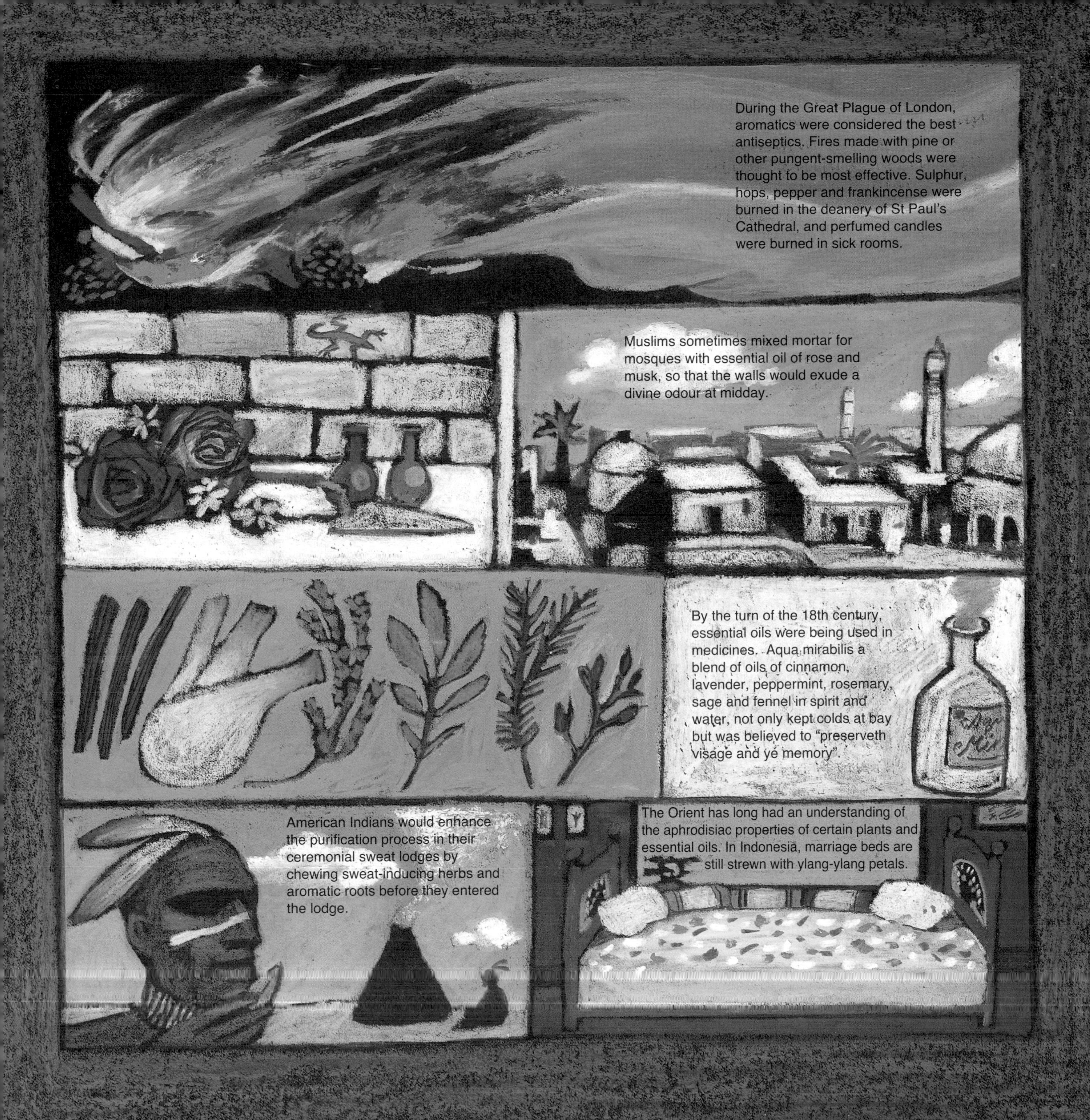

During the Great Plague of London, aromatics were considered the best antiseptics. Fires made with pine or other pungent-smelling woods were thought to be most effective. Sulphur, hops, pepper and frankincense were burned in the deanery of St Paul's Cathedral, and perfumed candles were burned in sick rooms.
Muslims sometimes mixed mortar for mosques with essential oil of rose and musk, so that the walls would exude a divine odour at midday.
By the turn of the 18th century, essential oils were being used in medicines. Aqua mirabilis a blend of oils of cinnamon, lavender, peppermint, rosemary, sage and fennel in spirit and water, not only kept colds at bay but was believed to "preserveth visage and ye memory".
American Indians would enhance the purification process in their ceremonial sweat lodges by chewing sweat-inducing herbs and aromatic roots before they entered the lodge.
The Orient has long had an understanding of the aphrodisiac properties of certain plants and essential oils. In Indonesia, marriage beds are still strewn with ylang-ylang petals.

The Ancient Chinese and the Japanese used scent to tell the time, with incense clocks. The clocks were candles whose wax was mixed with different essential oils in bands corresponding exactly to an hour of each day. At the change of every hour the scent in the air would change, so that you always knew exactly what time it was wherever you were. In the morning, stimulating scents were burnt, at noon, refreshing scents, and relaxing, sedative fragrances were used towards evening.

were also used by the priests in their role as psychiatrists, for treating depression, nervous tension and madness. Sweet flag, found in kyphi, was prescribed as an aphrodisiac, but also as a poultice for stomach troubles.

Lemongrass is widely used as an element of Ayurvedic medicine in the Indian subcontinent and is prescribed to bring down a fever.

The idea here was obviously for the essential oil to pass through the skin. Medical papyri show that while some remedies were swallowed, many were given in massage or as poultices, or else inhaled as fumigations; all are typical aromatherapy methods used today.

The Ancient Chinese had, if anything, an even more exquisite sense of the importance of smell. Their heightened awareness of the powers of essential oils meant they thought of different perfumes as different states of mind and used them to create harmonies of mood. An old Chinese maxim is "A perfume is always a medicine". Other ancient civilisations were similarly aware of the power of aromatics. The Assyrians used fumigations of cannabis to dispel sorrow. The Babylonians linked magical perfumes to astrological influences. The Indians built entire temples from sandalwood, which made the atmosphere permanently cool and meditative as well as keeping white ants at bay. Their tradition of perfume and aromatherapy is still very much alive.

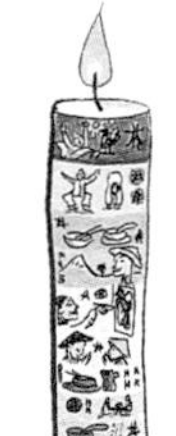

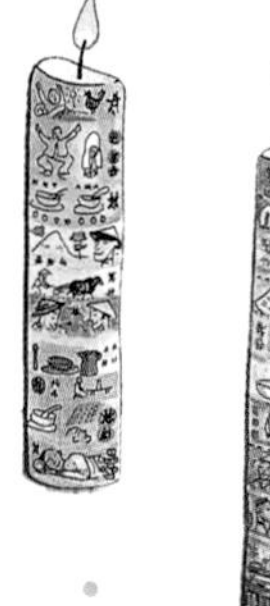

AN EXCESS OF SCENT

The Ancient Greeks used prodigious quantities of aromatic essences, learning from the Egyptians and importing a good deal from them too. Like the Egyptians, they considered perfume and aromatherapy as one; twin gifts of plants. Hippocrates, father of medicine, used many aromatics, detailing their use in his textbooks.

In Ancient Greece and Rome, aromatic baths and massage were a habitual part of everyday life. The basic cleansing function of the bath was only the beginning. For the Greeks, it was daily steeping in healthy aromatics that kept sickness at bay. Prodicus, a disciple of Asclepius, the mythical Greek physician god, noticed that athletes massaged with aromatic oils became more vigorous and developed beautiful skin. The Greeks used different oils to treat different parts of the body: thyme for legs and knees; mint for arms and back; Egyptian oil for the feet; marjoram for the hair and palm oil for the chest.

The Romans took their chief pleasure in the mood-altering power of scents and their sensual enjoyment. Scented ointments were rubbed on the feet of guests at banquets while elegant girls and boys offered alabaster fragrance jars. Nero had ivory joysticks in his dining-room walls which he could flick to release showers of rose petals, half drowning his guests. Scented wine with calming aromatics like rose and violet dropped into it was thought less inebriating.

In more recent times, Islam has embraced the poetry of fragrance to a much greater degree than Christianity. Perfume was one of three things Mohammed valued in this world. Today, Muslims from the Gulf scent their clothes with fumigations of an expensive aromatic wood called oudh. It purifies the air, deodorises, and apparently smells both celestial and cerebral.

THE WAY TO HEALTH

Hippocrates said that the way to health was to have a scented bath and massage every day. This simple and delightful advice has been ignored by mainstream doctors who prefer to prescribe a pill for every ill. As preventive medicine however, Hippocrates' advice is excellent. The benefits of massage for banishing the stress that is the root cause of the majority of modern ills are discussed in another chapter.

Hippocrates also recommended that both massage and bath incorporate essential oils. This was not simply to make them more enjoyable, but an integral part of the therapy. As massage encourages the flow of lymphatic fluids to eliminate toxins, essential oils help as they have the action of easing blood and lymph congestion. Oils inhaled in the bath soothe stress, or stimulate and refresh, depending on which are used, and treat aching muscles. And, of course, there are many other specific benefits depending on the oils.

The Japanese have retained a bath ritual that has something of the holistic benefits of the ancient world. They wash before getting into baths traditionally made of fragrant cedarwood, which is antiseptic, sedative, a good skin toner and which also strengthens the respiratory system. Into the water, they throw mixtures of aromatic medicinal herbs. They then soak and meditate in the plant-rich water, inhaling the essential oils. Clearly, the object is bathing therapy, not just getting clean. Like the Ancient Greeks and Romans, the Japanese enjoy bath houses where they can also benefit from a massage.

***Detox Bath:* add 2 drops geranium oil, 2 drops rosemary oil, 2 drops juniper berry oil and 2 drops lavender oil to your bath. Relax.**

THE ESSENCE REFINED

The usual method of extracting essential oils is distillation with steam. This involves heating the plants in big vats of water. Heat bursts oil sacs and, as the essential oils are the volatile parts of the plant, they rise up with the steam. They are then channelled along a pipe, which cools the mixture, causing it to condense, usually into a second vat. There, the oil and the water are easily separated and the oil floats to the surface.

Certain oils can simply be "expressed" or pressed from the rind. In the case of orange, this is sometimes still done by hand with natural sponges, which are then wrung out, releasing the oil. Maceration is another very old-fashioned method used for oils like jasmine and tuberose that change when heated. It involves steeping plants in oil or fat, or pressing them into fat smeared onto glass trays, so that they impregnate the fat. The flowers are replaced each day until the fat is saturated. But this is extremely time consuming and rarely used nowadays.

AROMATHERAPY FOR EVERYONE

Single essential oils form the basis of traditional aromatherapy. The vast majority of oils used sensibly and correctly do you nothing but good in almost every way, but essential oils can be strong medicine. They are highly concentrated, usually much more powerful than whole plant extracts, and should always be used with respect and care.

Because of their strength, essential oils are usually diluted in carrier oils for treatment - with the occasional exception of lavender - unless for inhalation. Misuse can lead to skin irritation and occasionally, more serious problems. For this reason, The Body Shop's oils are already blended at 3 per cent strength with grapeseed carrier oils so that they can be used without any worries. When using full strength oils, please follow the directions for dosage in massage and baths with care. Less, in the case of essential oils, is nearly always more.

If you would like some information on registered aromatherapists in your area, contact the International Federation of Aromatherapy, Department of Continuing Education, The Royal Masonic Hospital, Ravenscourt Park, London, W6 0TN.

QUINTESSENTIAL HEALTH

Using oils to boost your health is something learned with experience. If you are ill, it's a doctor you need, and possibly a qualified aromatherapist as well. However, a few essential oils in the first aid kit can be tremendously useful.

• Lavender is an oil that can turn itself into almost anything. It helps soothe minor burns and will help to prevent scarring and blistering. Lavender also helps heal stings and insect bites.

• Both lavender and camomile are good oils to use for children as they are mild and pacifying. Use half the normal amount of oil, diluted in a base of oil for massage or in the bath.

• Eucalyptus is so widely recognised for its effectiveness in clearing the respiratory system that it is available from pharmacies. When colds or flu threaten, rub eucalyptus, or a mixture of eucalyptus, bergamot and lavender, into the chest, throat and upper back night and morning, diluted in a little massage oil.

Aromatherapist Daniele Ryman suggests the following test to prove to yourself that essential oils are absorbed by the skin. Rub fresh garlic on the soles of a friend's feet. The essential oil (which, remember, is the aromatic part of the plant) will be detectable on his or her breath in a couple of hours.

Dr Jean Valnet, one of the modern pioneers of aromatherapy, recommended using essential oils to disinfect the air. His recipe was to vaporise several drops of thyme, lavender, pine and eucalyptus daily. You could try eucalyptus, lavender, juniper and bergamot in a bowl of hot water or on a cotton wool ball behind a radiator. Some essential oils are also very good for toning and reviving tired muscles: a massage and bath with rosemary for example, is excellent. Remember: oils act more slowly than conventional medicine so persevere.

Workaholic's Bath: fill a bath with warm water. Add 1 drop neroli, 2 drops lavender, 1 drop geranium. Relax and enjoy.

Different essential oils appear to be picked up and "fixed" by different parts of the body. Violet leaves tend to concentrate in the kidneys, rosemary in the intestines, sandalwood in the bladder, neroli and ylang-ylang are attracted to the nervous system, and this is where they have their chief effects.

Crushed juniper berries were used by the Ancient Egyptians as a cure for baldness. The Hopi Indians of North America rubbed Rocky Mountain juniper leaves on to the head to remove dandruff.

AROMATHERAPY FOR THE FACE AND SCALP

The Byzantines used myrrh and incense aromatherapeutically in fumigations to treat acne and skin impurities. Many oils are beneficial for the skin. If you are using single oils on your face, dilute them first in your favourite moisturising cream or oil. Use only a drop in a teaspoon of moisturiser (discontinue use if your skin feels itchy afterwards).

The following oils are recommended for various skin problems:

- for dull skin: lavender and rosemary
- for acne: lavender
- for reddened skin: soothe with camomile, neroli and rose
- for greasy skin: neroli.

Lavender and rose are two of the best oils for the skin. Lavender is cleansing and decongesting, rose is excellent for mature skin and dry skin. Shake two or three drops of the appropriate oil into a bowl of just boiled water, and give yourself a ten minute face sauna with a towel over your head to keep the steam in. Men whose skin feels sore after shaving should pat a little lavender oil into the area.

Essential oils are also good for the scalp. Rosemary stimulates the circulation and has an astringent action, and it's good for restoring the lustre to dark hair. Lavender and camomile will soothe an itchy scalp. Juniper is antibacterial and stimulating.

BRAIN FOOD

A study conducted by leading aromatherapist Robert Tisserand, in conjunction with an acupuncturist, found that 95 per cent of all essential oils tested had an effect on the acupuncture meridian most closely connected with the brain. Rosemary, basil and peppermint were the most active "brain foods".

It is their effect on mood and mind that gives essential oils their special fascination. The prospect of mood-altering essential oils has now gripped scientists and the fragrance industry's marketing men alike. Perfumes of the future, they say, will not just be pleasant or sexually suggestive, but will have specific mood effects. Warwick University's Olfaction Research Group has studied "brain maps" to see what happens when we smell different scents. Jasmine proved - surprisingly to the investigators, though not to aromatherapists - to have a brain-stimulating effect, and rose a sedating one. The study of odours' effect on the brain has been given the trendy title aromachology.

A CALMING INFLUENCE

Rosemary was used as a substitute for incense in Europe to aid prayers and meditations. In the Smell chapter, we saw how fragrance helps to quieten the "analysing" mind or cerebral cortex and stimulate the "freefall" limbic system. This banishes the banal and eases you closer to the state of meditation. The Islamic mystic Sufis urged their followers to think daily about the Prophet "in meditation and concentration, if possible, immersed in a perfumed, Elysian and supra-earthly atmosphere". When you are about to meditate,

NEROLI

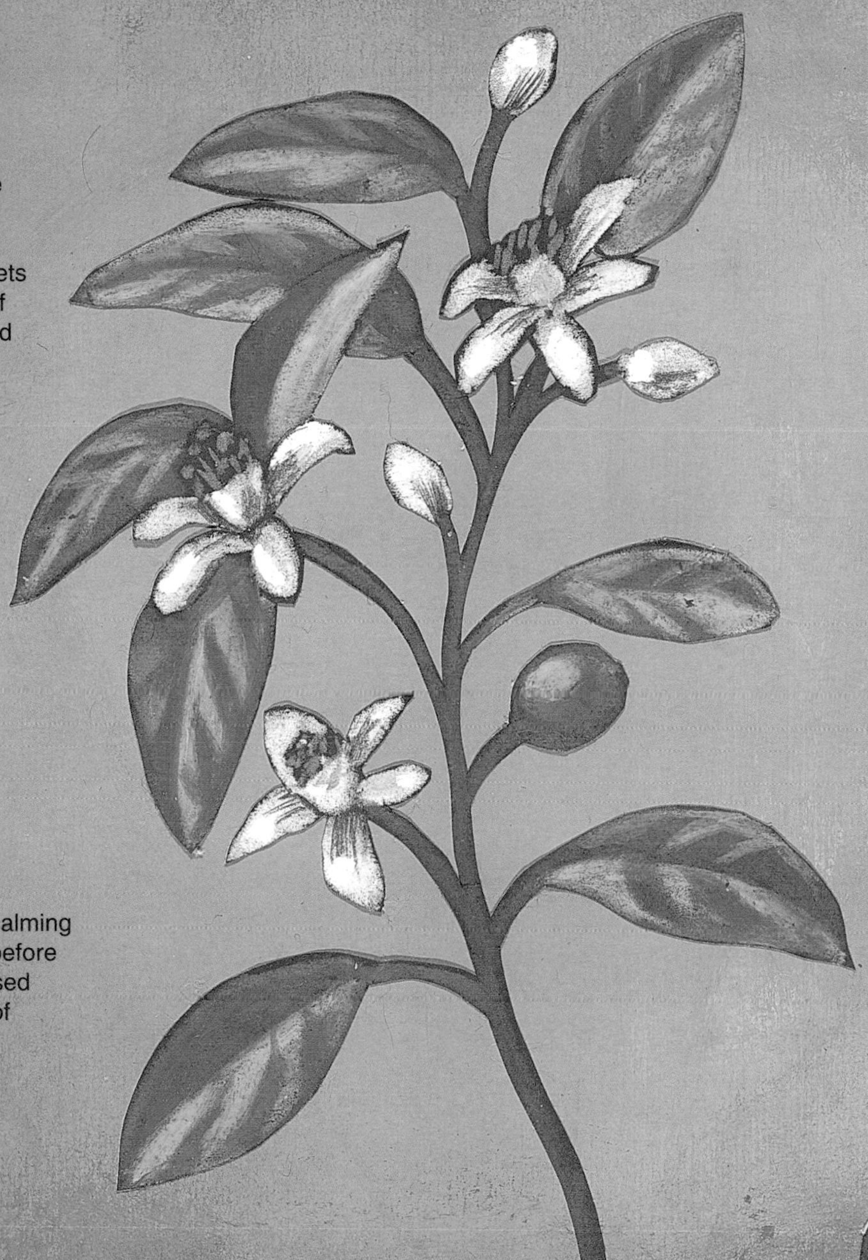

The best neroli oil is extracted from the blossom of the Seville or bitter orange, though sweet orange, lemon and mandarin blossoms are also used. It gets its name from Anne Marie, Countess of Neroli, who used the oil as perfume and to scent her gloves and bath water.

Neroli enjoyed a reputation as an aphrodisiac not because it stimulated but because it calmed any pre-performance worries (and therefore let the lovers frolic rather than fret).

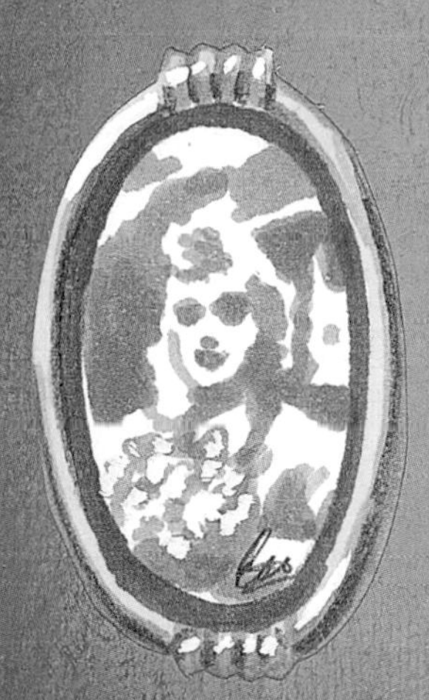

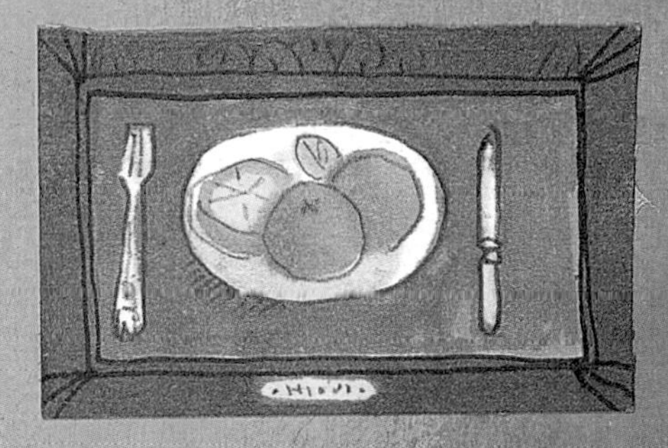

Neroli has always been valued for its calming properties. Its ability to reduce stress before an anxiety-causing event was recognised centuries ago in the traditional usage of orange blossoms in bridal bouquets.

Only recently have oranges been used as food. Their initial popularity in Europe was based on the ornamental appearance of the trees and the uplifting fragrance of the peel and blossom.

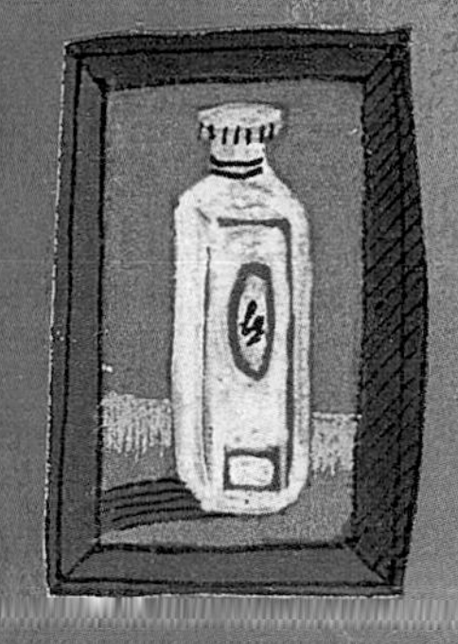

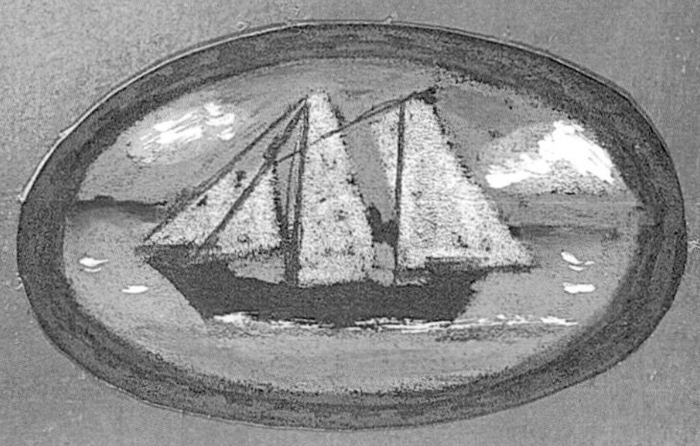

Neroli has traditionally been one of the elements of true eau de cologne. Perhaps it was its sedative properties that made it a hit with Victorian ladies tightly laced into their corsets - and with lifestyles to match.

The empire-building of, first, the Romans and then the Moors carried oranges through the Mediterranean and North Africa to Spain and Portugal. Christopher Columbus introduced oranges to the Western Hemisphere in the 15th century.

or otherwise want to make everyday worries evaporate, prepare by shaking a few drops of rosemary and lavender onto a cotton wool ball and tucking it behind a radiator, or shake a few drops into a bowl of steaming water placed by the radiator. You can also anoint your temples with this mixture. Above all, use oils you feel an affinity with for meditation.

If you get into a state, feel close to tears or an outburst of anger, pause and inhale a calming oil like lavender, rose or neroli to bring you very quickly back to yourself. Rose is a great comforter. The Greek physicians Galen and Celsus used aromatics like myrtle, sage and mint as remedies for hysterical convulsions. Inhaling a substance takes it immediately to the brain, where it works almost at once.

Senegalese women make belts from the tubers of the ginger plant, and wear them when they want to stimulate the erotic impulses of their men.

THE ESSENTIALS IN BRIEF

DO keep your essential oils in their dark glass bottles away from heat, light and moisture which generally have a damaging effect on them.

DO do a skin test on the inside of the wrist; leave for 24 hours and see if you react with any irritation. Not all oils agree with everyone.

DO remember that diluting an essential oil in a carrier oil will reduce any chance of irritation.

DO use small amounts. In some cases, oils will have the opposite effects to those specified if used in larger amounts. In a few cases, oils like basil can be toxic in large amounts.

DO consult a doctor before using essential oils if you have a tendency to epilepsy or if you are pregnant.

DON'T take oils internally.

Rose essential oil's regenerating powers on all kinds of skin, especially mature, wrinkled skin are well known. Apply nightly to clean skin to counter wrinkles, dryness, puffiness, clogged pores and generally to revitalise the face. A facial massage with rose oil is ideal for dry or mature skin. It also makes a wonderful, if expensive, hand oil.

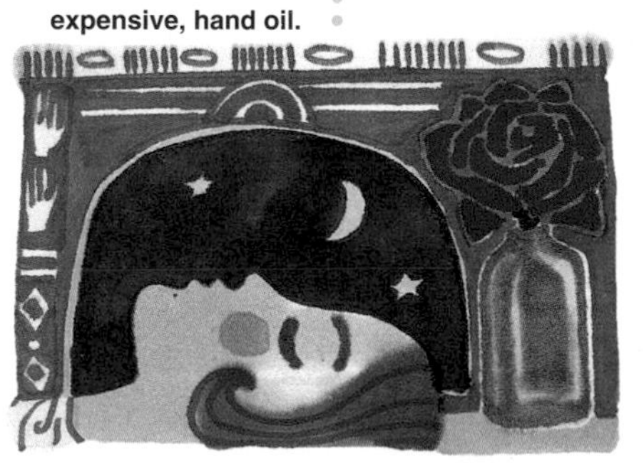

ESSENTIAL OILS AND PREGNANCY

Don't use essential oils in the first three months of pregnancy, to be on the safe side. A few oils are not recommended during any stage of pregnancy: for example, pennyroyal, wintergreen and sage. With a handful of others there is a low risk of inducing abortion, for example, basil, hyssop, marjoram, thyme, myrrh, rue, thurja, tansy, sassafras and mugwort. But after that initial three months, rubbing the tummy with 20 drops of lavender and 5 drops of neroli diluted in 50ml of a nourishing oil like sweet almond oil will help prevent stretch marks. Continue after the birth.

Babies have very delicate skin and essential oils are not recommended for them, though a very small amount of rose oil may be diluted in massage oil for the very young. Lavender, geranium and camomile are also gentle and effective for children. Use half or less of the normal amount diluted in massage oil, or in the bath for toddlers and older children.

SPECIALISED USES

THE EROTIC NARCOTIC

Essential oils that make you ready for love are often those that contain phytohormones or plant hormones, like clary sage, ylang-ylang and geranium. Rose, as we saw in the chapter on Smell, contains PEA, a chemical the body releases after sex that is known as "essence of post-coital bliss". Jasmine contains indole at the heart of its floweriness, a taint of flesh. Sandalwood is one of the best aphrodisiac oils, applied in a massage. It contains steroid molecules similar to testosterone, which drives libido in both men and women. It has long been used to stimulate desire. Oils that warm the skin are also considered sexually stimulating. "To lust as you please," wrote Caterina Sforza in her 15th century book *Experimenta*, "use white and black pepper and galangal."

In the sacred Hindu practice of Tantric sex, the object is to attain a higher plane of consciousness that brings union with God. In preparation, the woman's body is anointed in "the rite of the five essentials" to symbolise her role as the goddess Shakti and arouse all five senses. Jasmine is stroked into her hands, patchouli on her cheeks and her neck, spikenard is combed into her hair, and amber rubbed on her nipples. Saffron is applied to her feet, sandalwood to her inner thighs, and musk to her pubis. She is ready for love. Modern romantics can use essential oils with similar creativity, rubbing different oils into different parts, so that the whole body is constantly and variously stimulating to the nose.

Foot Bath for Tired Feet: fill a foot tub or bowl. Add 5 drops juniper berry oil, 3 drops rosemary oil, 2 drops lavender oil. Soak feet for 10 minutes.

ONE TO TRY AT HOME

The rule for aromatic aphrodisiacs is simple: use the ones you and your partner like. There will be a further interesting pay-off. Because of the connection between fragrance and memory, if you use a particular oil or blend of oils when you make love, your brain will come to associate that smell with sex. When you smell the oil in the future, it will powerfully trigger the memory and your body will begin to prepare itself for love, quickening your sexual responses.

- Oils of patchouli, frankincense and sandalwood are all known as aphrodisiacs.
- Ylang-ylang, a narcotically delicious essential oil from the Philippines, has a reputation for helping frigidity and impotence and, with its phytohormones, is also a natural euphoric. But it has a penetrating perfume; too much of it can bring on a headache.
- Vetiver is an earthy sexual stimulant good for both sexes, though women often find it especially alluring on men. Also known as "the oil of tranquillity", vetiver may help to calm any concerns about performance.
- Lavender's reputation as an anxiety soother might also be a help in this department.
- Neroli is one of the best sedative/antidepressant oils. Blend with geranium to create a receptive, warm mood.

CHASTITY SCENTS

Just as there are essential oils which will arouse ardour, so there are others reputed to cool it. These are probably not much use nowadays, unless you are going on a long trip away from the one you love. Even better, leave some behind for your lover to be sniffed daily while you are away. In previous centuries, chastity scents were particularly useful in monasteries. Essential oil of marjoram was considered a true passion killer, whatever its other benefits. Oils, especially those with a cool smell and businesslike antiseptic properties, were found to take the mind off the body: camphor, bay, saxifrage, niaouli (not the same as neroli) were all used in Eastern religions especially. Eucalyptus, lavender and rosemary were the Western equivalents.

MOOD KILLER

Above all, monks round the Mediterranean region treated themselves with applications from a tree called *Vitex agnus-castus* or the "chaste tree", a vervain plant that has a camphor-like smell. Chaste tree seeds stuffed into "neck girdles" or sachets immediately killed any unwitting influx of lust caused by the proximity of a beautiful woman. The pouch was raised to the nose and sniffed fervently for a minute or so. The Greek physician Galen recommended scattering chaste tree seeds under a wife's bed to keep her faithful. Coptic monks in Egypt still use meriandra leaves, which also have a camphor smell, to guard their chastity.

TOO MUCH OF A GOOD THING?

It should be emphasised here that an aphrodisiac fragrance will turn anaphrodisiac if used to excess. The Empress Josephine's inordinate love of musk, for example, sometimes worked against her. She went to the point of impregnating her boudoir's wallpaper with this throbbing odour. Having overdone it in preparation for Napoleon's return from battle on one occasion, she succeeded only in giving him a blinding headache - and the opportunity to deliver the legendary line: "Not tonight, Josephine." Napoleon immediately had the walls doused in lime and blanketed Josephine with his own favourite perfume, that of violets, which he later had planted on her grave.

The Sumerians lived between 4000 and 2000 BC. Somewhere during that time, one of them sent another a love gift, a vase of perfume, accompanied by a tablet engraved with the rubric: "This little vase contains 100 rose petals from my garden, but each petal expresses a thought of love for you." A hallmark message in the making from 6,000 years ago? Whatever the sentiment, the connection between eroticism and the rose was already established.

AROMATIC ENVIRONMENTALISM

Juniper, bay and lemon are tonics for the respiratory system and refresh the brain. Native Americans take steam baths of bay to clear the head, tone muscles and improve breathing

***Steam Facial for Normal Skin:* add 4 drops each of oils of lavender, geranium and bergamot to a bowl of hot water. Cover head, lean over bowl and steam face.**

Doctors at an American hospital found that when patients underwent a stressful test (Resonance Imaging) where they had to lie still in a claustrophobic tunnel for some time, spraying the tunnel with heliotrope proved more calming than giving them valium. In Japan, a major corporation is experimenting with "aromatherapeutic environmental fragrancing." Essential oils are dispersed into the air through the air conditioning to enhance not only the mood but the performance of workers in offices and factories. Conference room air conditioners emit lemon, jasmine and mint to improve alertness; reception areas release rose and camomile to soothe stress. The oils can be programmed to change throughout the day like modern-day incense clocks, releasing fresh aromas in the morning, siesta-zapping ones in the afternoon and relaxing oils after five o'clock.

AN EXCITING FUTURE

Some scientists are sceptical of the essential oil studies, saying that people will always respond positively to any fragrance they like, and that the impressive results of the Japanese experiments are due to this, not to specific properties of specific oils. But the Japanese remain staunch. In one test they conducted, the Keypunching Room Study, lemon essential oil reduced workers' error rate by 50 per cent, though it also slowed them down: lemon initiates an alert yet relaxed state. For some scientists, the jury is still out. Nevertheless, the idea of being able to inject a stream of anxiety-reducing essential oils like camomile, bergamot and neroli into the atmosphere to bring down the stress levels that contribute so greatly to modern man's ill-health is an exciting one.

"Perfume will always help you along the way of wisdom" was a maxim of the Ancient Chinese writer, Chiang-tse. Certainly, keeping a phial of geranium or rosemary oil on your desk to be sniffed from a tissue when the brain is exhausted or bored is a healthy step towards helping banish fatigue and concentrate the mind. You can also stop work for a few minutes and rub one of the oils onto the temples, nape of the neck, back and palms of the hands and the solar plexus to completely refresh yourself. Rest for a few minutes and then resume work.

And if you need a quick energy boost before a big night out, try putting a few drops of uplifting geranium oil in a hot bath. Then soak for half an hour. Geranium was once regarded as a great healer and was planted around cottages to keep evil spirits away.

A-ROOM-ATHERAPY

The Ancients knew how to shape their environments with fragrance. The Egyptians burned scented oils - a lamp found in the tomb of Kha at Deir el-Medina still contained the remains of fat along with odiferous material. Since remote times, the Japanese have left scented cones to smoulder in bedrooms and built whole rooms of costly and therapeutic cedar so that every breath is cool and easy in summer, and healing and gently antiseptic in winter.

• To alter the atmosphere subtly, sprinkle a few drops of your favourite relaxing or stimulating oils in a bowl of water and place the bowl near the fire or a radiator. Light citrus oils make a refreshing change from chemical air fresheners.

• You can also use an aroma pot. Shake a few drops of undiluted essential oil into the pot and hang it up near the doorway of a room so that the aroma is perceptible as you walk in. The volatile molecules seep out through the terracotta.

• Shake up essential oils in water and spray them through a dispenser - this is useful to fumigate a room that has a bad smell. Try bergamot and eucalyptus. Sprinkle a few drops onto a carpet to combat unpleasant post-party odours.

• Eucalyptus is not only a great stimulant to body, mind and easier breathing. It also makes a great insect repellant. Try it in a dispenser (as above).

• Scent your surroundings as protection against bacteria: add a few drops of peppermint oil to a bowl of warm water and place it on a table away from the window. Or drop them on a piece of damp cotton wool placed on a radiator.

THE BODY SHOP ESSENTIAL OILS

Some essential oils are very powerful, even when diluted to the correct strength. Pregnant women and people with epilepsy should use a small selection of oils with caution. Please refer to our product labels.

REVIVING OILS	HOW TO USE	FREQUENCY	PROPERTIES AND USES
EUCALYPTUS	In bath; forehead, throat and chest massage; inhalation	As often as needed Daily	Cooling and uplifting. Can help clear the head and focus the mind. Good for oily, combination skins.
GERANIUM	In bath; body massage facial massage	Daily	A refreshing oil good for oily skins. An effective insect repellant. Could possibly irritate sensitive skin.
BERGAMOT	In bath; body massage facial massage; inhalation	Daily	A reviving, cooling oil great for summer. Good for oily skin. Effective insect repellant. Could possibily irritate sensitive skin.
ROSEMARY	In bath; body massage forehead and scalp massage; inhalation	As often as needed Daily	Helps clear the head and revive the body. Has a toning and astringent effect on skin. Can help condition dry, flaky scalps.
JUNIPER BERRY	In bath; body massage scalp massage; inhalation	Daily	Wakes up a tired body and mind. Great as a scalp tonic. Gives your spirits a lift.

RELAXING OILS	HOW TO USE	FREQUENCY	PROPERTIES AND USES
CAMOMILE	In bath; body massage facial massage	As often as needed Daily. Nightly	Good for dry, sensitive skin. Very soothing, especially for children. Helps relax the body at night
NEROLI	In bath; body massage facial massage; inhalation	As often as needed Daily. Nightly	Relaxing and soothing, helps to unwind after a stressful day. Helps condition dry and sensitive skin.
YLANG-YLANG	In bath; body massage scalp massage	Daily. Nightly	Has a relaxing and soothing effect on the emotions. Skin softening for both oily and dry skin. Good tonic for the scalp. Said to contain aphrodisiac qualities!
LAVENDER	In bath; body massage facial massage	As often as needed Daily. Nightly	A versatile oil that is valuable for most skin conditions. Can help you gain a good night's rest. Great after sunbathing to soothe over-exposed skin. (Just add a few drops to your bath)
ROSE	In bath; body massage facial massage	As often as needed Daily. Nightly	Moisturising for dry, sensitive or mature skin. Has a soothing effect on the emotions and can help promote easier sleeping. It has a wonderful fragrance and can be worn as a perfume.

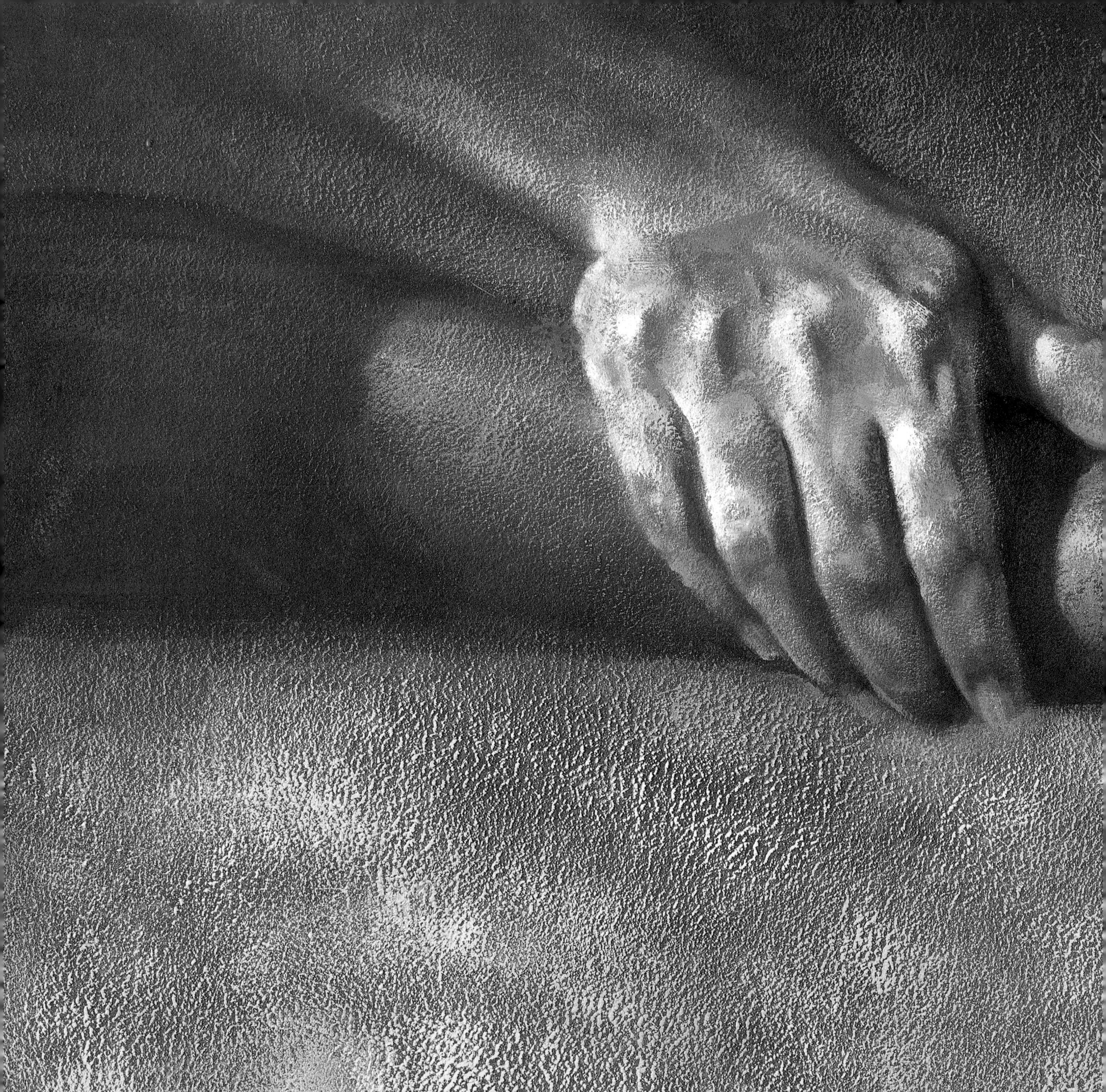

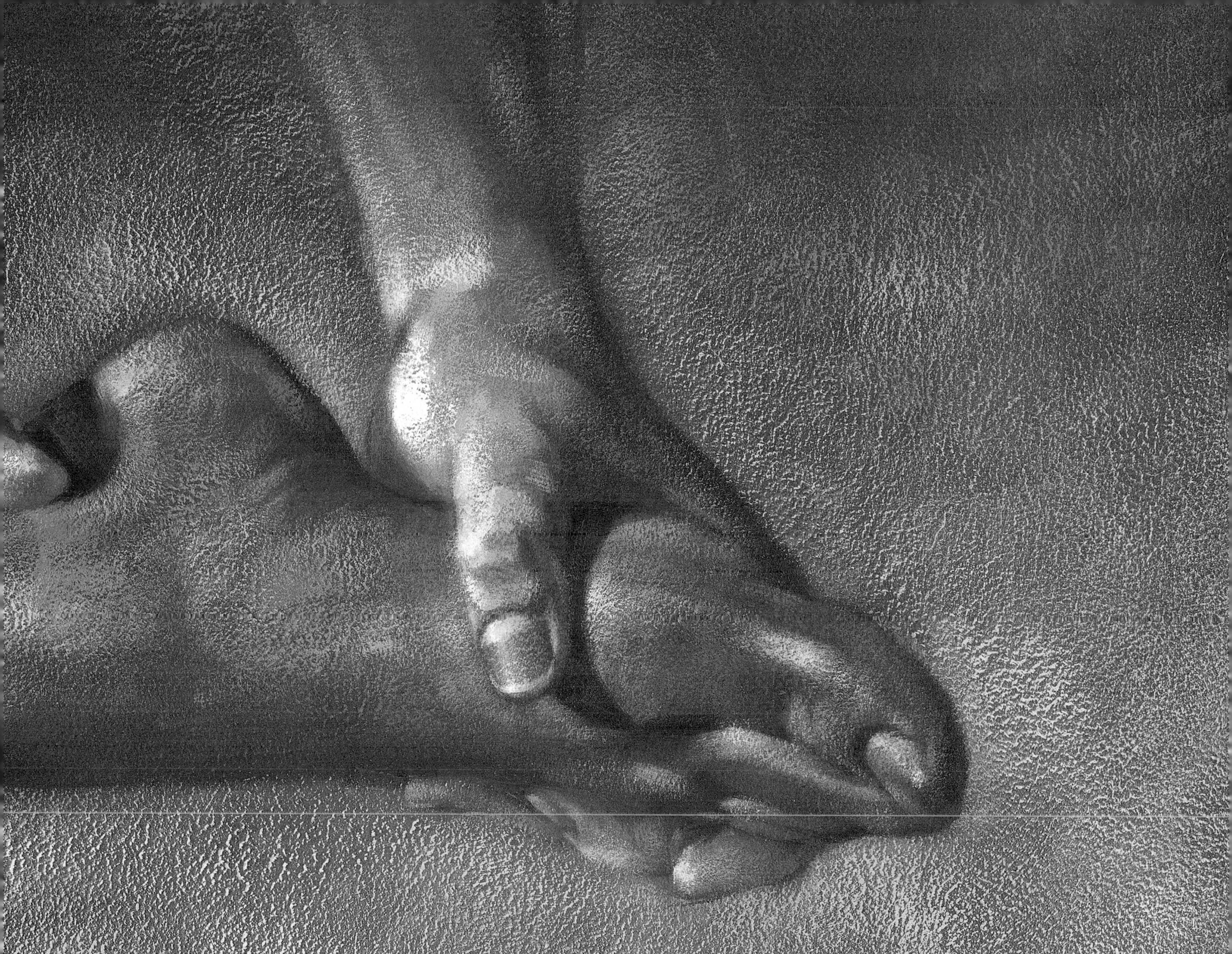

MASSAGE

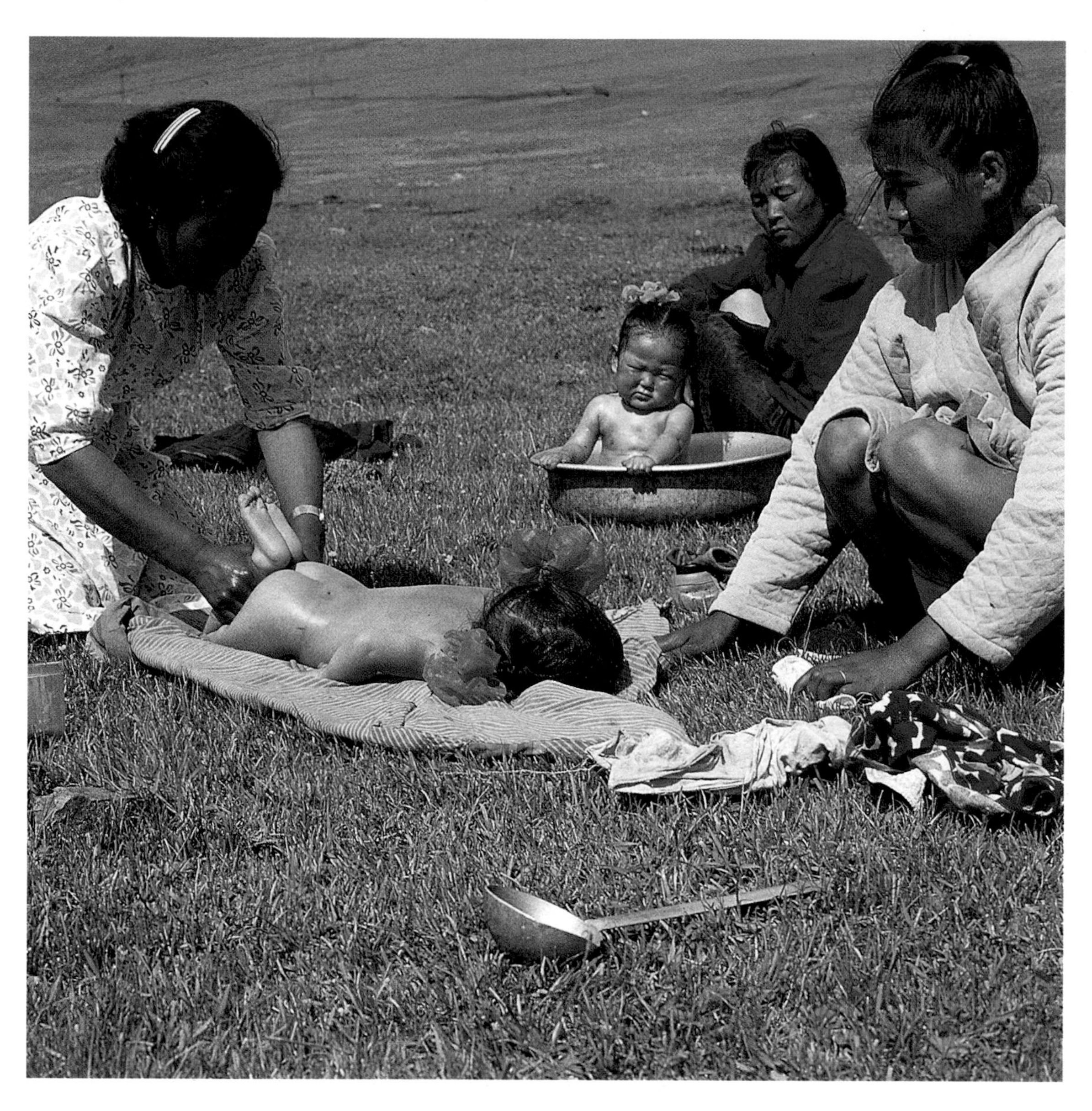

Mongolia is just one Asian country where massage is used to help bring sickly children back to health.

massage

Nineteen months after she was born in 1880, Helen Keller contracted a disease that left her deaf, dumb and blind. Her world was formed out of two neglected senses: smell and touch. "Touch brings the blind many sweet certainties which our more fortunate fellows miss, because their sense of touch is uncultivated," she wrote. "When they look at things, they put their hands in their pockets. No doubt that is one reason why their knowledge is so often vague, inaccurate and useless."

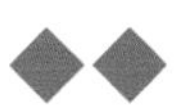

We know we need food and shelter to survive. But most of us don't realise that touch is as important. It is a biological necessity as well as a physical pleasure. Regular massage is one way to put us back in touch with our bodies and the bodies of those around us.

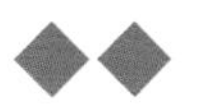

Recently, cognitive psychologists have come to question the linear, one-dimensional type of intelligence that our outlook is based upon, agreeing with Helen Keller that downplaying the sense of touch limits the richness of our perception. Logico-mathematical intelligence, the standard by which all intelligence is measured in the West is, after all, not the only kind, but simply one intelligence among many. What about the musical intelligence of the composer, the bodily-kinetic intelligence of the dancer, or the bodily-intuitive intelligence of the massage healer? Why is one superior to another? Psychologists are now arguing that by changing our sense bias away from the vision dominated towards the touch orientated we could reconcile mind and body and overcome many of the psychoses that are part of modern urban living.

Once, we didn't think of mind and body as separate entities. We were our bodies. The medieval church preached that the body was a microcosm of the universe and therefore sacred. Autopsies were forbidden because they breached this sacred wholeness and doctors had to rely on grave robbers to bring them dead bodies for dissection, under pain of excommunication.

In many societies, the holistic philosophy still holds true. In tribal cultures, the individual feels his body to be part of a greater organism - the social body of the tribe. Among the Nyinban of Northwestern Nepal, for example, an entire community will take turns at regularly massaging an expectant mother. They do this because they believe that an anxious mother is bad for the health of the village as a whole.

Western thought, however, has led us to see ourselves as superior minds incarnated - if not incarcerated - in inferior bodies. The resulting mind/body split has led to the isolation and alienation that characterise post-industrial Western society. We have lost the tribal sense of belonging. And because we don't consider our bodies to be the "real" us, we yield responsibility for them to "expert" others.

Other cultures have their own traditions of healing touch too. In Mexico, Zinacanteco shamans hug patients to help them recover the lost part of the soul, "to get in touch with it".

This is particularly evident in the field of medicine. When we are ill, we invest our doctors with complete responsibility to heal us. In a shaman-led tribal society, by contrast, it is the patient who must assume responsibility for getting well. The concern of the shaman, or priest-doctor, is health in the broadest sense. He heals your body, because in so doing he heals the tribe, the greater body of which yours is a part. Our doctors simply prescribe a remedy for a given ill, but a shaman gives a diagnosis that aims to tell someone in social and spiritual terms why they originally became sick.

The problem of the mind/body divide is an absorbing one for modern philosophers, sociologists and psychologists. But one down-to-earth solution presents itself literally close at hand. Massage reawakens our bodily awareness. Whether we are massaging or being massaged, it puts us back in touch with our bodies and the bodies of others around us. Massage is a powerful tool which will help us discover non-sexual bodily intimacy, and so re-integrate our senses.

MASSAGE: THE NURTURING TOUCH

"Touch is a language that can communicate more love in five seconds than five minutes of carefully chosen words," writes Phyllis K. Davis in her book on touch therapy *The Power of Touch*. She puts forward an excellent case for increasing the amount of touch in families. Too many years of pop psychology and disturbing cases of child abuse have pushed us deeper into fear of touch. Compare this to India where a young girl will come home from school and give her uncle a caring massage. Perhaps it's the Christian tradition which has fostered a fear of bodily pleasure. Since touch can bring pleasure as well as comfort it became tarnished with sin. But Davis points out that, normally, we can all tell immediately if a touch is nurturing and healing, or if it is sexual.

Other societies value touch more than we do. Among the Wolof of Senegal, when a visitor is received into the family compound, he or she is handed a baby, often before a single word is exchanged. The intention is for the baby to mediate the relationship between the adults, expressed with the potent gesture of touch. Touching is the medium of companionship between them, regardless of gender, and is used with the same unaffectedness as verbal communication in Western society.

Touch is something that is, sadly, nearly always denied the old. They quite literally lose touch. But we must not let that happen. The elderly need to be held, hugged and massaged as much as the rest of us.

A HANDS-ON PAST

Touch has always been linked with healing. Cave paintings from 15,000 years ago show the healing touch in action. Christ is said to have healed with a touch. This practice, known as the laying on of hands, is still used today by faith healers. Ancient Chinese, Indian and Egyptian manuscripts contain numerous references to massage as a therapy for preventing illness and promoting healing. Massage is a central part of the Ayurvedic system of medicine, which dates back to 1800 BC and is still thriving in India. In the oldest known medical treatise, written in China in about 2700 BC, the following advice appears:

"Early morning stroking with the palm of the hand, after the night's sleep, when the blood is rested and the tempers relaxed, protects against colds, keeps the organs supple and prevents minor ailments."

The Ancient Greeks and Romans were great fans of massage. The daily routine of the Greeks always included a visit to the gymnasium, for social intercourse as much as a workout. After exercise, they were rubbed down with oil, which was then scraped off with a special instrument. Greek physicians prescribed massage as a cure for melancholia (depression), asthma, digestive problems and sterility. Galen, the Greek doctor to the Roman emperors in the second century AD, wrote 16 books about massage and exercise. And Julius Caesar was massaged daily to relieve neuralgia.

MASSAGE MEDICINE

Research shows that the healing power of touch may be connected with the key part it plays in forming attachment bonds and associated feelings of pleasure and good health in childhood. At the University of Maryland Medical School and the University of

Pennsylvania School of Medicine, doctors have discovered that the heart beat of patients who are touched and whose hands are held changes for the better. This is true even when they are in a deep coma or paralysed.

Massage seems to work on that part of us where mind, body and spirit connect. It is a holistic form of healing. The nurturing aspect of touch is as important a part of the therapy as the physical benefits of stroking the muscles and stimulating the circulation. Our bodies are more deeply integrated with our minds than Western schools of thought have allowed us to believe. Massage is now beginning to be used in hospitals because of its power to help patients recover. This is a return to what was normal practice in the 19th century when doctors still took the time to massage patients as part of their treatment.

> ***Do you know how to relax? The de-stressing effects of a good massage can give us a valuable glimpse of what it really means to unwind.***

"HIGH TOUCH"

In this century, as the obsession with technology grew, massage was lost as a medically valued treatment. But as "high tech" crept into every aspect of our daily lives, it was inevitable that "high touch" would enjoy a renaissance as a reaction. And science can back up what many of us instinctively know: massage helps heal.

Dolores Krieger, a professor of nursing at New York University, has pioneered a method in hospitals known as Therapeutic Touch. This is a development of the laying on of hands, using the hands to direct human healing energies. Krieger has come up with hard evidence to support her claims for touch's healing powers. Tests have shown that it has a positive effect on haemoglobin (which delivers oxygen to tissues) and on brain waves.

Besides, if we accept the premise that anything up to 90 per cent of all illnesses may be stress related, then any method of relieving stress as effectively as massage does is guaranteed to improve our general condition. Like a natural antidepressant, massage can soothe and uplift the mind at the same time. This effect can be greatly enhanced by the use of aromatherapy oils (see Aromatherapy chapter). It triggers metabolic and chemical changes in the body that promote healing. Pleasurable tactile stimulation releases endorphins, natural body hormones that control pain and enhance our sense of well-being.

In 1983, a study of psychiatric patients in West Lothian in Scotland proved that 30-45 minutes of massage a day were more effective than large doses of drugs in alleviating chronic tension and anxiety and associated muscular pain. Three out of five of the patients stopped taking drugs for these symptoms after receiving massage.

TOUCH - A BARE NECESSITY

Each of us is born with two hungers: food hunger and what scientists are now calling skin hunger. Touch is the first sense to develop inside the womb. A foetus' skin can sense touch at just nine weeks. During its nine months inside the mother, it is constantly rocked and massaged by her body. At birth, it is deprived of this constant reassuring contact.

Until the 1930s, the death rate for babies under one year old in American foundling hospitals was nearly 100 per cent. They died from a condition known as marasmus, from the Greek for wasting away. Then a Dr Fritz Talbot visited a children's clinic in Germany where he saw a fat old lady shuffling around with babies clinging to every part of her. The clinic director explained to him that if a baby still didn't improve after they had done everything they could medically do for it, it was handed over to Old Ana. She simply carried the babies around with her. They always thrived. When Talbot returned to America, he introduced the idea of mothering into foundling institutions. The infant death rate instantly decreased.

What Talbot had discovered was the importance of touch. Recent studies have shown that a premature baby which is massaged for 15 minutes three times a day in its incubator gains weight 45 per cent faster than others left alone. The massaged babies don't eat more, their weight gain is due solely to the effect of touch on

At a maternity hospital in Cambridge, England, researchers found that stimulating a premature baby's skin by laying it on a lambswool blanket enabled it to gain an extra 15 grammes a day. This has helped scientists understand the tradition of swaddling a baby, or securely wrapping it in bands of cloth at birth. Swaddling can reassure very young babies by making them feel they are still held in the protection of the womb.

their metabolism. They are also more active and responsive, show more control over their emotions and have fewer health problems. In one experiment, the nervous systems of massaged babies developed more rapidly and they were discharged from hospital an average of six days earlier.

Experiments by one American neurologist proved that licking and grooming by the mother rat is an instinctive massage which stimulates production of the growth hormone in her pup.

START THEM YOUNG

It was once thought that breastfeeding bound mother to child in the primate family to which humans belong. But startling research in the 1950s revealed that touch is a more important factor than food to a baby primate in forming attachment. A researcher studied infant rhesus monkeys who were taken away from their real mothers and each given two wire-frame surrogate mothers. One of the "mothers" provided milk, the other was covered with terrycloth and provided touch. Surprisingly, the baby monkeys bonded with the touching mother, not with the feeding mother. Touching has since been shown to be crucial to the development of normal socialising in humans too.

Anthropological studies of body contact in different cultures have found a correlation between low levels of infant touching and high levels of violence. Societies that don't have a lot of body contact with their children, and prohibit premarital sex also show tendencies such as slavery, castration fears, sexual disabilities and warlike attitudes. Societies who are loving and touching with their children but prohibit premarital sex are non-violent. Societies that have less physical contact in their child-rearing practices, but allow premarital sex are also non-violent. The study seems to indicate that it's never too late to feed the skin hunger people feel as a basic need, though it's clearly preferable to start as young as possible.

A child needs most skin contact in its first year. Research shows that children in America are touched more in their second year than their first, and girls are touched more than boys. What would happen if these biases were to change? If we fed the basic skin hunger babies are born with, would the result be happier, better-integrated children who felt loved, reassured and less inclined to alienation and violence in later life?

Other cultures are streets ahead of us in this respect. We carry our babies home from hospital in baby-carriers rather than wrapping them in a shawl and hugging them to our bodies. Once home, they are exiled to cots, often isolated in another room; when we take them out into the wide world, we send them out ahead of us in push chairs. The touch factor is severely rationed. A Kung! mother in Botswana, by comparison, carries her baby in a curass, a sling that holds it at her side. The infant is in touch with someone at least 90 per cent of the time.

RECIPES FOR BABY CARE

In Morocco, a newborn child is welcomed into the world by hands eager to hold and reassure it. In the first week after birth, the baby is never left alone, for fear a jinni or demon will take it and substitute one of her own children in its place. Everyday, the mother is massaged with henna, walnut bark and kohl to stimulate her recovery. The child is also massaged daily with various concoctions, such as butter mixed with henna, or henna, sugar, alum, marjoram, mint, mastic, water and oil. Whenever the child cries, protective hands reach for it and hold it in the lulling smoke of burning incense.

In India, mothers regularly massage their children, and teach their daughters how to do the same. Among the Zinacanteco of Mexico, embracing is a symbolic action performed by parents and godparents so that the child does not lose its soul. Nyinban children in Nepal are massaged twice a day with mustard seed oil and breast milk until the age of two. Western women may share the same level of maternal devotion, yet they rarely manifest it so diligently. But massage is one of the simplest and most mutually gratifying ways to build a bond between parent and child.

Before you learn to massage your baby, simply try to increase the amount of touch you give it. Hold it naked against your bare chest, covering both of you with a shawl or blanket if it's cold. Many Western babies never experience this most fundamental form of touch with their mothers. Spend time cradling, rocking and gently stroking your child all over.

New parents, uncertain of how and where to touch their newborn baby, can gain enormous confidence by learning the techniques of massage. In time, the movements become intuitive.

AVOCADO

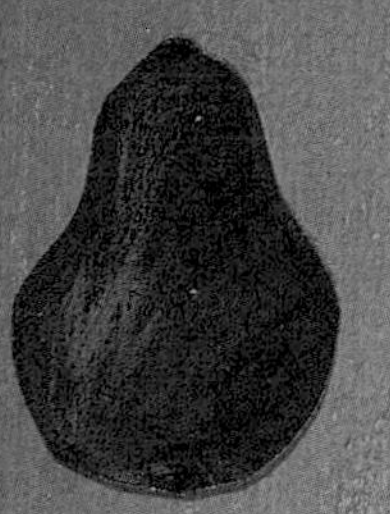

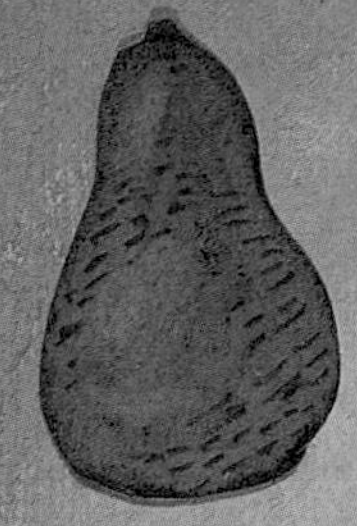

The avocado is an evergreen tree native to the tropical New World. Its green to dark-purple fruit is properly known as an avocado pear because of its shape.

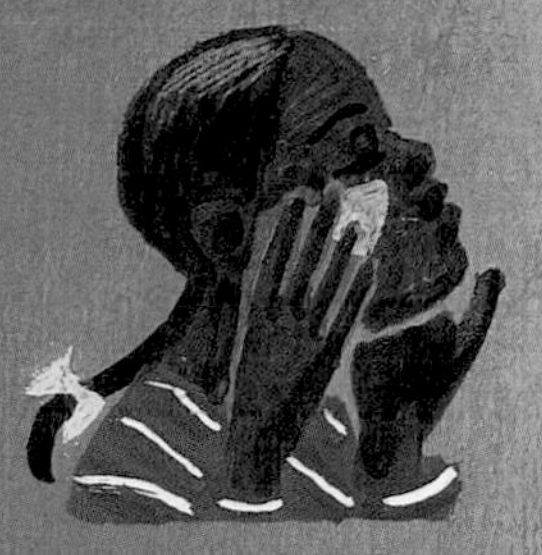

For at least 400 years, South American and Mexican women have used avocado as a moisturiser to protect their skins against the effects of the sun.

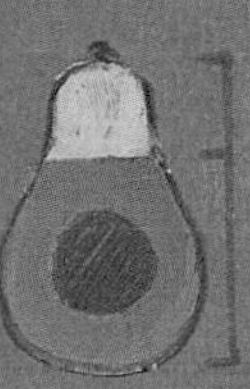

The soft greenish flesh of the avocado is 75 per cent unsaturated fat and up to 25 per cent oil. It is high in vitamins A, B and C and rich in linoleic acid, an essential fatty acid which helps skin to retain moisture. Products formulated with avocado oil are therefore ideal for dry skins.

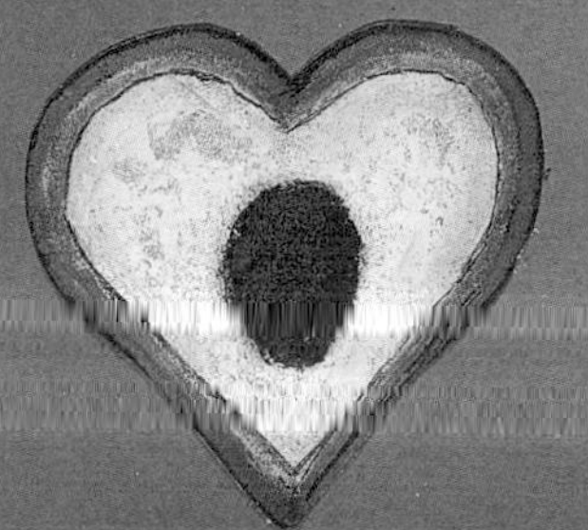

The Aztecs called the avocado love food due to its reputed aphrodisiac properties

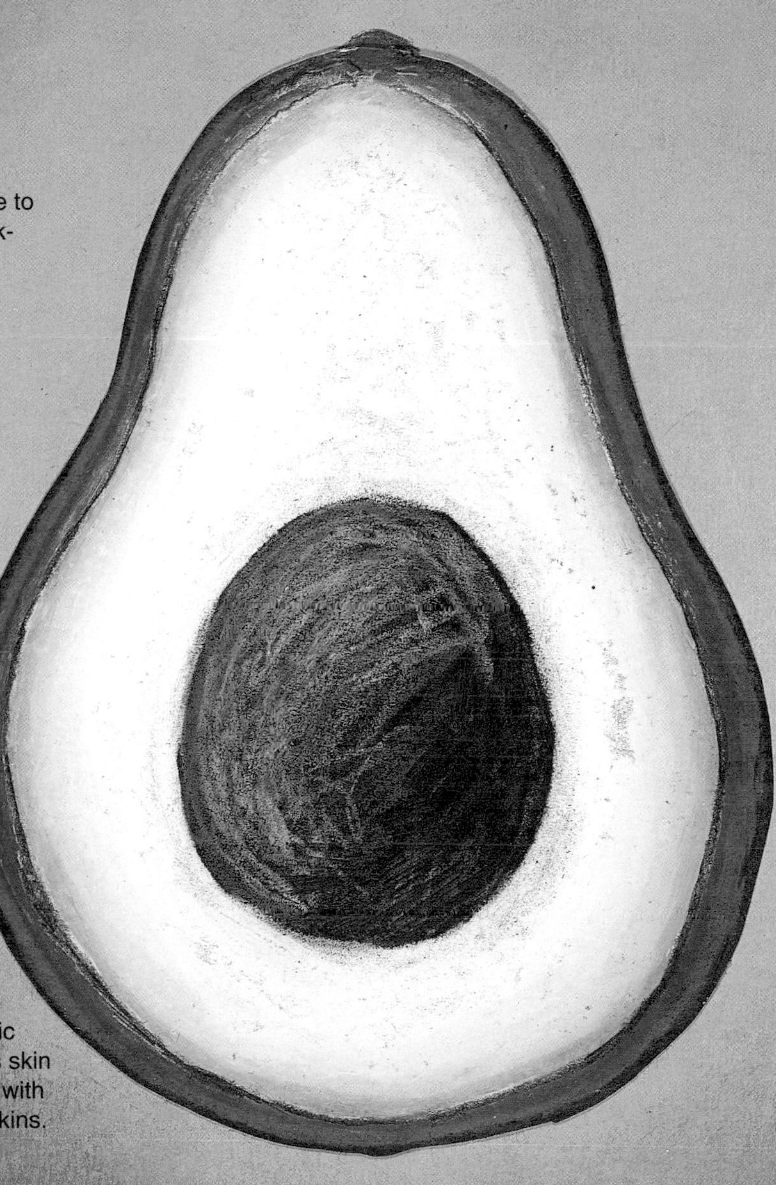

Here's a face mask to try at home:

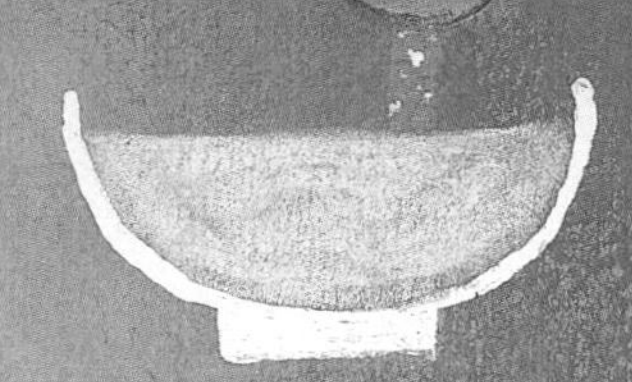

1. Finely pulp half an avocado, then add 2 tbsp almond oil.

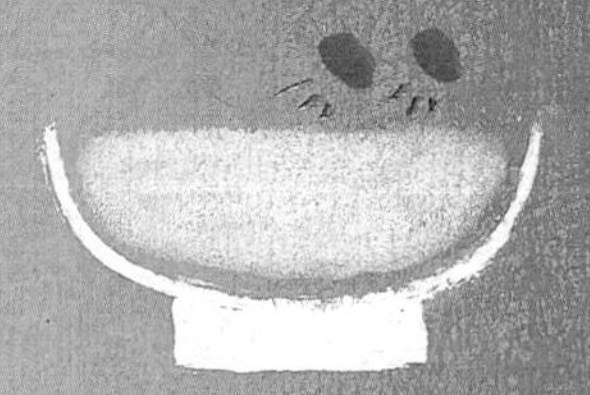

2. Pierce vitamin E capsule and squeeze contents into the avocado mixture.

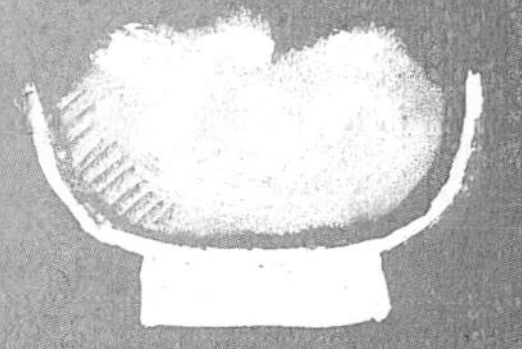

3. Lightly whip 3 tbsp heavy cream and mix thoroughly with the avocado.

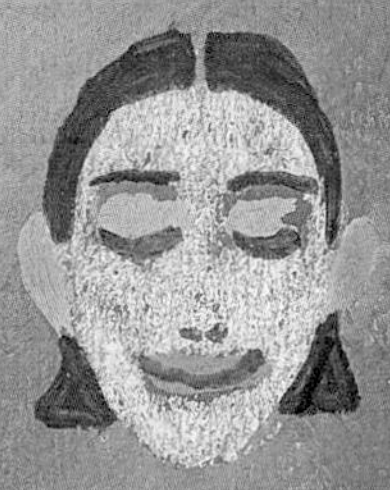

4. Spread the mask over the face, avoiding the eyelids.

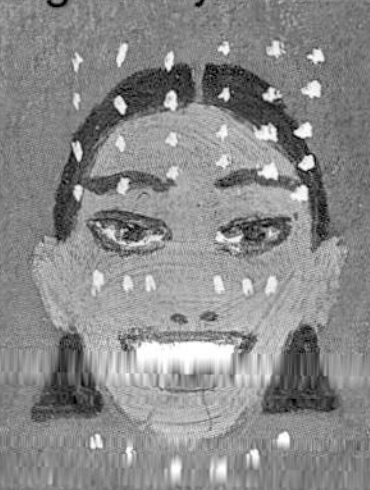

5. Leave on for 10-15 minutes. Rinse off with warm water.

MASSAGING YOUR BABY

• Before you start a massage, make sure you are both warm. A good time to massage a baby is after its bath.

• Wear soft, natural fibre clothes.

• Relax your hands by stretching and shaking them.

• Prepare the baby's skin with a silky coating of baby powder or a very light oil, such as almond.

• The baby can lie on its tummy on the floor, in bed, or lie against your chest as you lean back in a chair.

• Begin by gently stroking your baby's arms, legs, back, tummy and chest. Touch in a light, soothing way.

• Stroke the baby's tummy. Put one hand on each side of the tummy and slide them back and forth - not too firmly - in a criss-cross motion. Now stroke clockwise around the belly button, one hand following the other. Lift one hand over the other arm as you cross to keep the motion smooth.

• Experiment with strokes your baby likes, making sure you use flowing rhythmic movements. Try to make the massage symmetrical - don't just do one leg! Only massage your baby for as long as you both are happy. 10-20 minutes is ideal. Often, a massage before bed will soothe and help it to sleep easily.

Massaging should be exquisitely gentle - a baby of a few weeks needs only a feather-light caress - it is the touching all over that babies love. Be careful around the leg and umbilical cord and never try to extend the legs and arms too firmly.

Russian mothers are taught how to massage their babies in order to stimulate the development of their nervous systems. In California, doctors have ingeniously placed premature babies on mini-waterbeds that rock them like a mother's womb.

The result has been babies who sleep more soundly and are better tempered.

DIFFERENT TYPES OF MASSAGE

Given the healthy, uninhibited attitude of many Oriental cultures towards massage, it's not surprising to discover that modern massage methods have their origins in the East. Shiatsu, for example, has been practised for centuries in Japan. The complicated system, which is built around energy pathways and pressure points, is based on the principles of traditional Chinese acupuncture, but over the years it has been enriched by Western techniques of manipulation, such as osteopathy and chiropractic.

Reflexology, a specialised massage for the hands and feet, is gaining acceptance as a means of diagnosing and treating a variety of minor ills. Paintings discovered on the walls of a physician's tomb in the Valley of the Kings indicate that reflexology, or something very like it, was practised by the ancient Egyptians in 2330 BC. However, it is likely that the method stems from the kind of pressure-point therapy that has been used for thousands of years in the Far East. These are complex techniques which require practice and commitment, but we should not let this deter us from experimenting with natural, untaught methods which can be equally beneficial.

SHIATSU

This is the Japanese interpretation of Chinese acupuncture; it also incorporates the principles of other massage techniques. Most Shiatsu is based on 12 basic Chinese acupuncture meridians; the energy is referred to as chi, and the pressure points, of which there are some 365 over the entire body surface, are called tsubos.

The points easiest to locate lie on either side of the entire length of the spine, along the so-called bladder meridian. Using the "soles" or pads of the thumbs, not the tips, apply firm pressure to the point and hold it for 3-10 seconds before releasing. You will know when you have found a pressure point or tsubo because it will feel slightly tender. Starting at the top of the spine and working downwards, touch on the points between the shoulder blades, to stimulate circulation and help to relieve anxiety, distress and insomnia. The points in the middle-back region are concerned with digestion, those in the lumbar region (lower back) influence the kidneys and help to control water retention. Working down the spine stimulates the spinal nerves which supply all the internal organs, and almost every point on the back influences the supply of energy to the other meridians

Other pressure points, which should be easy to find, run across the tops of the shoulders; working these helps to relieve stress and tensions and soothes headaches and colds. Moving down to the hips, apply pressure to points close to the "sacral dips" or dimples on either side of the spine; this is especially soothing and relaxing for women, and helps to relieve period pains. The bladder meridian continues down the back of the legs. Pressing the points at

REFLEXOLOGY

This increasingly popular alternative treatment is based on the concept that the body is divided into ten zones of energy which can be manipulated to prevent or treat physical and mental problems. Taking the foot as a paradigm of the whole body the reflexologist massages reflex points on the feet which correspond to internal organs elsewhere in the body. The idea is to stimulate these organs so they function healthily, clearing any energy blockages and helping the body relax along the way. The massage itself may be gentle or deep, depending on what degree of blockage the reflexologist finds.

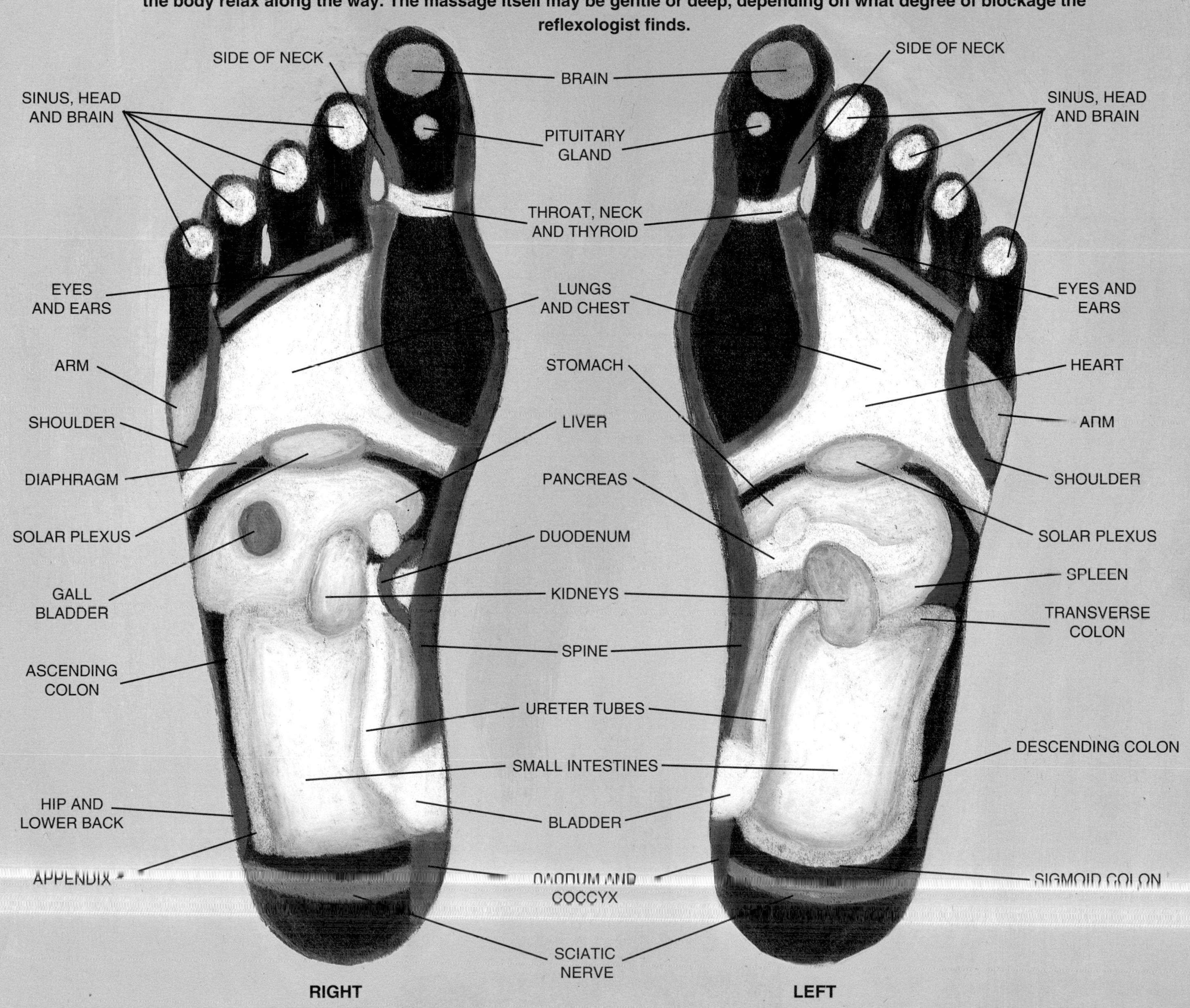

PALMISTRY

Soothsayers and mystics look at our hands to determine individual characteristics and map out our lives. Palmistry is about more than the lines that crisscross both our palms. It also calls for an analysis of the shape of the whole hand, including fingers and joints and the state of the nails. But for the purposes of this diagram, we're simply offering you an introduction to the main junctions of the hand and what they can represent.

LINE OF HEAD
LINE OF HEART
LINE OF FATE
LINE OF THE SUN
AFFECTION LINES
LINE OF LIFE
TRAVEL LINES

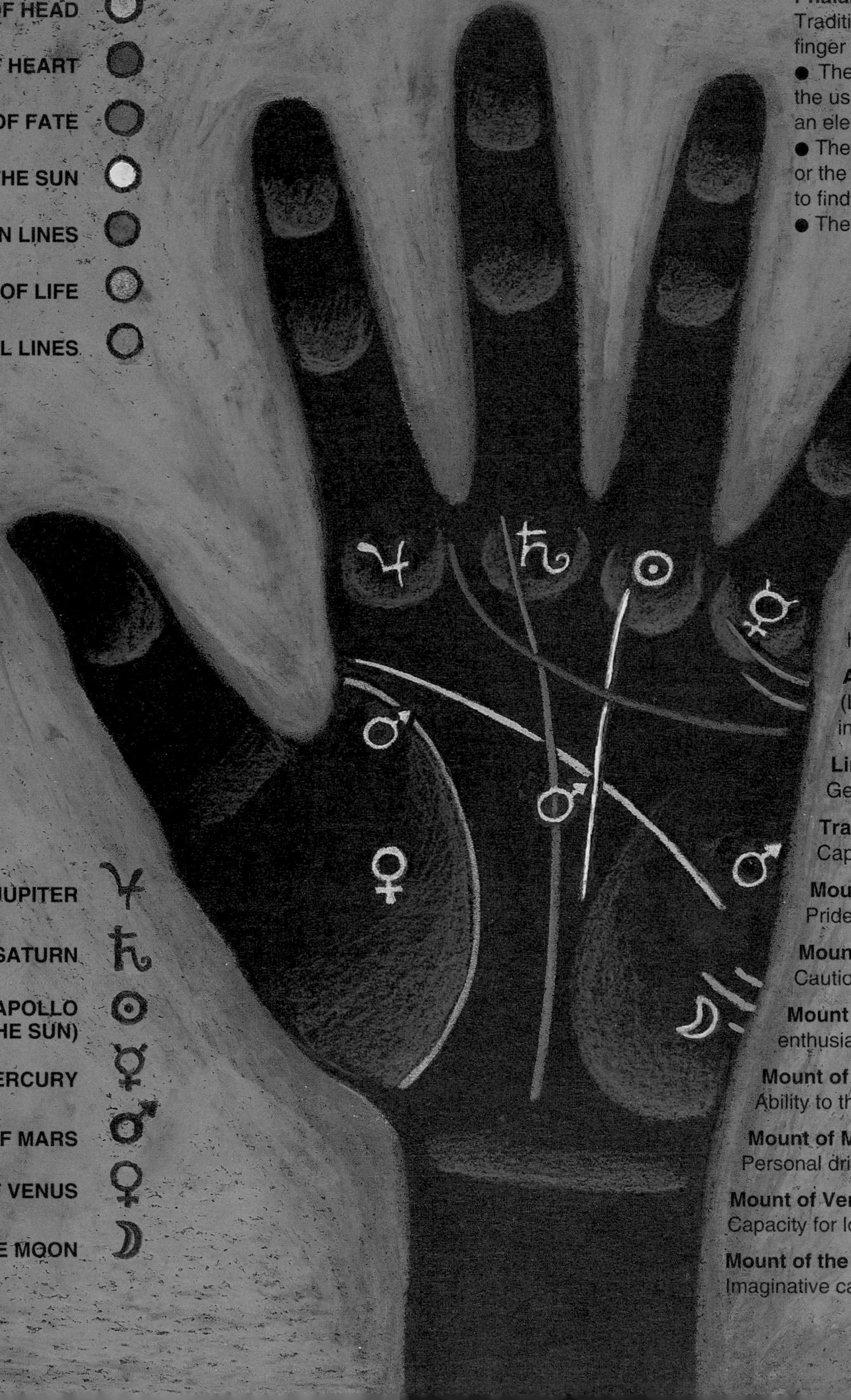

MOUNT OF JUPITER ♃
MOUNT OF SATURN ♄
MOUNT OF APOLLO (MOUNT OF THE SUN) ☉
MOUNT OF MERCURY ☿
MOUNT OF MARS ♂
MOUNT OF VENUS ♀
MOUNT OF THE MOON ☽

Phalanges
Tradition has it that the three phalanges of each finger represent the Three Worlds:

- The first (higher) phalange stands for Soul, or the use of one's intellectual capabilities to achieve an elevated state.
- The second (middle) phalange represents Mind, or the practical application of one's mental abilities to find constructive solutions to life.
- The third (lower) phalange stands for Body, or material interests geared towards immediate gain.

Line of Head
Intelligence, reasoning concentration, memory

Line of Heart
Emotional state, physical conditions dependent on the heart

Line of Fate
(Line of Saturn) How chance affects your life and career

Line of the Sun
(Line of Apollo) Potential for success and happiness based on a personal talent

Affection Lines
(Lines of Marriage) Close relationships, including family

Line of Life
General health and vitality

Travel Lines
Capacity for enjoyment of travel or exploration

Mount of Jupiter
Pride, ambition and leadership abilities

Mount of Saturn
Caution, reticence, love of solitude

Mount of Apollo (Mount of the Sun) Artistry, enthusiasm

Mount of Mercury
Ability to think quickly especially in career matters

Mount of Mars
Personal drive, persistence, ability to endure

Mount of Venus
Capacity for love and affection

Mount of the Moon
Imaginative capabilities

the back of the knees can relieve emotional strain and release tension in the knees.

Six different meridians run the length of the arms. By working the points at the top of the arm and in the crease of the elbow, you can encourage the elimination of body wastes, which is helpful for treating blemished skins, and also improves circulation, respiration and digestion.

REFLEXOLOGY

The precise origins of reflexology are unknown. It is a type of pressure-point massage for the hands and feet which probably evolved from a massage technique practised thousands of years ago in China. For the purposes of reflexology, the body is divided into ten different zones, five on each half of the body. Any organ, gland or part of the body occurring within a particular zone will have its reflex in the corresponding zone of the hand and foot. If an area of the hand or foot feels particularly tender, the pain, to a trained reflexologist, will indicate tension or congestion in some part of the body which lies within the same zone. The theory is that by working a point on the hand or the foot that corresponds to a certain part of the body, such as the eye, liver or stomach, its function can be affected.

A thorough hand and foot massage is a marvellous way of reviving anyone who is tired or jaded. Such massage will also work to release congestion in the body resulting from stress, bad diet, lack of sleep, an alcoholic evening, etc. Reflexologists claim that they can treat ailing organs and glands by working the feet and hands, and at the same time discover which parts of the body are not functioning as efficiently as they might be. You can use reflexology as an antidote for many everyday problems. It is not necessary to incorporate it in a full body massage; simply work the particular reflex points for 30 seconds or so, two or three times a day or whenever the need arises.

WHY MASSAGE?

THE BENEFITS OF HAVING A MASSAGE

The overwhelming benefit of being massaged is that it reduces stress, which is a root cause in up to 90 per cent of all diseases. This makes it excellent preventive medicine. In addition, massage:

- boosts circulation.
- stimulates the lymphatic drainage system. Lymph is the medium in which toxins are drained from the body and runs in its own channels. It relies on muscle contraction in order to flow along, and this is helped by massage.
- improves your performance in most athletic activities and helps soothe aching muscles afterwards by speeding up the elimination of lactic acid build-up.
- increases body energy and well-being.
- feeds skin hunger, getting us back in touch with our bodies.
- soothes muscles and undoes knots of physical tension stored in places like shoulders and neck.
- helps release emotional tensions along with physical tensions.
- can speed the healing of tissue. It's particularly useful in this way for a mother after birth, when tissue is slack.
- can help overcome insomnia.

THE BENEFITS OF GIVING A MASSAGE

If you are giving a massage, don't imagine that all the benefits are flowing one way, from you to the person being massaged. Research has shown that massage is very soothing and calming for the person giving it, and your blood pressure will go down.

There are spiritual benefits too. You are learning to nurture another person, and there's no reason to limit that nurture to your partner in life or your baby. Massage your mother, your sister, your friends, your grandmother. It's a caring gesture that can only benefit you too.

INTUITIVE MASSAGE

There's no mystery to massage. Anyone can do it and everyone should learn. Perhaps the first kind of massage to learn should be intuitive massage, which teaches you to tune into another person's body and their needs without worrying too much about technique. The one rule is not to continue doing anything that hurts.

BEFORE YOU BEGIN

A good time to start is after a bath, before bed. Ideally, your partner should lie on a large table, just below waist height, but the floor will do just as well. Whatever surface you are using, it should be padded with a couple of

In Nigeria, the moment a Bornu baby is born, it is held and stroked by all the birth attendants who first heat their hands over hot coals. How's that compared to being held upside down and slapped on the bottom?

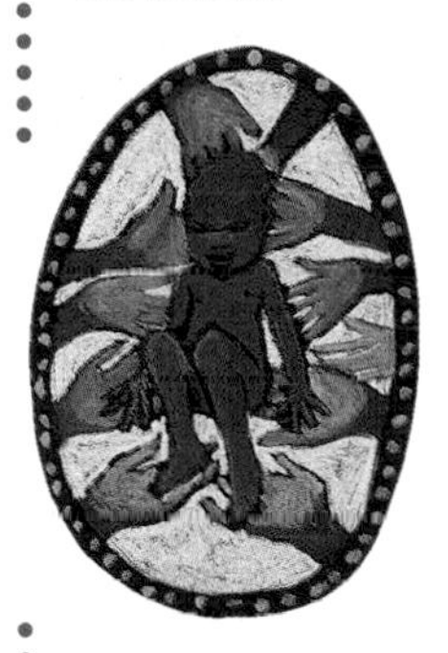

Dr Frederick Leboyer promoted the idea of baby massage in France. His technique was as follows: let your hands slowly travel up the baby's back, one hand following another like waves. One hand begins a stroke as the other ends it. Do this very, very slowly.

HOW DO YOU LIKE TO BE STROKED?

A typical Swedish massage employs several techniques which aim to soothe tension and promote relaxation, boost blood and lymph circulation, improve muscle tone and flexibility of the joints, and to revive flagging energy levels.

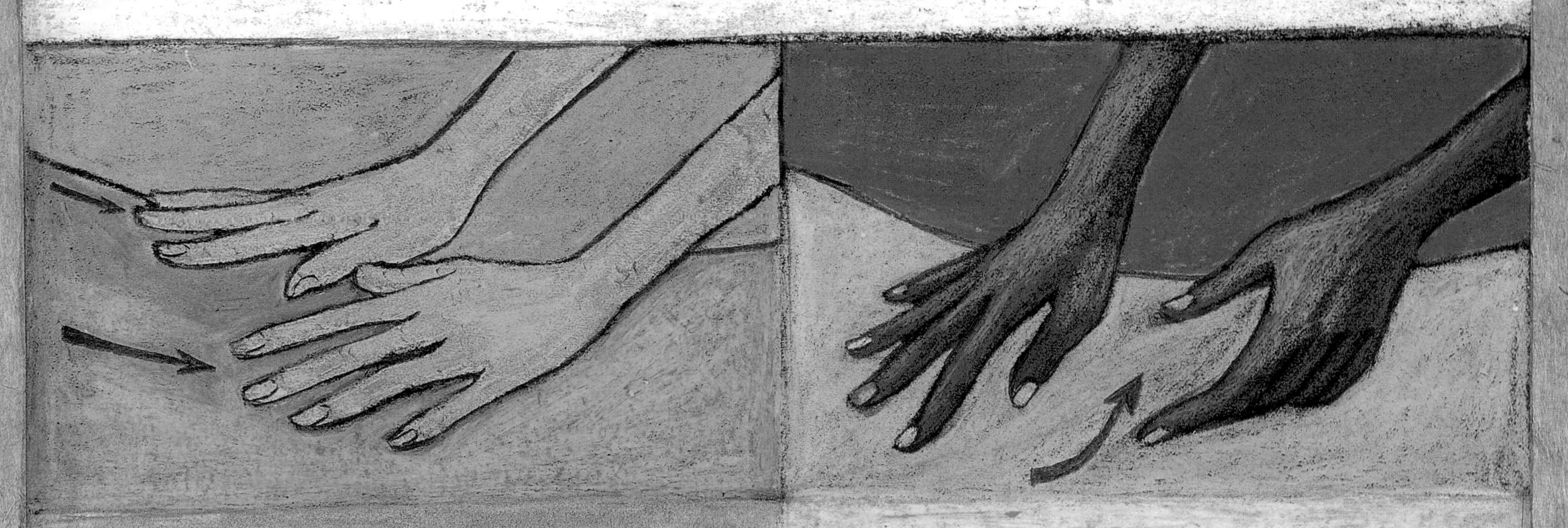

EFFLEURAGE

A long stroking movement which introduces the sensation of touch to the skin. Glide both hands over the skin applying a constant, even pressure on every part of the body. Use slow gentle movements. Effleurage warms and relaxes, while stimulating the blood circulation and lymph flow throughout the body.

TAPOTMENT

Also known as percussion, this is the action usually associated with massage - cupping, slapping and chopping with the hands. Use on the back and along backs of legs. Properly performed, with the wrists loose and flexible, the movements should be fast, invigorating and never painful. Good for improving muscle tone and firming sagging skin.

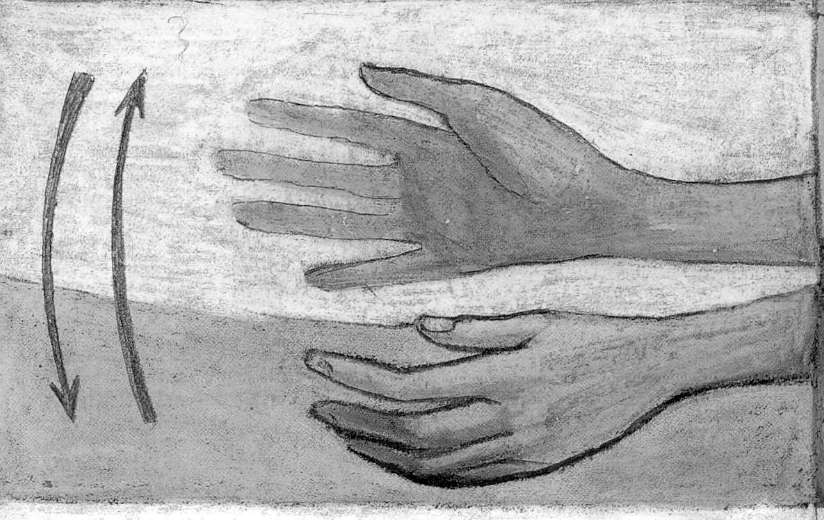

PETRISSAGE

The rhythmic lifting, squeezing and rolling of muscles with the hands. Take hold of the flesh between thumb and fingers and pull the body as well as on the muscles. Use firm movements. Petrissage pumps nutrients through the muscles and drains away wastes while acting on the deeper blood and lymph vessels.

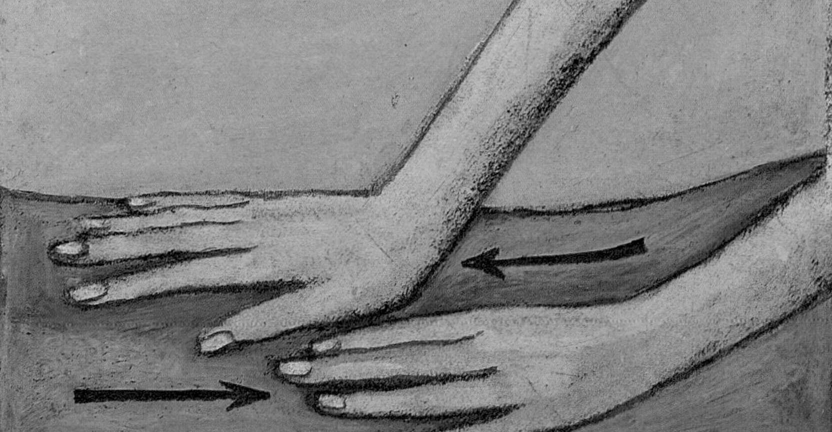

FRICTION

A rapid oscillating movement that is a useful stroke for stiff joints. Place the palms of the hands on the particular area of the body and with even pressure rub them back and forth energetically. Use firm movements. Friction increases the blood supply to internal organs.

blankets for comfort. Don't be tempted to give a massage on a bed; few mattresses provide the necessary support for muscles during a brisk massage.

Make sure the room is warm as the body tenses when it is cold and this is counterproductive. The person giving the massage usually feels much warmer than the one being massaged, so you may want a blanket or a few towels to cover up parts of the body while they are not being massaged. The feet, particularly, may need to be covered. A few small pillows or cushions can be useful. When your partner is lying on his or her back, a small pillow under the hollow of the neck, another under the knees, and possibly another under the ankles can aid relaxation. When your partner is lying on his or her stomach, a lightly-padded pillow under the abdomen may feel comfortable. Low lighting and gentle ambient music are an aid to relaxation.

Centre yourself for the massage with a brief meditation. Here's one: imagine warm golden light being breathed in through the top of your head, and breathed out down through your arms and into your partner. After a few moments, rest your warmed hands on your partner. Spend some time becoming aware of how your partner needs to be stroked. Keeping your eyes shut can sometimes help.

When gliding your hands over your partner's limbs, imagine you are pulling negative energies out of his or her body. Intuitive masseurs shake their hands occasionally during a treatment to get rid of any negative charges they are pulling from the body. At the end of the session, for the same reason, they wash their hands and arms. Afterwards, let your partner lie under a warm blanket and sleep.

MASSAGE BODY PARTS

BACK

- Start from the buttocks and stroke lightly up the back. As the skin warms up, apply firmer pressure.
- Follow with friction, then petrissage. There is little flesh on the back, but you can squeeze and knead the shoulders, hips and buttocks.
- Work the pressure points (see reflexology) down the spine and over the shoulders and hips.
- Follow with tapotment; be gentle on the back, energetic over the buttocks.
- Finish with effleurage.

LEGS

Massage and finish the back of one leg at a time:

- Stroke lightly down the leg and firmly back up to the buttocks to encourage the flow of blood and lymph.
- Use friction on the ankle joint and over the back of the knee.
- The pressure points can be worked now if desired.
- Follow with petrissage and tapotment, and end with stroking down to the foot.
- Work over the whole foot with firm circling thumb movements. Concentrate on the soles where the reflex points lie and try to break down any gritty crystalline deposits.
- Rub the foot briskly.
- Stroke up the leg, over the back to the shoulders, let your hands rest here for a moment, then ask the person to roll over.

ARMS

Massage one arm at a time:

- Holding your partner's hand in your left (or right) hand, stroke lightly from the shoulder to the wrist, then firmly back up to the shoulder, first on the outside, then on the inside of the arm.
- Let go of the arm and follow with petrissage, working up the arm from the wrist. Be gentle on thinly fleshed, sensitive areas, and use both hands to squeeze and knead the flesh of the upper arm.
- Work the pressure points if you like.
- Stroke down the arm and over the hand.
- Massage the hand in the same way as the foot, with particular attention to the palms, using firm circling movements with the thumb. Grasp each finger between thumb and forefinger and pull from the joint to the fingertip working the knuckles as you stroke over them.
- Stroke the whole hand several times.

CHEST AND STOMACH

- Stroke down the neck, then out towards the shoulders. Move from the neck down over the collarbone

• Almond oil can be used for babies and for massaging the face. It was commonly used for massage in Imperial Rome.
• Wheatgerm oil is soothing and good for post-operational scars as it is high in vitamin E.
• Mustard seed oil is most common in the Indian sub-continent and is an excellent all-round massage oil.
• Coconut oil is used in the West Indies.
• In Malaysia, pregnant women massage coconut oil onto their abdomens - they say it helps the baby to descend.

MASSAGING THE SCALP AND HEAD

A scalp massage has a solid physical *and* psychological payoff. The thin layer of muscle which covers the skull tightens when we get tense. This can cause headaches. It also restricts the blood supply to the hair follicles, so they can become under-nourished which affects the condition of the hair. A regular scalp massage will not only alleviate feelings of anxiety, it can also preserve, even improve, the lustre and feel of your hair.

Self-massage is easy - you can do it when you're shampooing. If you are massaging a friend's head, the best position is sitting on a chair with your friend on the floor in front of you leaning against your knees. Are you sitting comfortably?

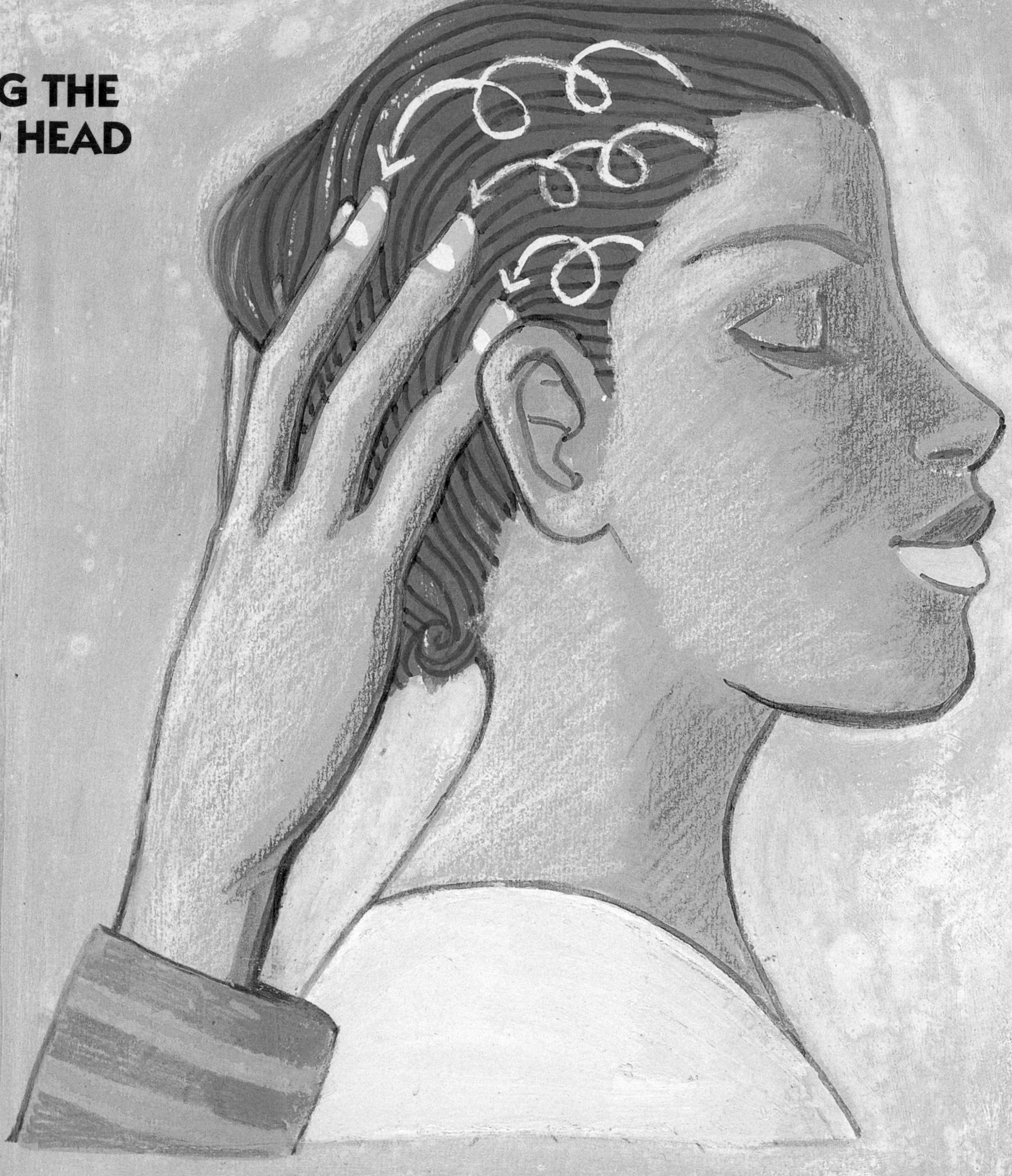

1. Stroke lightly from the forehead, over the top of the head and down to the neck. Repeat, starting from the temple and stroking over the ears. Follow with firmer stroking movements.

2. Using thumbs and fingertips, make small but firm circles all over the scalp. Start at the forehead and work back over the whole head. Pay special attention to the areas around the ears and at the base of the skull, where tension often builds up.

3. Move the skin around as much as possible - this will help relax the scalp muscles.

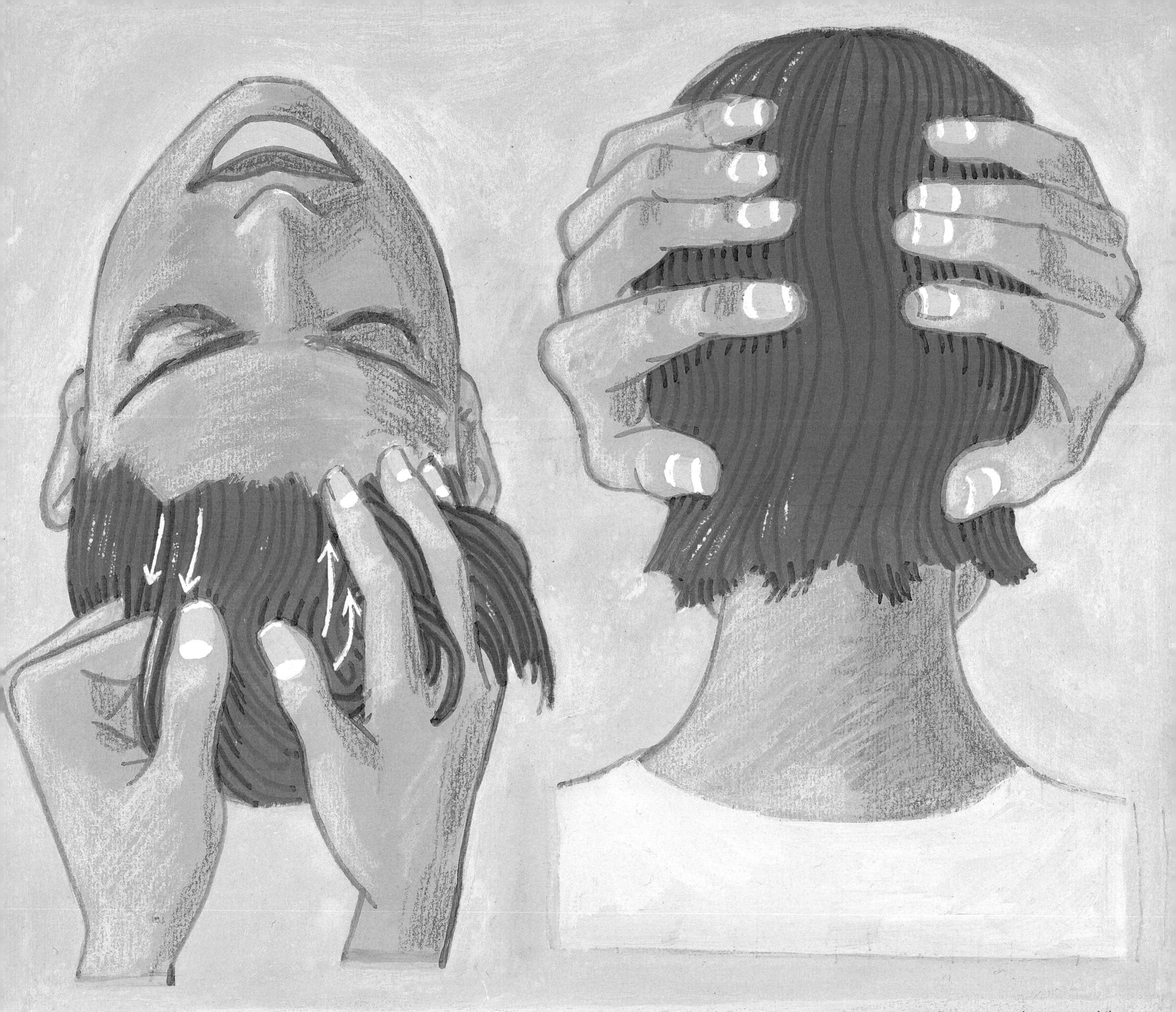

1. Stroke the hair gently, then grab a handful and pull towards you (It won't hurt if you grab it at the roots).
2. Release the hair, then glide your fingers through it.
3. Build a rhythm, pulling with one hand, gliding with the other. It will feel like you are pulling out all the tension.

1. Position your hands on either side of the head, with fingers over the ears and the heels of your hands by the temples.
2. Gently press your hands inwards and hold for a couple of seconds
3. Slowly release pressure, glide hands up the sides of the head and gently off the top.
4. Repeat several times.

to the chest, lightly at first, followed by firmer strokes.

• Follow with friction over the entire chest area if you are very familiar with your friend; otherwise skip the chest and stroke lightly down over the ribs towards the stomach.

• Using the palm of one hand stroke firmly over the abdomen in a clockwise direction several times.

• Follow with petrissage; knead and squeeze the flesh round the waist and hips.

• Stroke slowly and firmly from the stomach up the rib cage; glide back down and repeat several times.

• Finish by gently stroking the whole area.

• Massage the front of the legs in the same way as you did the back of them.

On his voyage in 1779, Captain Cook recorded how his excruciating sciatica was cured when 12 Tahitan women massaged him from head to toe.

FACE AND HEAD MASSAGE

This is an easy massage that everyone will love. Give it to someone who is tired or has a headache. It is also good for an old person who is deprived of skin touch, but may be embarrassed by the idea of a body massage.

• Use a rich moisturising cream or oil. Let the person to be massaged lie down on her back. You can put a small cushion in the hollow at the back of the neck if necessary. Kneel behind her head.

• Begin by pouring some lotion into your hands, then rubbing them vigorously together so that they are warm. Place your hands over the face for a few moments, then draw the hands up and into the hair.

• Start at the throat and sweep up over the chin and jaw area. Move up in slow sweeping motions over the sides of face to the temples, then on to the hairline.

• Now stroke from the centre of the face outwards to the temples.

• Place your hands on either side of the forehead, with fingers pointing in to the centre of the forehead. Draw outwards towards temples with middle fingers, working your way gradually up the forehead towards the hairline. At the end of each stroke, sweep fingers down the side of the face then down the side of the neck. This will promote lymphatic drainage, which relieves headaches.

Massage your scalp for ten minutes twice a day and you should notice a real improvement in the condition of your hair.

• Sweep down to just under the cheekbone and press the heel of your hands in under the cheekbones quite firmly for a few seconds.

• Place index fingers under the jaw and loosen the muscles with short sliding strokes of the thumbs along the jawline. Work from the centre of the chin to the sides of the face.

• Now massage all round the mouth area in small circular motions.

• Pull your hands up over face and draw the hair back once more. Use your fingers to make small circles all over the scalp quite firmly. Now stretch the neck by putting your hands behind the neck and gently pulling the neck towards you keeping the head dead straight on the shoulders.

• Don't forget to massage the ears. In Shiatsu they are considered very important mirrors of the whole body and said to look like an embryo lying upside down in the womb. Rotate them, holding onto the lobes and pulling gently downwards.

• Finish by pressing both hands, one on top of the other, on the forehead and hold pressure for a moment. Release very slowly.

D-I-Y MASSAGE

Most people think of massage as something that is done by others instead of a do-it-yourself performance. It is naturally more relaxing to lie back and let someone else do the hard work, but we can still benefit greatly from massaging ourselves. There are certain areas such as the back that are difficult to work properly, though some massage tools come in handy. In order to reap the full benefits of massage it must be done regularly, like cleaning the teeth, and unless you have a generous partner or friend, that means doing it yourself. Try to find half an hour extra and include massage in your daily routine.

One of the best times to fit in massage is during a shower or a bath. Instead of oil to lubricate the skin, use a fast-foaming liquid soap to reduce the friction between your hands and the skin. Any of The Body Shop's fruit body shampoos are ideal. Use a Body Buddy or Sisal Body Scrub Mitt for effleurage and to slough away dead cells.

After bathing, the skin is warm and the muscles relaxed; this is a perfect time to indulge in petrissage, friction and tapotment, even while watching television. There are other occasions when massage is, if not essential, beneficial and relaxing:

- After a particularly stressful day: it releases tension before this has a chance to manifest itself in the muscles.
- When you are utterly exhausted: it will cleanse the body of the chemicals that cause fatigue; a quick massage is a better and safer pick-me up than a cup of black coffee or a stiff drink.
- Whenever the skin looks puffy; this is a sign that the lymphatic system needs a little boost.
- After a day spent sitting in an aeroplane, train or in the office. It can substitute for the exercise you missed, helping to stimulate the flow of blood and lymph and leave you feeling refreshed and revitalised.
- When feet are tired and aching, soothe them by rolling each one back and forwards on a Footsie Roller - a great way to unwind.

Manual lymph drainage, a gentle massage technique useful in dealing with cellulite, also helps with sports injuries.

CELLULITE AND MASSAGE

Cellulite is a French term given to the fatty deposits which form beneath the skin and result in a lumpy, "orange peel" effect when flesh is pinched.

The condition is influenced by a combination of elements. Overeating and lack of exercise can cause a build-up of excess fat cells. Collagen fibrils, irritated by the accumulation of toxic waste, then wrap themselves around these cells, effectively locking the fat and the toxins away. Other factors, such as sluggish circulation and insufficient drainage of the lymphatic system, can also exacerbate the problem of cellulite.

Massage cannot actually break down the lumpy fat commonly found in the thighs and buttocks, but the manipulation of taut muscles does stimulate the circulation and encourages the mobilisation of lymph fluid. This carries toxic waste to areas of the body where it can be easily removed, helping to speed up cellulite removal.

So, massage can have a beneficial effect on the elimination of cellulite and the slimming process in general. By its very nature, massage heightens bodily awareness, entailing the removal of clothing, and a certain degree of intimacy with a partner from whom it is impossible to hide the shape and condition of one's figure. Working muscles in often neglected areas of the body, massage reminds us to carry ourselves erect, and often improves bad posture. This is a problem for many slimmers, whose low opinion of their own figure can cause slouching, and a general desire to conceal the body with which they are so dissatisfied.

Dieting alone is not sufficient to achieve the permanent removal of cellulite; nevertheless, calorie intake must be lowered in order to mobilise excess fat from the cells. Remember to include plenty of fresh fruit and vegetables in your diet, as they are high in fibre and have a cleansing effect on the system.

The liver is the organ primarily responsible for neutralising toxins within the the body. Try to avoid overloading it with fatty and creamy foods, or chemical additives, caffeine and alcohol, all of which can prevent the liver from functioning efficiently, prompting toxic build-up and cellulite formation. By stimulating the lymphatic and circulatory systems, massage tones the skin, and smooths the appearance of the flesh. This, in turn, can boost the confidence level of the slimmer, and inspire a healthy, body-conscious frame of mind.

MASSAGE FOR CELLULITE

Combined with a balanced diet and regular exercise, massage is a vital factor in ridding your body of cellulite for good. The following massage is designed principally to promote lymphatic drainage, but will also accelerate blood flow through the tissues:

- Using one of The Body Shop's Body Brushes, brush

Touch is an intelligence in itself. German philosopher Immanuel Kant called the hands "the visible part of the brain", implying that our physical senses are in no way inferior to our intellectual understanding. We must learn from other cultures the way to integrate the senses, so that tactile awareness carries the same significance as visual perception.

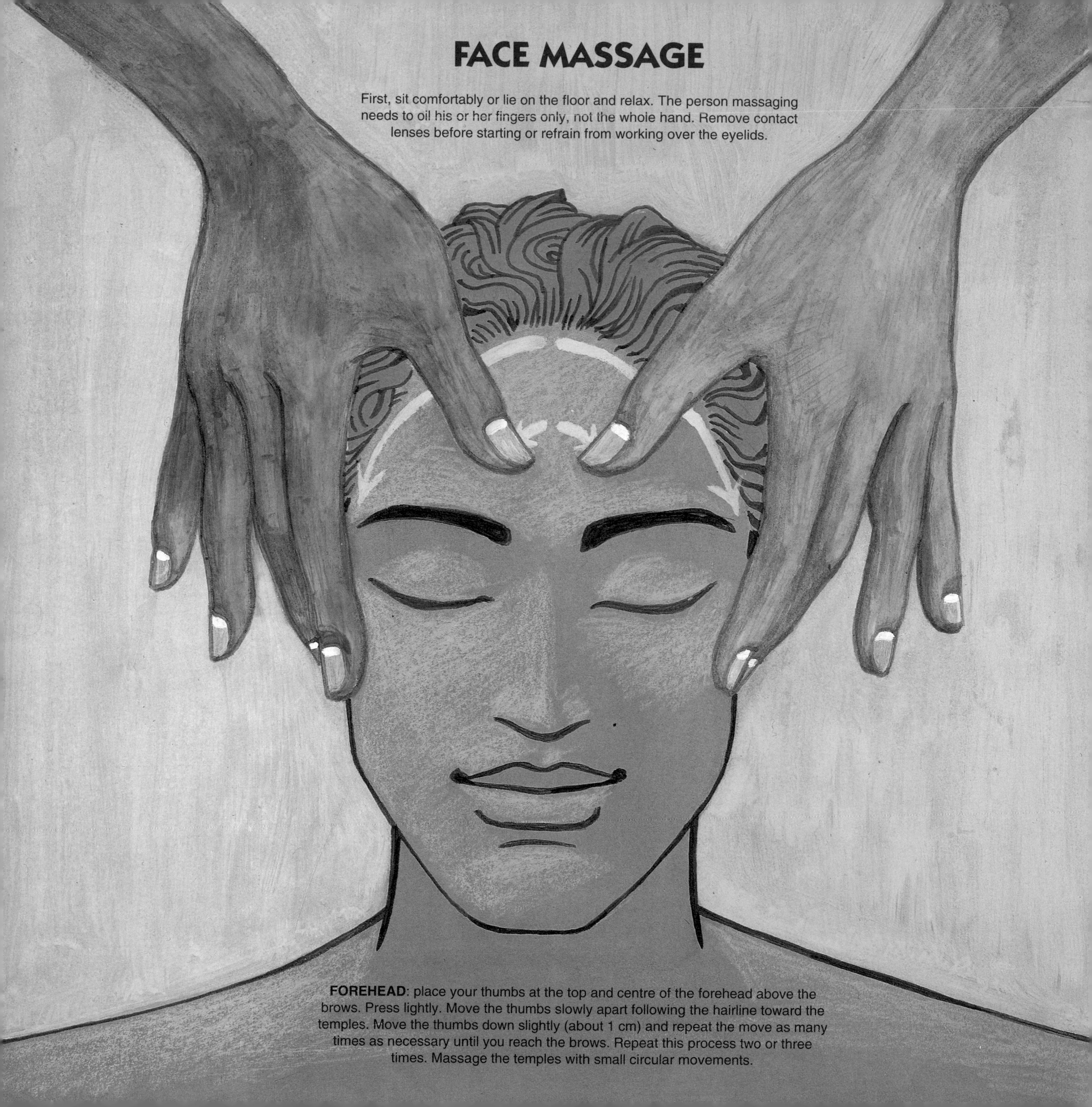

FACE MASSAGE

First, sit comfortably or lie on the floor and relax. The person massaging needs to oil his or her fingers only, not the whole hand. Remove contact lenses before starting or refrain from working over the eyelids.

FOREHEAD: place your thumbs at the top and centre of the forehead above the brows. Press lightly. Move the thumbs slowly apart following the hairline toward the temples. Move the thumbs down slightly (about 1 cm) and repeat the move as many times as necessary until you reach the brows. Repeat this process two or three times. Massage the temples with small circular movements.

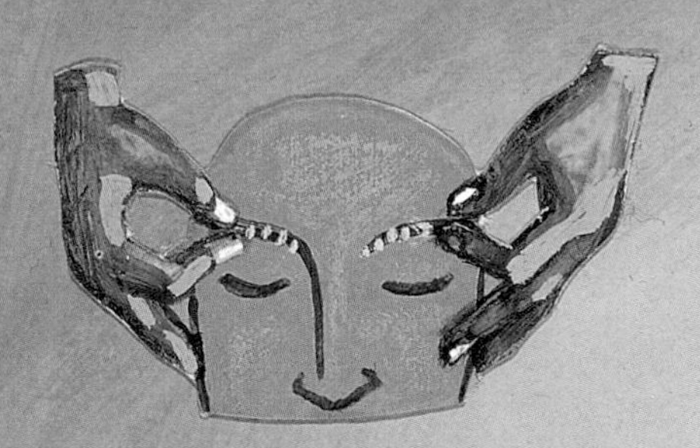

EYEBROWS: place the thumbs at the inner end of the brows and start here. Using the thumbs, press firmly and follow the brow bone ending with an upward movement towards the temples. Also, pinch lightly along each brow.Repeat several times.

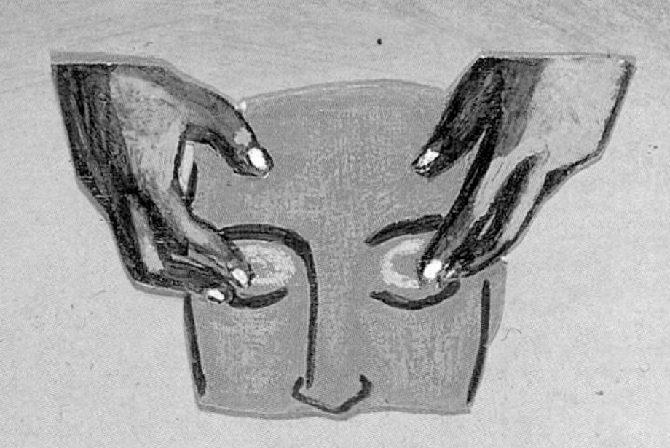

EYES: with two fingers, gently stroke eyelids several times from the inner to the outer corners of the eyes. Then, gently massage eyelids several times in small, circular movements. Move fingers along inner side of brow down outer side of eyes, underneath eye along the bone and up inner side of eyes back to inner brow. Repeat.

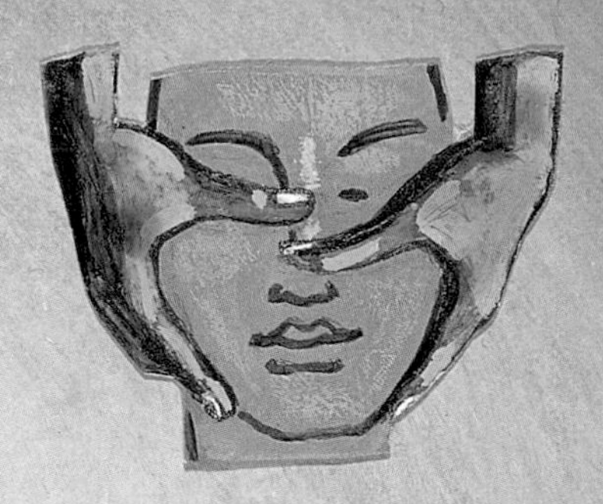

NOSE: using the thumbs alternately, stroke down bridge of the nose from top to tip. Repeat several times. Then lightly squeeze tip of the nose between the thumbs and index fingers. Sandwich the nose between the thumb and index finger at the top of the nose and move down gently. Use the index fingers to make small circular movements on either side of nose.

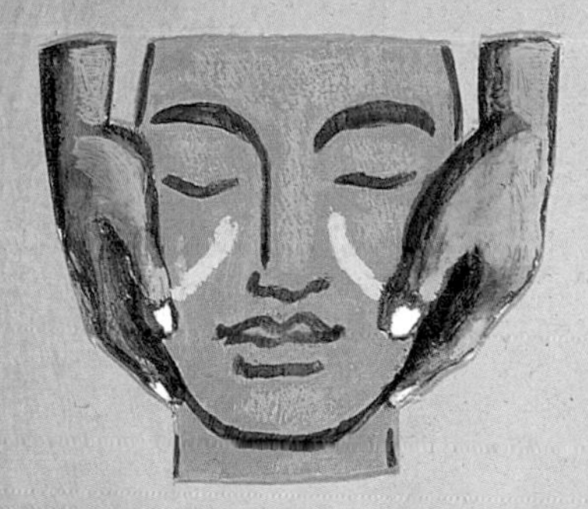

CHEEKS: beginning just under inner corners of eyes, stroke thumbs across cheekbone to the hairline above the ear and off the head. Repeat stroke in strips, moving down face - below cheek-bone, above upper lip and below lower one. Massage cheeks in gentle, circular movements. Place heels of hands on either side of nose, with fingers pointing toward ears. Now slowly part hands, gliding firmly over cheeks towards ears.

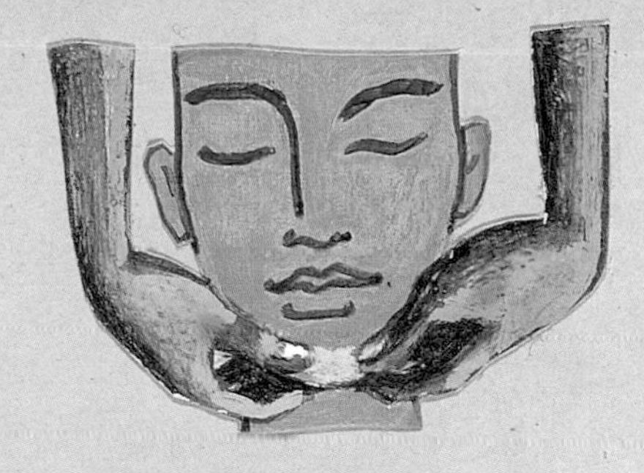

CHIN: hold the point of the chin between the thumbs and index fingers and squeeze along the whole chin.

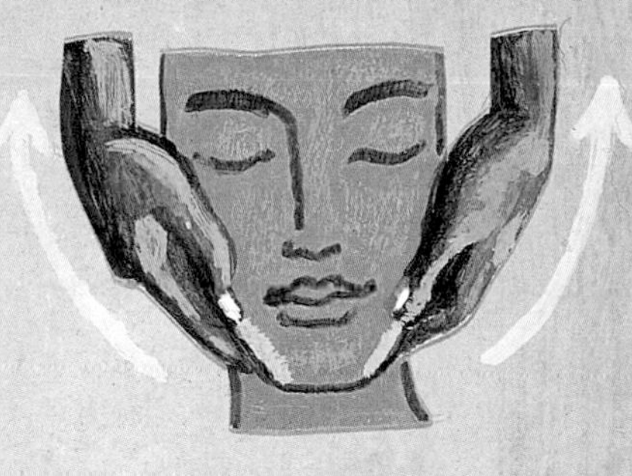

JAW: hold the rim of the jawbone at the chin, then draw your hands slowly apart, squeezing right along the jawbone as far as the ear lobe. Use the index fingers and massage in small circular strokes along the jaw line up to the ears.

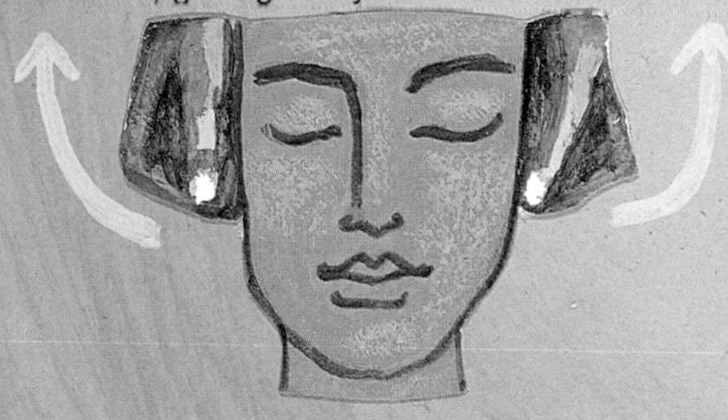

EARS: pull the earlobes gently outwards between the fingers and heels of the hands, stretch gently and hold. Then squeeze (pinch) all around the ears with the fingers and thumbs.

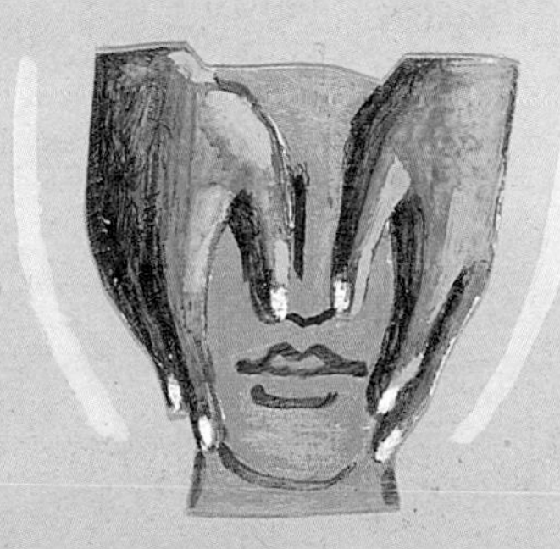

HEAD: cup your palms over the eyes with the thumbs on either side of the nose. Remain there for a moment, allowing the eyes to rest within the darkness of the hands. Fingers first, slide the hands smoothly down over the face, across the cheeks and under the ears to the back of the neck. Without stopping, pull the hands up the neck and, cupping the hands under the back of the head, draw them towards you coming slowly off the top of the head and then the hair.

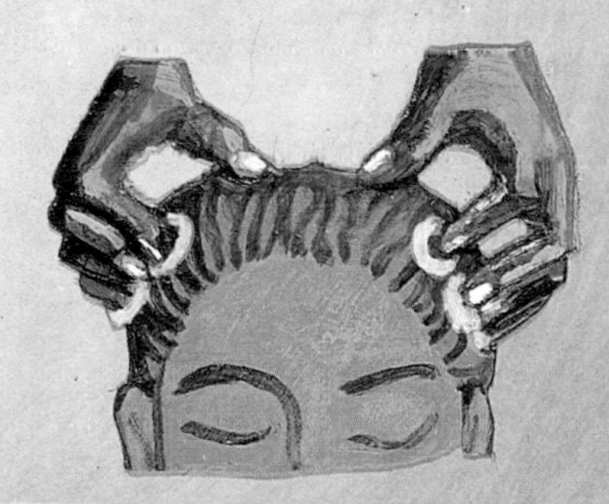

SCALP: massage using small circular movements with the fingers.

Although it is possible to massage without oil (talcum powder is one alternative), you'll find oil gives the best "slip". Before giving a massage, have plenty of oil or lotion ready. A light vegetable oil makes a useful lubricant - The Body Shop's Body Massage Oil contains pure soyabean oil, good because it is slow to be absorbed. When massaging dry skin, you may want something with a little extra moisture such as Rich Massage Lotion or Mango Body Butter.

from the tips of the fingers up the arms using long sweeping movements and firm but not hard pressure.

• Then brush down the neck, across the shoulders, and down the breasts.

• Sweep down the back and down the tummy and finally work from the toes, up the front and back of the legs and up over the buttocks.

• Do not rub back and forth or use circular movements.

During a bath or shower, work the affected areas with a Body Buddy; the specially moulded nodules encourage the softening of collagen fibrils and increase fat mobilisation without the need to apply too much pressure. These problem areas tend to be painful to the touch, and they bruise easily if zealously attacked.

After a bath, when the skin is warm and the muscles relaxed, massage the cellulite with your hands using some of The Body Shop's Cellulite Massage Oil:

• Begin with the effleurage technique to stimulate circulation.

• Then take hold of the flesh with both hands and squeeze, first with one hand, then with the other, working over the whole area.

• Clench your hands and push the knuckles into the skin, twisting them around at the same time.

• Finally, stroke the area again with a Body Buddy, always working towards the heart.

OFFICE HEADACHES

Work over the pad of the thumb (from the knuckle joint to the tip), concentrating on the area closest to the forefinger which is confusingly known as the outside. Treat both hands.

MID-AFTERNOON FATIGUE

This can be alleviated by stimulating the adrenal glands. To locate the appropriate point, trace a straight line across the palm beginning from the point at which the thumb joins the hand. Drop another imaginary line from the join of the first and second finger. Where these lines meet you will find the adrenals. Treat both hands.

Because nerves branch out all over the body from the spine, a good back massage works wonders for the whole nervous system.

INSOMNIA

If you are unable to sleep because of tension or racing thoughts, of have trouble unwinding, it may help to work the solar plexus reflex point, which can be found at the centre of the palm. Press the point for between 30 seconds and one minute. Treat both hands.

PERIOD PAINS

Two points on the feet can be worked in order to relieve period pains. They correspond to the uterus and the ovaries; the reflex point for the ovaries is on the outside of each foot, just below and to the back of the ankle bone. The uterus point lies on the inside of each foot, almost directly opposite the ovary reflex points. The uterus can also be reached by pressing on each side of the Achilles' tendon, the hard ligament at the back of the ankle.

INDIGESTION

A meal consumed too quickly can cause gas to build up in the colon. This puts pressure on the spleen, diaphragm and heart, often resulting in bloating and heartburn. The colon, heart and spleen all lie in the zone corresponding to a band running along the outside of the left foot. Start from the little toe and work along the bottom of the foot towards the heel.

WORKAHOLIC'S BACKACHE

At the end of a working day spent over a typewriter or desk, the chances are that your back will ache. Treat the spinal area whose reflex points run up the inside of each foot; begin with the big toe and work along the foot towards the heel.

COLDS IN THE HEAD

Perhaps the most unpleasant aspect of a cold is congestion of the sinuses; it brings a dull aching headache that clouds the ability to think. Catarrh can be encouraged to drain from the tissues by working the sinus reflex points. They are found on the pads of all the toes except the big toes.

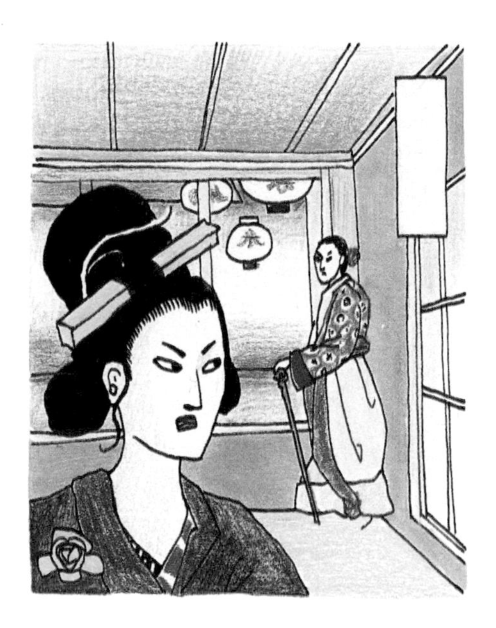

An old Oriental story tells of a woman who despaired of her mother-in-law, a crotchety old battleaxe with whom she shared her house.

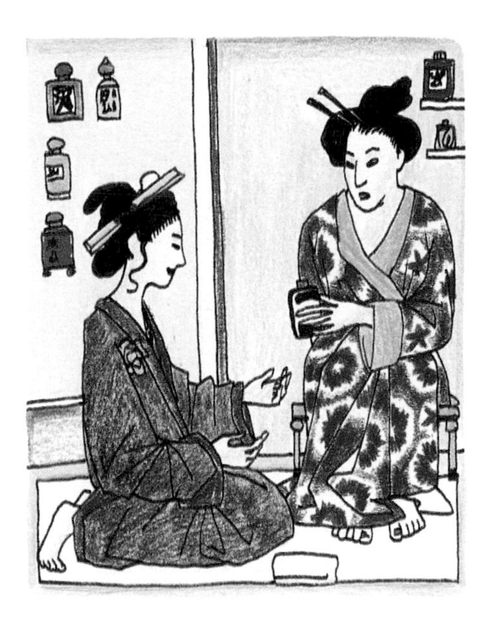

Full of hate, the wife went to the local wise woman and asked her for some poison with which to kill her mother-in-law.

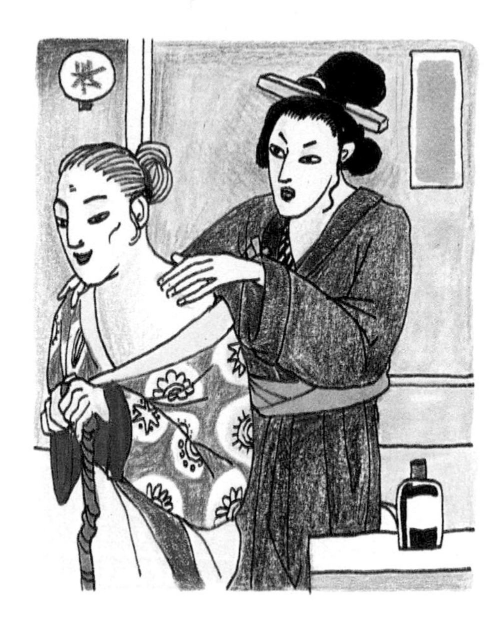

The wise woman thought for a while and then produced an aromatic ointment. "Massage this ointment into her skin every day," she said, " and in three months' time, she will be dead."

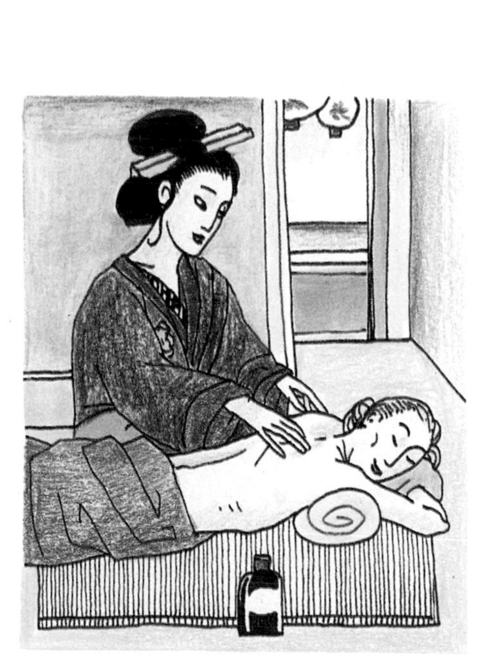

Delighted, the woman went home with her prize. Four weeks later, she came running back, pale and in tears.

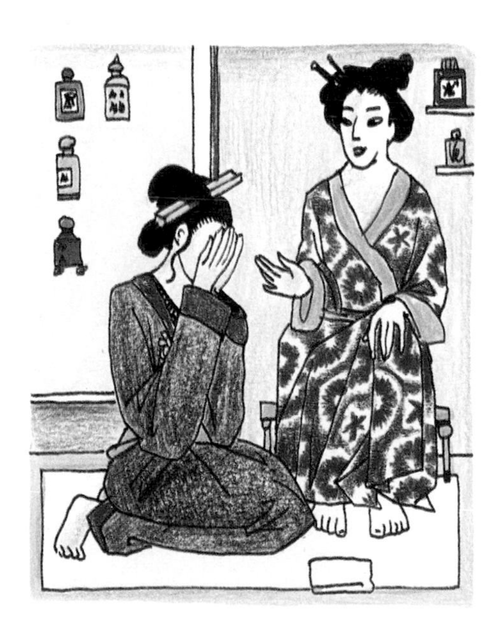

"The antidote," she sobbed, "I must have the antidote. I've realised that I don't want her to die." The wise woman smiled. "You have it," she said.

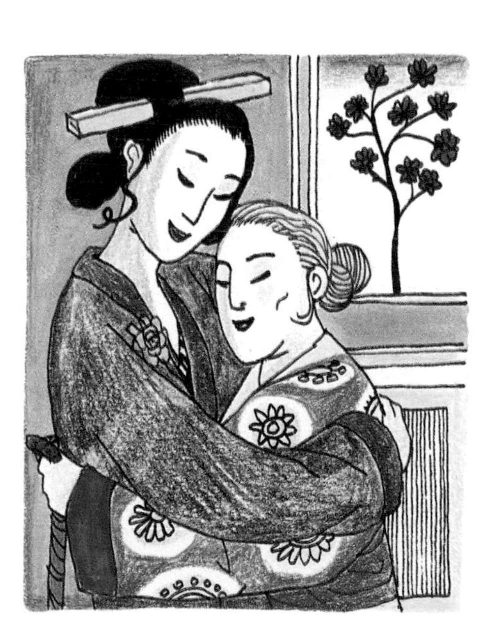

"The potion I gave you is harmless. By massaging your mother-in-law every day you have come to know her and to love her, and she has grown grateful to you. You cannot massage someone and continue to hate them."

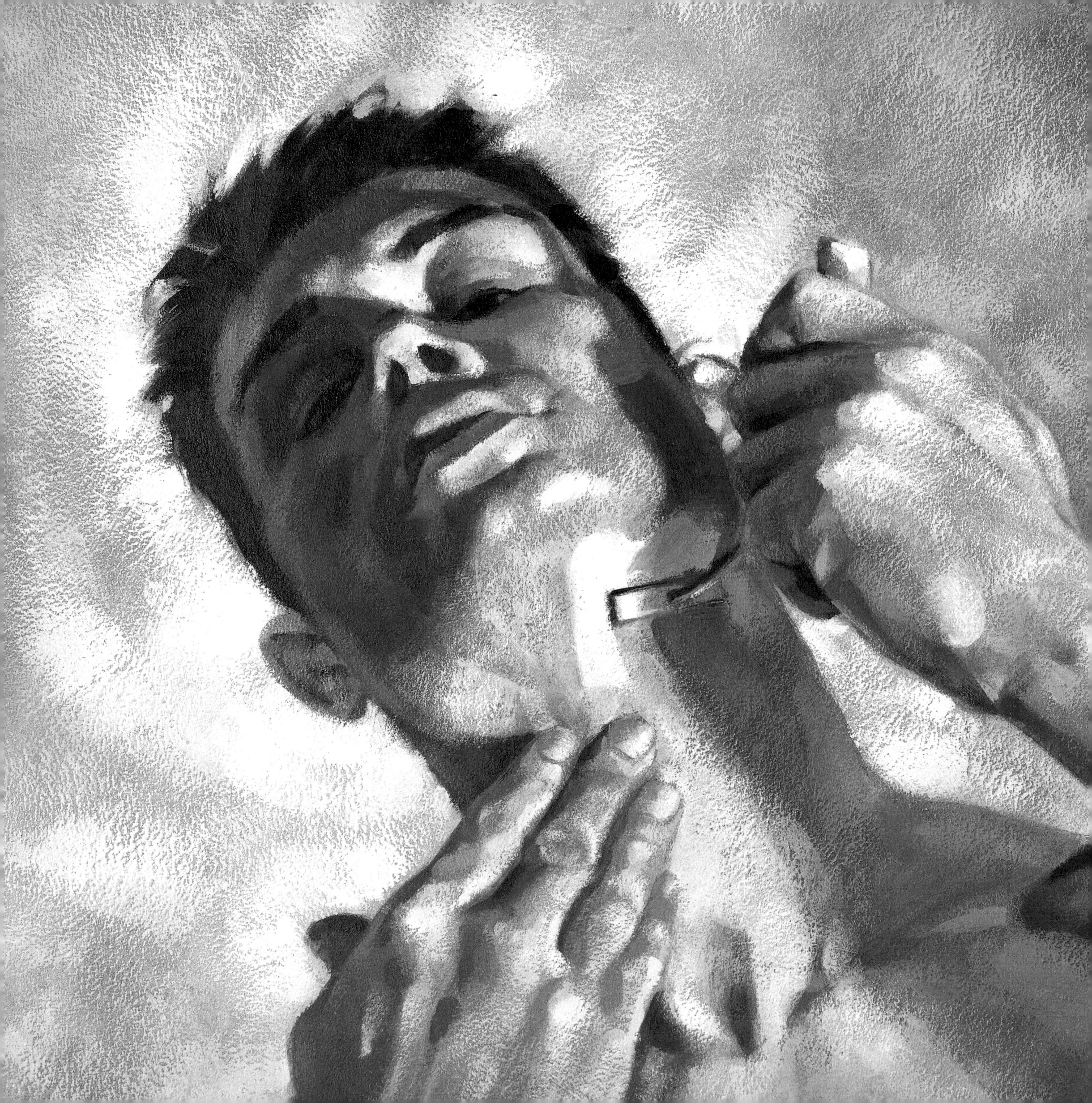

MEN

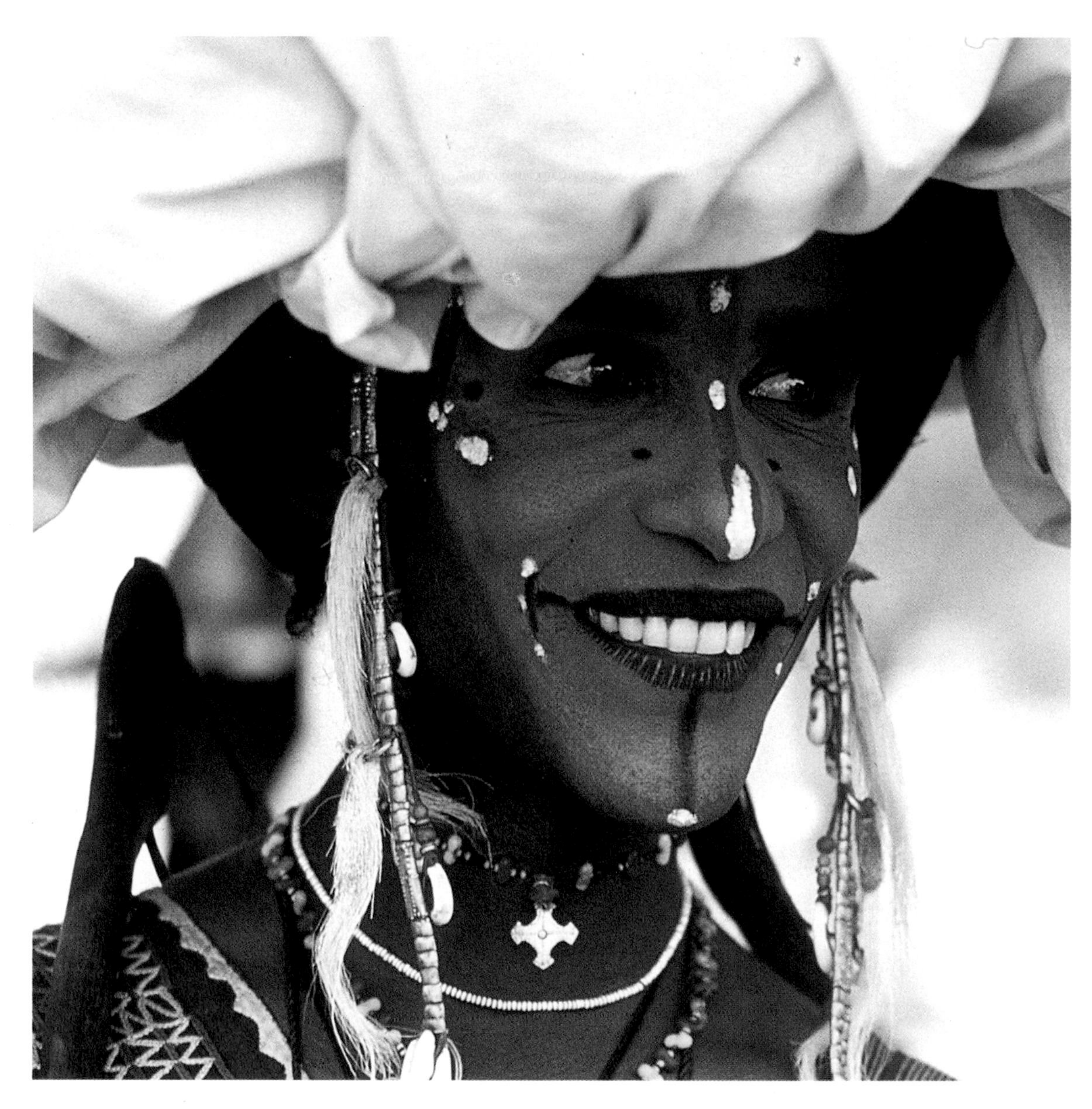

Cosmetic beauty is a male matter for the nomadic Wodaabe of West Africa - it's a significant component of the charm they value above all other assets.

men

Odd, isn't it, to look back in time and see how often beauty was a strictly male preserve? It was, for example, the Greek Herodotus who, in the 5th century BC, advised the Egyptian goddess Atsositou about a beauty mask of apricot pulp, dates and coconut milk. Not only is this one of our earliest extant beauty tips, but it was given by a man.

But Herodotus was only following the lead of his countrymen. Men in Ancient Greece were generally very serious about their pursuit of physical perfection. For them, it was an aesthetic exercise. As much as they valued physical strength, they also sought an ideal look. On special occasions, they'd have a manicure, pedicure and their hair done at the barber's. Whilst they exercised, they were hoping to attract sculptors and painters looking for inspiration. Women didn't get a look in.

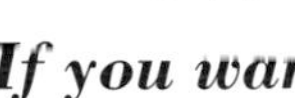

If you want to pay modern man a compliment, just tell him he's successful. Complimenting him on his appearance is liable to make him uncomfortable, even in this day and age.

OBJECTS OF BEAUTY

Dedication to their appearance was for the Greeks a simple way to broadcast their natural superiority over the animal kingdom, since animals couldn't spend hours working on their skin, hair or physique. The Greek male believed that in developing his body, he was cultivating his mind. His ideal was *aidos*, a combination of dignity and modesty, and his public work-outs in the nude, which to us seem anything but modest, were earnest efforts to display *aidos* unadorned.

A variant of the same concept can be found with the males of the nomadic Wodaabe tribe in West Africa today. Like the Greeks, they view the pursuit of beauty as a socialising bond between people. In addition, they see it as the most effective corollary of the charm that is their greatest social asset. At their ceremonial gerewol dance, charm wins young Wodaabe males a lover, recognition by their elders and social status. In their efforts to be the most charming, the men will spend several hours a day in the period leading up to the gerewol swapping make-up tips, working on their wiles, enhancing in every way possible their natural assets. At the actual ceremony, they flutter and flirt in all their painted glory like the most winsome Southern belle, but not for a moment is their masculinity compromised. It is just that, as with the Greeks, beauty is a male domain.

The early Christians found this idea hard to take. For men as well as women, attention to the physical self was tainted by pagan associations. Even the Renaissance man believed body care was a sin. But what he shared with his "pagan" antecedents was a love of display. Quite as much as his forebears in Ancient Rome, the Renaissance courtier gloried in exaggerated style; ruffles, silks, velvets and codpieces turned him into a human peacock. For several hundred years, the courts of Europe were crammed with daintily powdered, bewigged show-offs, with effeminacy almost a token of the upper classes. Then came history's most famous dandy, George "Beau" Brummell. As the friend of England's Prince Regent in the late 18th century, Brummell used clothes as a painter uses oils: as the raw material of a living art. But such obsession with appearance became socially unacceptable in the reign of Victoria, when the sombre style of her consort Albert set a tone that was to last for the rest of the 19th and much of the 20th century.

As many as 50 per cent of all men over 24 years old have fine or thinning hair. Hair can start to recede in men as early as 17.

But men were still the keepers of beauty secrets. Catherine de' Medici, queen of 16th century France, relied on one René de Florentin for her perfumes. Three hundred years later, Hitler determined the beauty regimen of his mistress Eva Braun. And after World War Two, it was men - Payot, Stendhal, Dior - who launched the classic French cosmetic houses. It is a fact that most of the famous fashion houses, past and present, have been driven by males.

Some evidence that World War Two helped men relax their dress code: in 1939, American men bought 27 million felt hats. By 1985, that number was less than 5 million.

BEAST OR BEAUTY?

The rather puritanical traditions of our own culture dictate that appearance is something men appreciate in others, rather than in themselves. The same kind of gender stereotyping says a man is more attractive when he's busy, a woman when she's idle. Therefore, if a man looks better when he's active, his looks aren't as important. So men are engaged in a constant struggle between being seen to care about the way they look, and being seen not to care. It's a dilemma - after all, it was the Beast that Beauty loved, not the handsome prince.

It's easy to see how this confusion affected society. Men became materialistic: "Judge me by what I have, not by what I am." And the great cultural myth - that power equals sex appeal - gained more credibility, alongside that curiously enduring phenomenon that blesses the ugly man, the short man, the bald man and the hunchback with a perverse sexual charisma. You can run a line from the Frog Prince through Quasimodo to Aristotle Onassis and Pablo Picasso.

So how did concern about looks work its way back onto the male agenda during this century? World War Two may have helped by loosening society's stays, getting all those good old American boys off the farm and out into a world they would otherwise never have seen. They became a whole new market to be targeted by advertisers. For example, toiletry sets were an excellent gift idea for the man in service. When the soldiers came home, they still wanted their gift packs of toiletries and scented colognes.

THE SKIN-DEEP MAN

But men proved hard for the cosmetics industry to address as a group and it was a long slow slog from 1945 to 1975 when the beginnings of the fitness movement heralded the kind of narcissistic attention to self that would offer the cosmetics industry endless opportunities to appeal first to women and eventually to the reluctant male market. The secret was leisure time. As that increased and there was less call on the primal male attributes such as strength (so necessary during wartime), it became just as important to look like a man as act like a man.

Judging a book by its cover is something we're always counselled not to do. But in the last decades of the 20th century, appearances count, not simply because to look good is to feel better about yourself, but also because careers depend on projected competence. Today men exercise, diet, even subject themselves in growing numbers to cosmetic surgery to maintain a semblance of capability for as long as possible. Their role model might be the property developer who increased his business after he lost 2st, switched from off-the-peg suits to a tailor and started using a moisturiser.

THE SAMSON SYNDROME

So modern men have found out what it feels like to be an object, judged on appearance the way women have always been judged by men. Unsurprisingly, men's worries about baldness have surged as a perfect correlative to women's insecurities about ageing.

If the media can be blamed for promoting idealised and

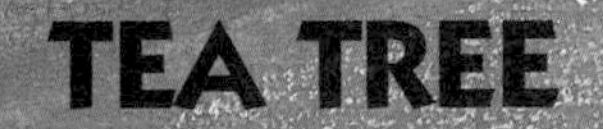

TEA TREE

The tea tree (Melaleuca) is found in parts of South East Asia, Australia and New Zealand. It is a tough little shrub that flourishes where other plants can't grow.

Australia's Aborigines have used tea tree oil for over 40,000 years.

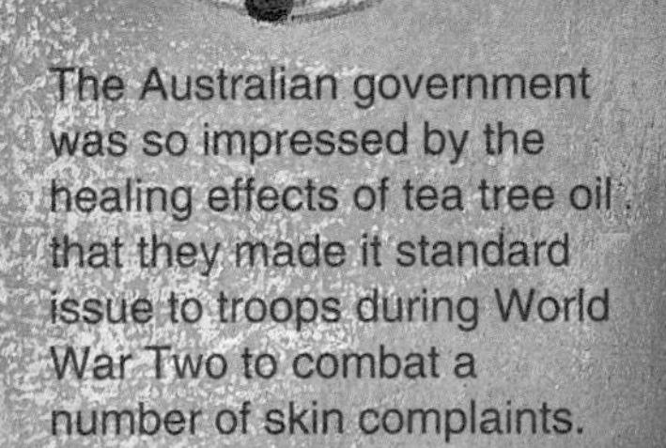

The Australian government was so impressed by the healing effects of tea tree oil that they made it standard issue to troops during World War Two to combat a number of skin complaints.

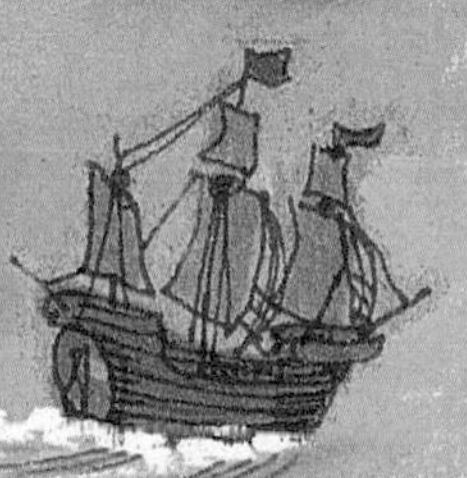

When Captain Cook reached Australia on his exploration of the Pacific in 1768-79, his botanist Joseph Banks found the Aborigines using the leaves of the Melaleuca to make tea. That's how the plant got its English name.

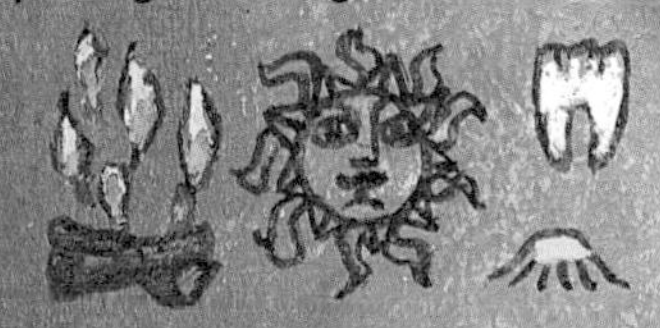

In Australia, tea tree oil has a wide range of germicidal and fungicidal applications. It is used to treat burns, sunburns, pimples, boils, stings, toothache, gum infections, cuts, sore throats and athlete's foot.

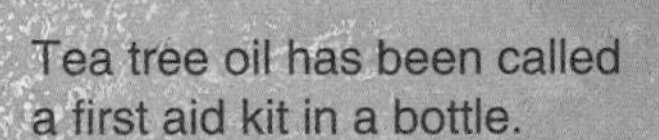

Tea tree oil has been called a first aid kit in a bottle.

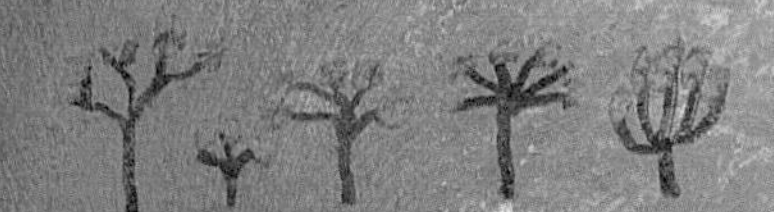

There are over 180 species of tea tree but only the oil steam-distilled from the leaves of one particular species (Melaleuca alternifolia) is used commercially. It occurs naturally only in Northern New South Wales.

Though tea tree oil is not a good moisturiser, its valuable properties as a deep cleanser and antiseptic make it especially good for oily or problem skins and irritated scalps.

10 STEPS TO THE PERFECT SHAVE

The average male will spend a few thousand hours of his life in pursuit of the perfect shave: smooth, close, quick with no nasty stings or nicks. That's why men, otherwise notoriously resistant to the charms of skin-care products, are more easily seduced if such products include the word "shave" in their name.

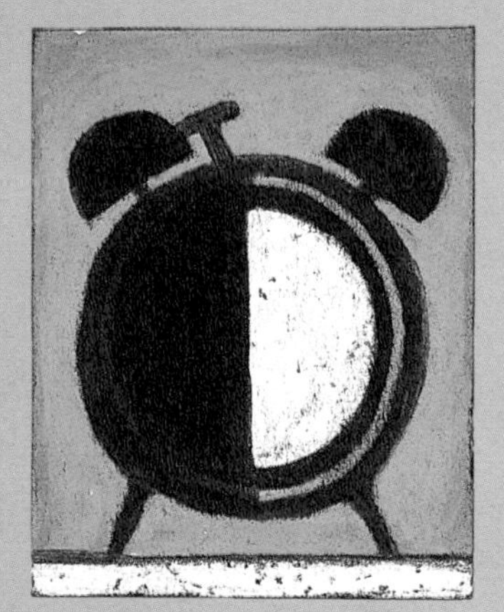

1. Wait at least half an hour after you get up in the morning before shaving. This allows facial muscles to tighten and gives whiskers a chance to stand away from the skin.

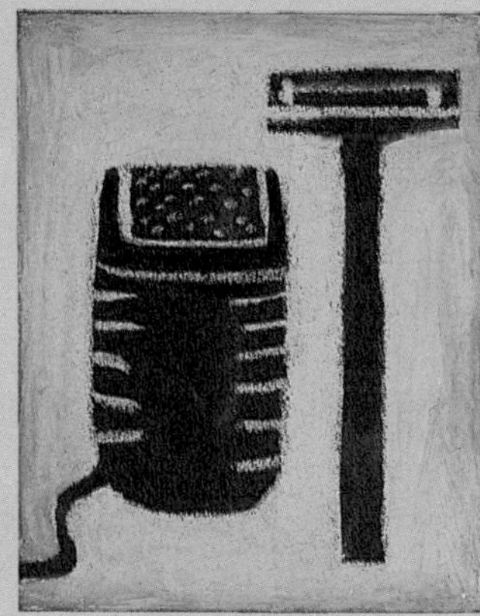

2. Wet shaving is kinder to the skin, though on a regular basis it may be irritating to men with dry or sensitive skin. They could consider alternating electric and wet shaving.

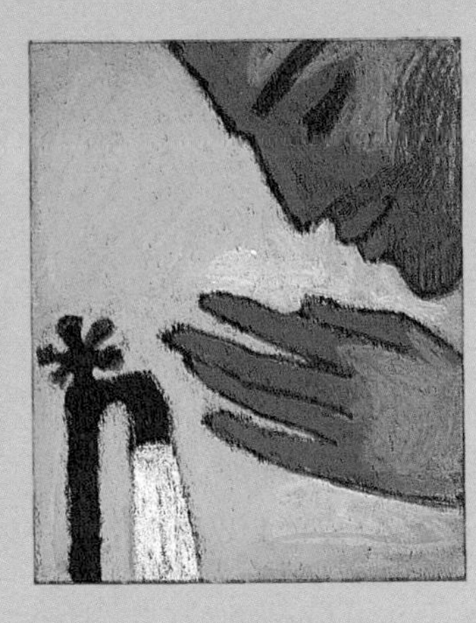

3. The texture of beard hair is like that of copper wire - always soften with warm water before shaving. That's why it is often a good idea to shave in the shower.

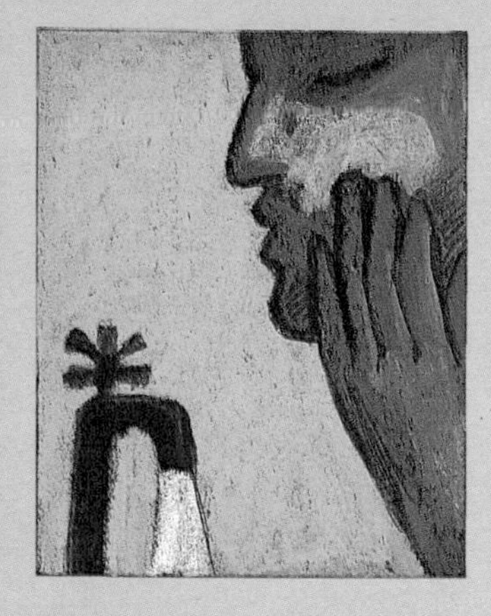

4. Use that two minutes to massage the face with gentle soap or face wash. Cleansing is essential to rid the skin's surface of grime that can block pores and lead to spots. Then rinse.

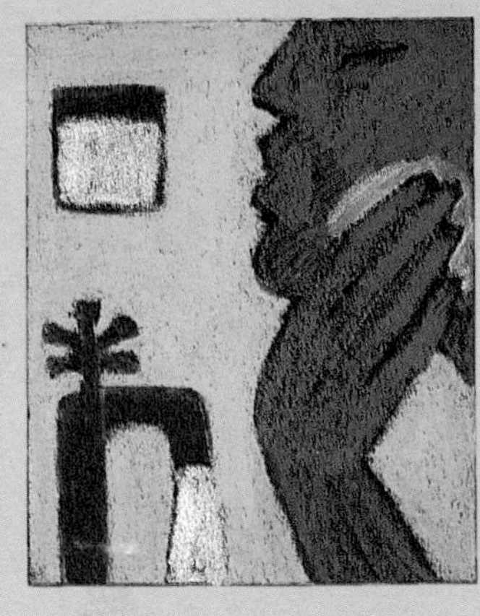

5. Now you can add a secret ingredient. Dead skin cells can make the skin's surface uneven, leading to nicks and sore spots after shaving. Why not try a face scrub at this point to smooth the skin? Rinse again.

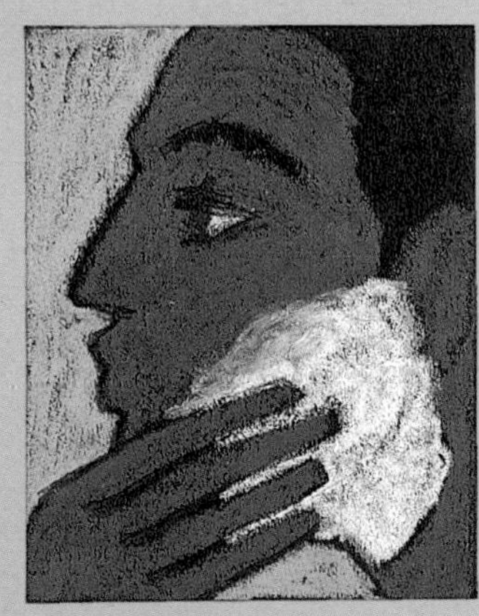

6. Massage in shaving cream to lubricate skin and soften beard. The secret of a good shave is in the quality, rather than the volume, of the lather.

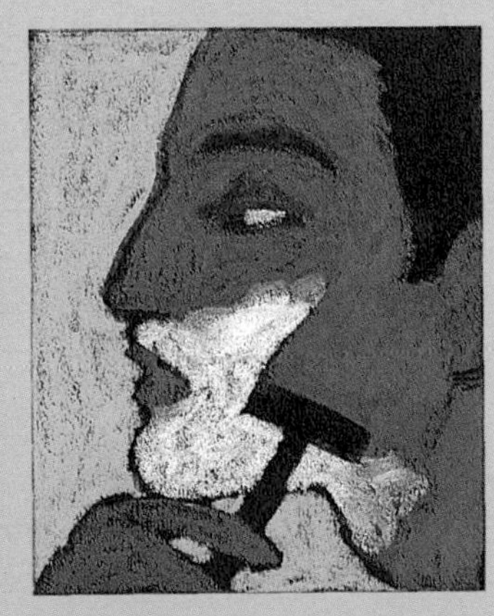

7. Shave the jawline and cheeks first, then the neck, upper and lower lips and lastly the chin, where whiskers are thickest. Always shave with the grain, in the direction of natural beard growth.

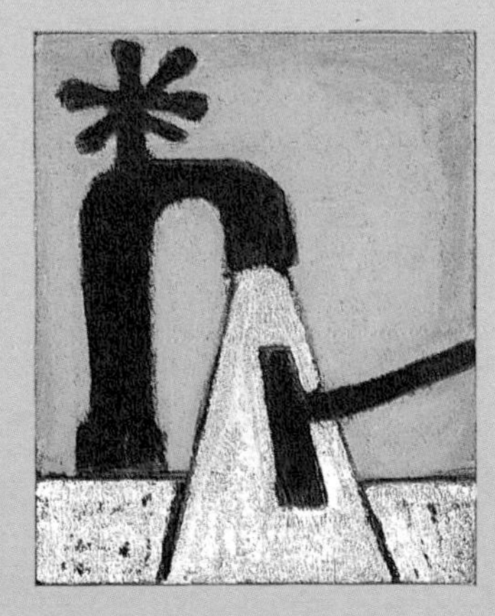

8. Rinse your razor often to prevent clogging. Avoid undue pressure with the blade. Don't rush. Shaving can remove three skin layers, so don't shave over the same spot several times.

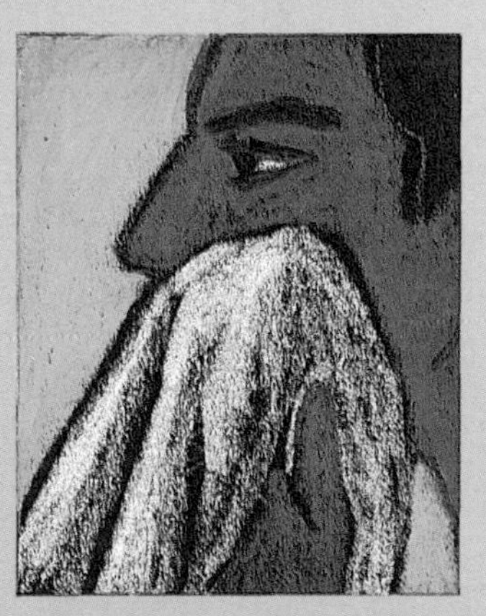

9. After shaving, splash your face with warm water. Gently pat dry with soft, clean towel.

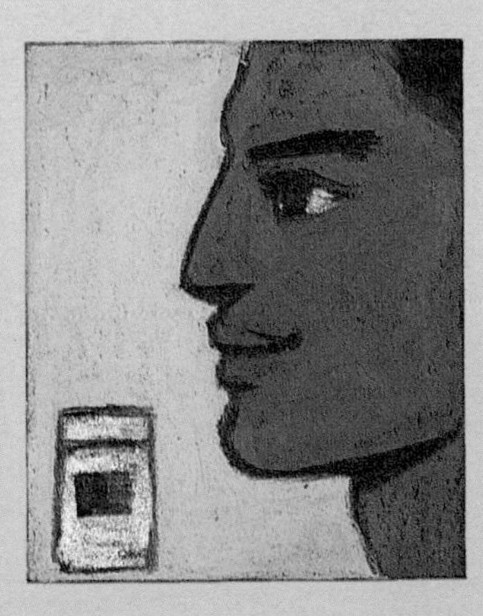

10. Moisturise or - if you feel moisturiser leaves your skin too oily - apply an after-shaving gel.

unattainable images of womanhood, the same criticism can be levelled at the depiction of men. To be sexy, a man should be tall, in good shape, with a good head of hair. That holds out little hope for the average man. As many as 50 per cent of men over 24 years old have fine or thinning hair. And hair can start to recede at 17. Men make it easier on themselves by generally seeming to be more comfortable about the ravages of time than women. It's that old saying - character on a man is wrinkles on a woman. Still, many men would have to concede that they channel their vanity into keeping their hair on their heads for as long as possible.

Roman soldiers used pumice to keep their cheeks and chin smooth. Men in the South Seas clipped their whiskers between two pieces of flint.

Man has subjected himself to horrendous indignities in pursuit of perpetual hair, culminating in a 1983 ban by the Food and Drug Administration in America on the sale of artificial hair fibres for scalp implantation. Fibres of such synthetic materials as polyester, modacrylic and polyacrylic, as well as natural human hair, were being processed for implantation. In 21 cases, the fibres could not be removed and the patients' scalps remained permanently disfigured.

To demonstrate that an ingredient is a hair restorer, it must be proven that the active ingredient gets to the root and stimulates hair growth. Leaving aside artifice, the simple fact is that, once the hair shaft emerges from the scalp, there is nothing that will influence its growth. For men, there are two causes of baldness: stress and genetics. Despite the magic potions and miracle cures, there is absolutely nothing you can do about the second process, bar try to slow it down. Male pattern baldness, alopecia androgenetica, is genetically programmed like colour or texture. Researchers know it is inherited from the female line. And they know that the follicles are still under the skin in bald men. What they don't know is how to stimulate them to grow again once they have been deprogrammed. As yet there has been no breakthrough.

NOT NECESSARILY A LOSING BATTLE

So far, stimulating the scalp by massaging it with a scalp oil or an aromatic oil and using a zestful shampoo to help increase the blood supply to the beleagured follicles, seem the most viable options for slowing this traumatic process. And there's time - male pattern baldness occurs over a long period.

- Treat your hair gently - never use a metal-toothed comb. Try a plastic one instead.
- Avoid too much brushing and, if possible, don't brush wet hair.
- Dry hair is much stronger. Brush before you wash and you'll loosen dead skin and stimulate blood circulation.
- A regular scalp massage encourages blood circulation in the scalp, and will also help alleviate the tension that can contribute to hair loss. (See Hair chapter for details.)

Actually, there is one way to head off baldness but it is rather extreme. Men go bald because of a high level of the male hormone testosterone in the blood, hence the received belief in the sexy he-manliness of bald men. One guaranteed way to maintain a full head of hair is to seal it in its youthful glory - by castration. Eunuchs and castrati have no need to produce testosterone so they never go bald.

There are all sorts of ancient "cures" for baldness: sadly none of them work. The Ancient Egyptians used to put lettuce on their heads, the Mongols used yoghurt and one old wives' remedy was to powder the head with parsley seeds three times a year before going to bed.

MEN AND FRAGRANCE

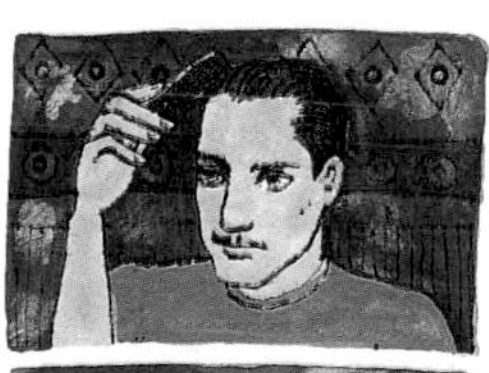

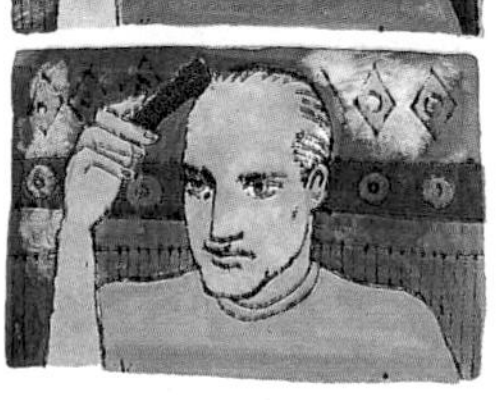

For millennia, men gloried in scents. Alexander the Great had the floor of his home sprinkled with scented waters, and fragrant resins and myrrh were burned on censers to perfume his clothes. Louis XIV was renowned as the sweetest-smelling monarch in Europe. He had all his shirts scented with "aqua angeli". Aloes wood, nutmeg, cloves, storax and benzoin were simmered in rose water for 24 hours, then water of jasmine and orange flowers and a few grains of musk were added. The king's shirts were rinsed in this solution. A quarterly bill shows that Chardin supplied Napoleon with 162 bottles of eau de cologne (essential oils of neroli, rosemary and bergamot dissolved in grape spirit).

Some 93 per cent of British men shave daily. The average man removes 25ft of whiskers in his lifetime.

Again, it was those sober Victorians who put paid to such "vanities". That they have steadily crept back into favour reflects a general trend in society towards a more sophisticated sense of self. Fragrance becomes one more tool in the creation and projection of self-image. As the

A SHORT HISTORY OF THE SHAVE

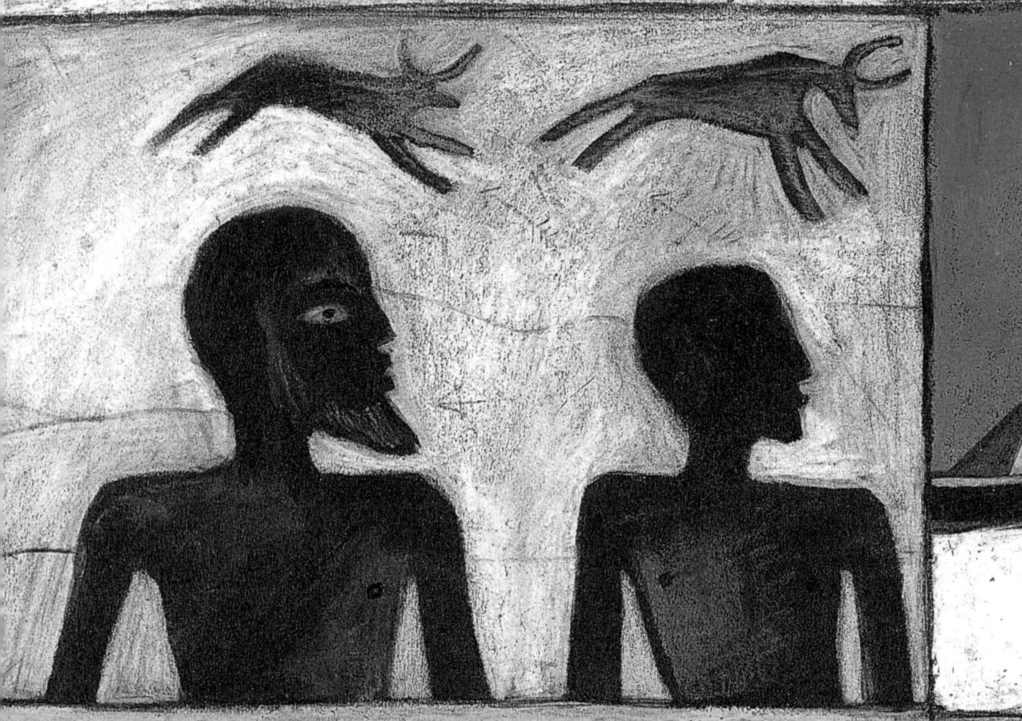

Cave drawings from 20 000 BC show bearded and beardless men. Sharpened flints and shells - the first razors - have been found in gravesites.

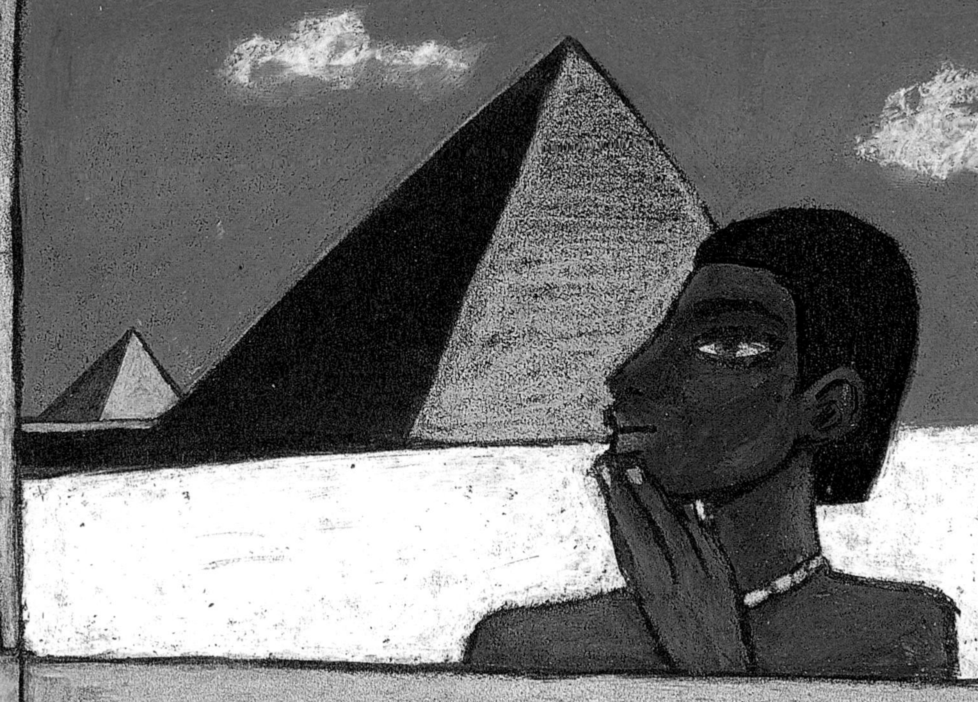

In Ancient Egypt a clean-shaven face was a status symbol. Pharaohs were buried with their bronze razors.

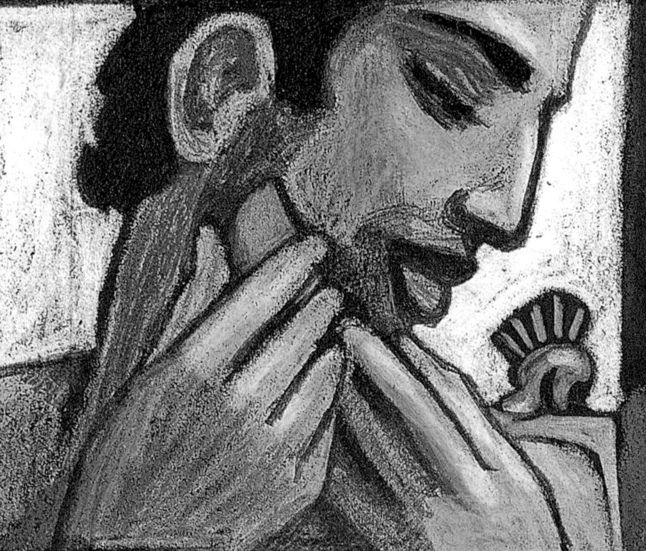

The Greeks shaved daily. The Romans thought a daily shave was effete, but legionnaires used pumice as well as razors to keep their cheeks and chin smooth: a beard got in the way during battle. (Barba, Latin for beard, gives us our word barber.)

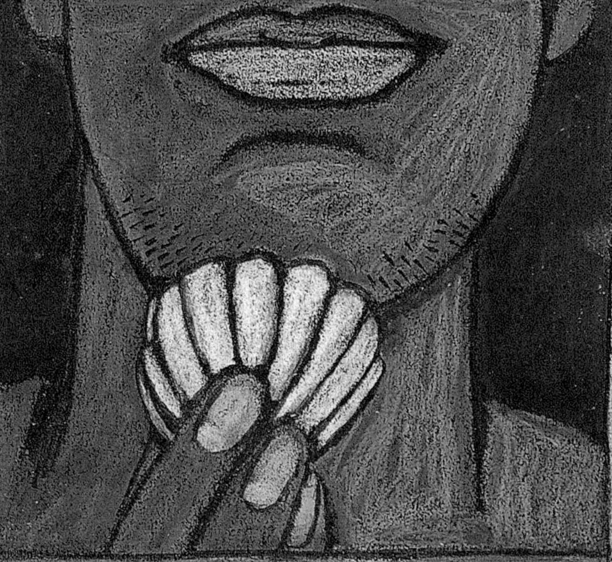

American Indians plucked their bristles out one by one, using clam shells as tweezers. In the South Seas men used two pieces of flint.

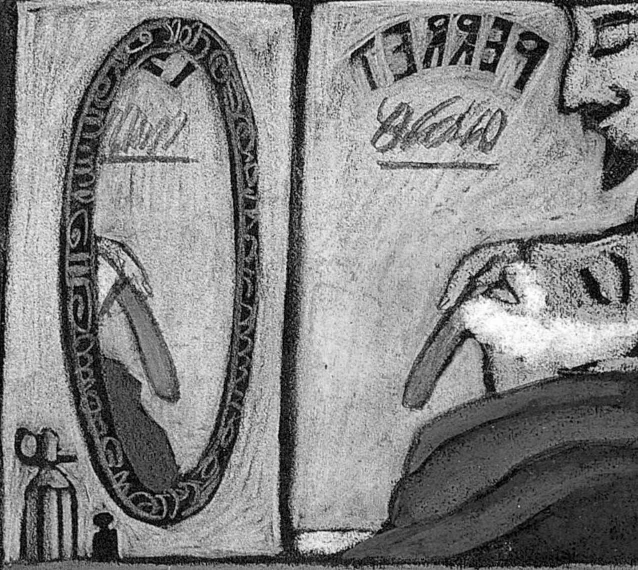

In France in 1762, a professional barber, Jean Jacques Perret, designed the first safety razor with a metal guard along one edge of the blade to prevent nicks and cuts.

General Ambrose Everett Burnside, commander of the Union Army of the Potomac during the American Civil War, was famous for his bushy side whiskers, which started a trend. Originally known as "burnsides", they somehow suffered a linguistic about turn around 1900 to become "sideburns".

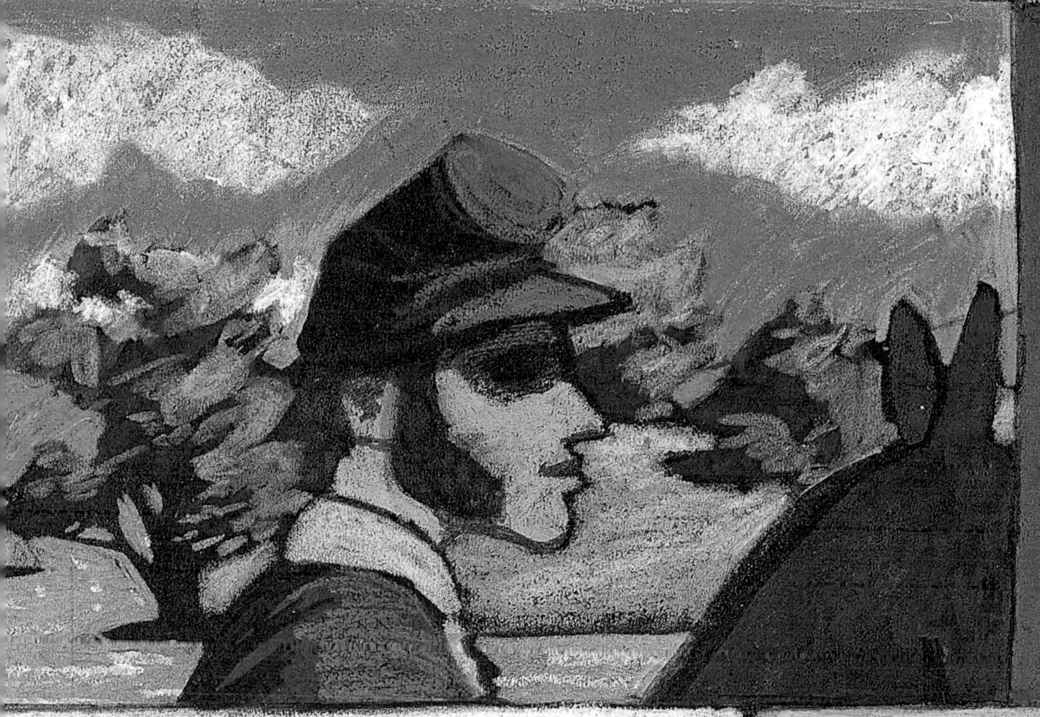

It occurred to a travelling salesman-inventor named King Gillette that a disposable blade would be a convenient solution to the time-consuming routine of razor-sharpening. In collaboration with a professor at the Massachusetts Institute of Technology, Gillette developed such a blade, which went on sale in 1903.

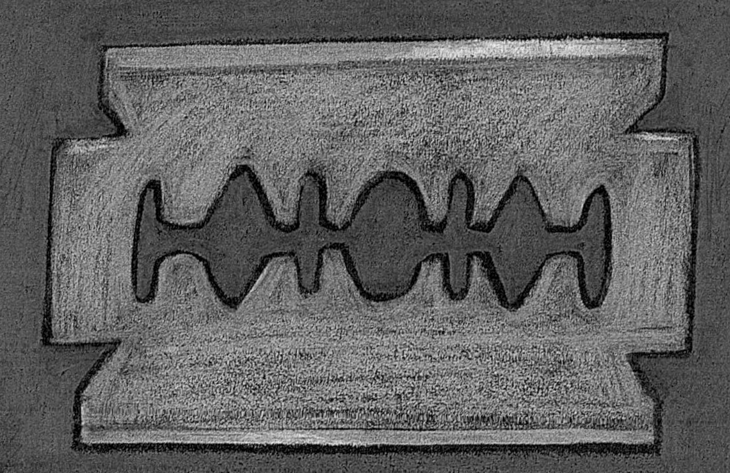

When America entered World War One, the US government ordered three and a half million razors and 36 million blades from Gillette, enough to keep the army clean shaven and to introduce men from all over the world to his invention.

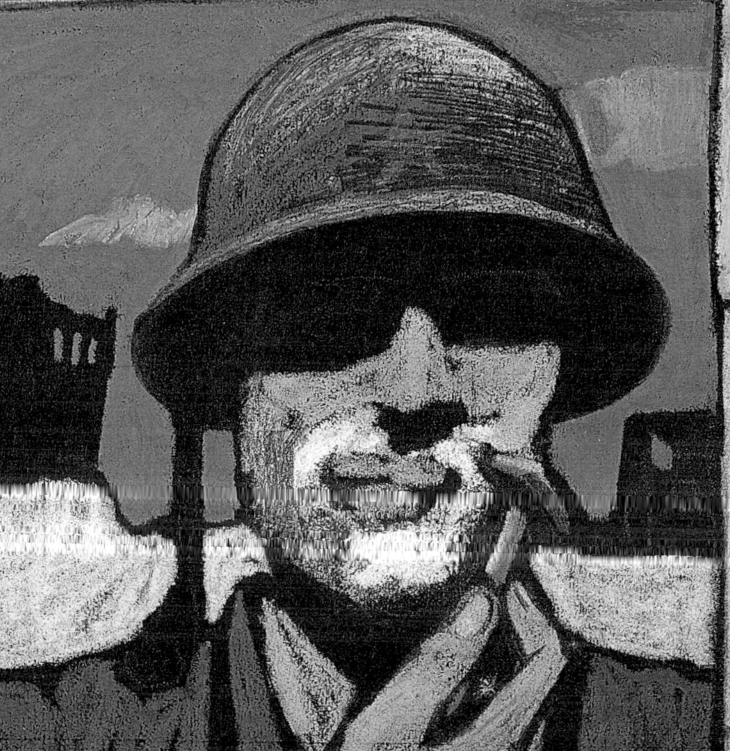

Soldier Jacob Shick had no complaints with his Gillette razor - except when there was no water, soap or shaving cream. He decided the solution was a dry razor powered by an electric motor. It took, him five years to invent one small enough, and he finally launched his new product in 1931, with a $25 price tag. That first year, he sold 3,000. Six years later, he was selling almost two million a year.

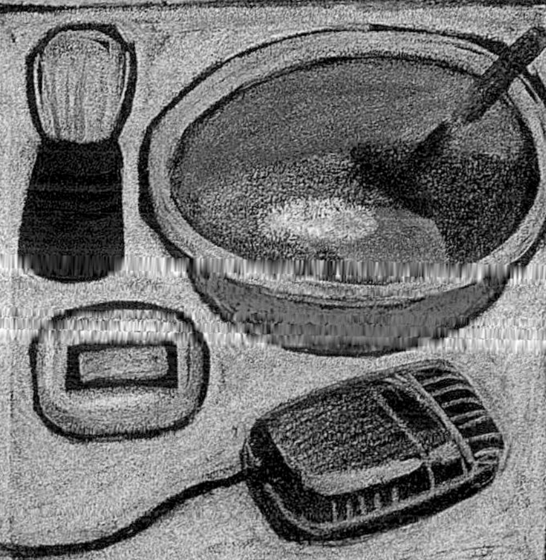

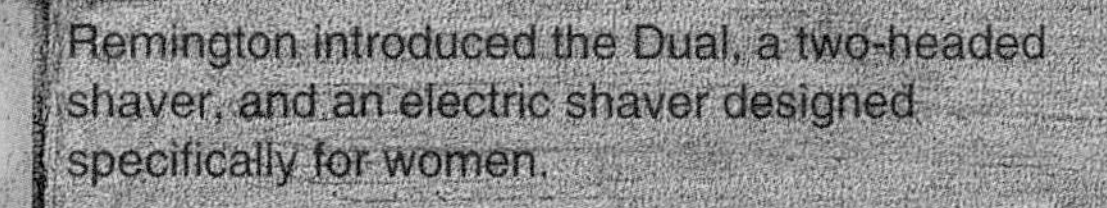

Remington introduced the Dual, a two-headed shaver, and an electric shaver designed specifically for women.

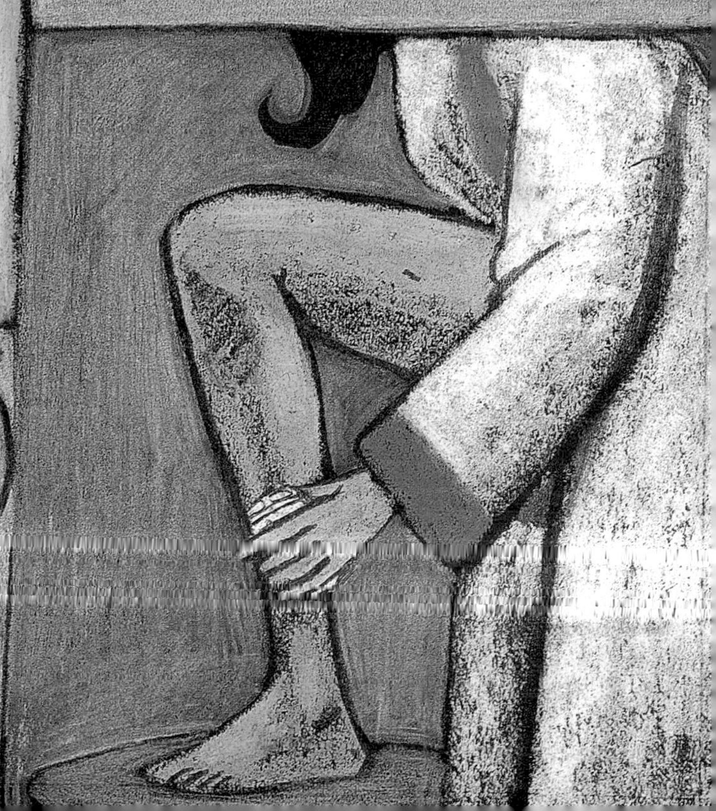

American Fragrance Foundation discovered, men choose a fragrance according to how they'd like to be perceived, rather than how they actually are. And there is always that underlying primal concern - a 1991 poll taken by the Fragrance Foundation found that 21 per cent of male respondents claimed to wear fragrance as an attractant to potential partners.

Swordsmiths produced the first straight razors for dangerously close shaves. A prototype of the safety razor was created in 1762 by a French cutler.

In the Swinging Sixties and Seventies, cosmetics companies obviously felt subtlety was a no-no when they made their appeals to the male market. Among American product names from that period are: Sweat, Balls and Below the Belt (a deodorising powder spray for the groin).

For all that, men still feel most comfortable with the unambiguously masculine association of the shave. Male fragrance is sold as "aftershave". Perish the modern male who wears perfume, but give him something scented to use after shaving and there's no holding him down. By the mid-1960s, when the cosmetics industry decided men were an under-exploited market, they were already using more fragrance in terms of total gallonage than women . In fact men have always used more fragrance than women. In the bad old days the macho men of the Wild West would buy lilac water by the gallon to improve their chances with frontier women.

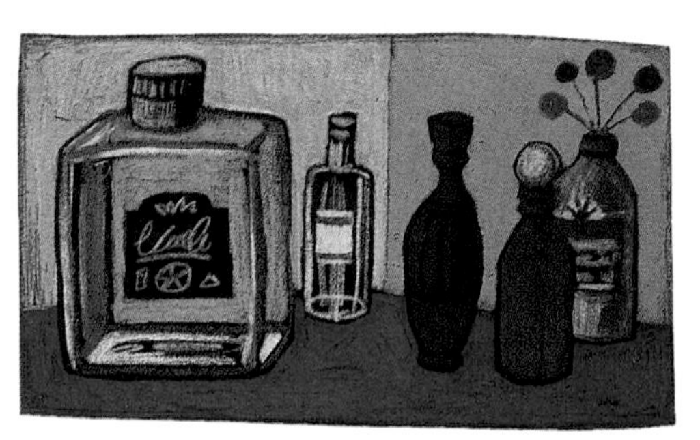

HOW TO GET THE SCENT WITHOUT THE STING

Aftershave is essentially formulated in the same way as the eau de toilettes favoured by women, but the difference lies in application. Where eau de toilette is designed for dabbing on or lightly misting the skin in certain areas, aftershave was customarily promoted as something to be splashed on newly shaved skin, the aftershock seen as "toning" or "bracing". Which was just another way of saying it stung like blazes. No wonder, given the alcohol content of more than 80 per cent. And as it stung, it was drying out the skin which made no sense at all. Surely it's more logical to apply a soothing, moisturising balm or gel. It certainly feels much more gratifying. And it just isn't true that aftershave closes pores.

Because of their alcohol content, aftershaves and eau de toilettes are taboo for Muslims. But they can use headier, heavier, alcohol-free essential oils.

So if you use aftershave, don't apply it to newly shaved skin. Splash it on the back of your neck, or anywhere else you would apply eau de toilette. But remember - dabbing it behind the ears could be severely drying because the skin there has no oil glands.

VIVE LE DIFFERENCE!

Men's skincare products are often just women's products repackaged, with any feminine scent removed and a manly musk added. That in itself is a comment on the subtlety of the differences between men's and women's skins. But it is safe to say that men's skins are generally thicker and oilier, so they age better. Also, the daily shaving routine acts as a valuable exfoliant, keeping skin cells ticking over at a healthy rate.

Why not also try using a face scrub as a daily exfoliant on the back and shoulders where skin is oiliest?

ADULT ACNE - A PARTICULAR MALE PROBLEM

Long considered a trial of adolescence, acne increasingly affects the mature male: up to 25 per cent of men in their twenties, and up to 10 per cent of men in their thirties. Though the precise trigger for adult onset acne hasn't been identified, it is widely believed to be multifactorial, with stress and pollution among the leading suspects.

Acne is caused by abnormal amounts of sebum (oil) secretion in the skin's tiny hair ducts. Such over production is triggered by an abnormal response to the hormone testosterone. In adult women, its main effects are counteracted by oestrogen. Men have no oestrogen and therefore tend to suffer more from widespread chronic acne.

DON'T think that stripping away all facial oils will solve the problem. That simply stimulates the sebaceous glands to produce more oil.

DO look after yourself, since stress is a major factor: a good diet, plenty of sleep and regular exercise will help.

DO get rid of blackheads without scarring with a blackhead remover.

DO gently cleanse the face with a calming, absorbing product such as an oatmeal cleanser. Use two or three times daily. Keep bacteria to a minimum by not fiddling with your face during the day.

DO see a doctor if acne persists.

MEN'S SKIN- AND HAIR-CARE GUIDE

SKIN TYPE	DRY	NORMAL	OILY
CLEANSER	Glycerine and Oat Facial Lather	MM Face Wash Passion Fruit Cleansing Gel	Pineapple Facial Wash
SOAP	Aloe Soap	MM Soap	Vitamin E Soap
FRESHENER	Honey Water	Cucumber Water	Eldorflower Water
MOISTURISER	Aloe Vera Moisture Cream	MM Face Protector	Aloe Gel
EXFOLIATOR	Glycerine and Oat Facial Lather	MM Face Scrub Japanese Washing Grains Honey and Oat Scrub Mask	Blue Corn Scrub Mask Japanese Washing Grains
FOR TROUBLE SPOTS	Sage and Comfrey Blemish Gel	Sage and Comfrey Blemish Gel	Sage and Comfrey Blemish Gel
HAIR PRODUCTS	Banana Shampoo and Banana Conditioner Jojoba Oil Conditioning Shampoo and Protein Cream Rinse	Shampoo & Conditioner in One Seaweed and Birch and Light Conditioner Tangerine Beer Shampoo and Light Conditioner	Ice Blue and Light Conditioner Frequent Wash Grapefruit Shampoo and Light Conditioner

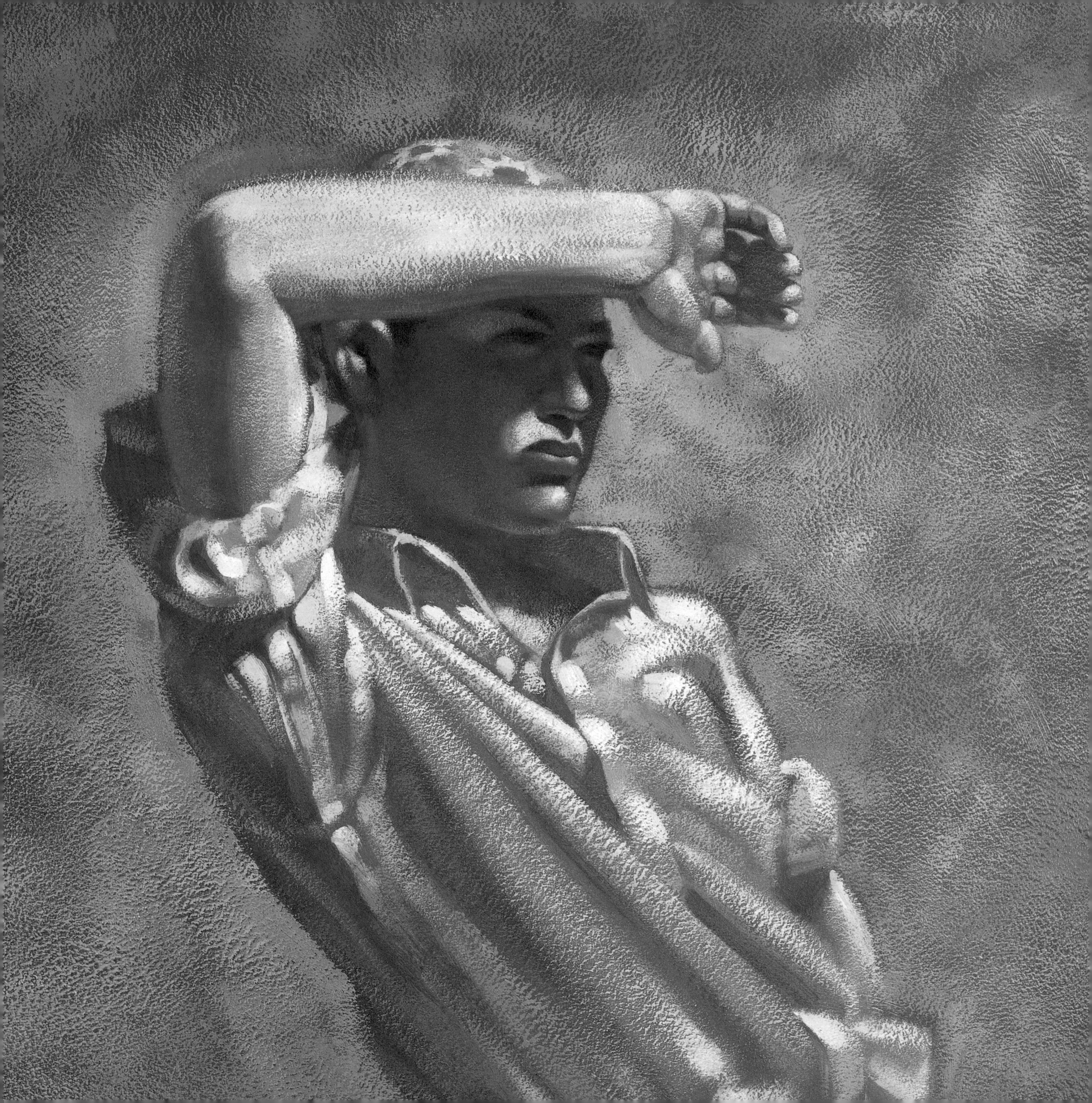

SUN

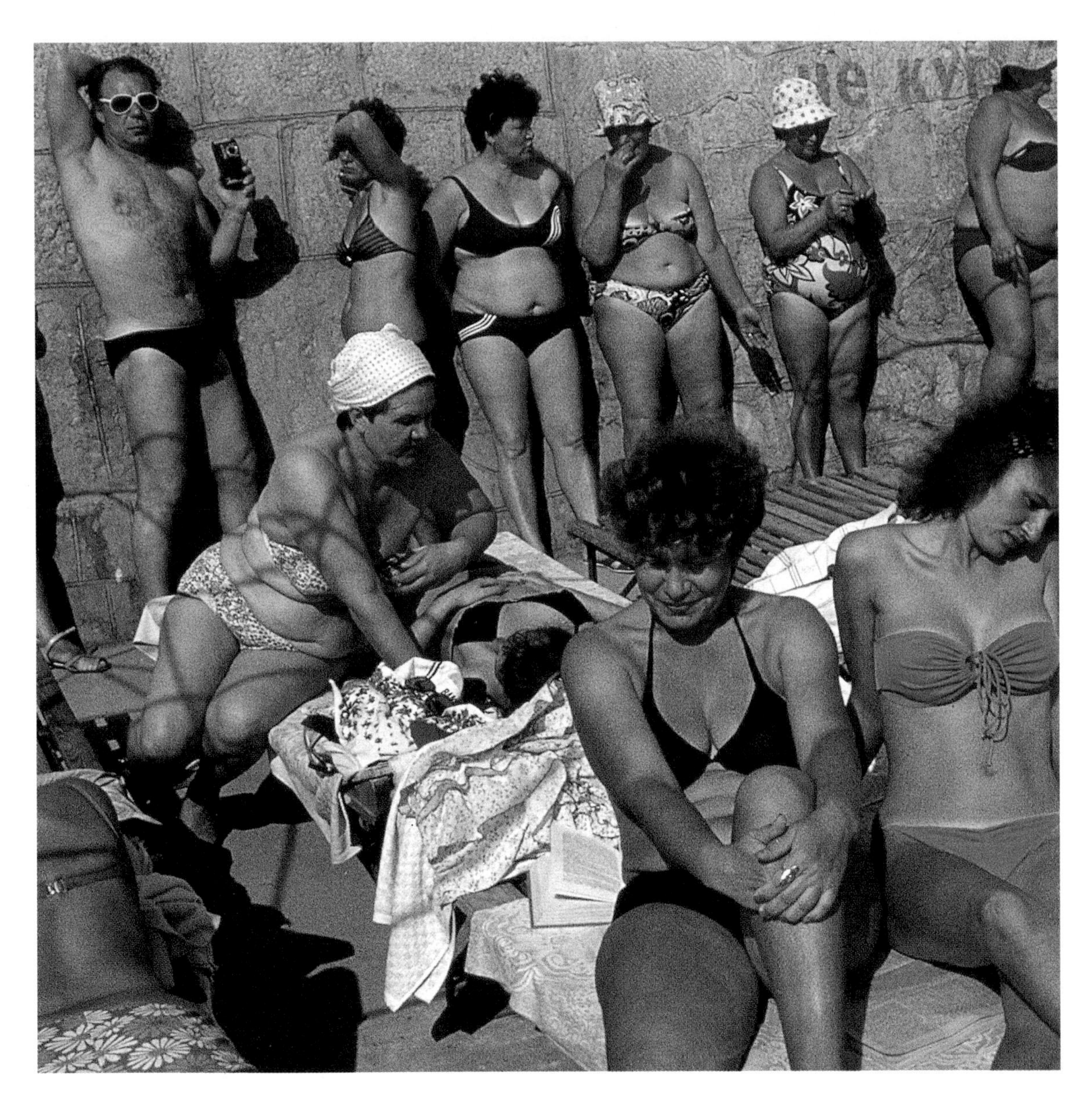

Try telling these sun-worshippers in the Ukraine that exposure to solar rays is dangerous - it feels good and it's free!

sun

Most people love being in the sun - and in moderation it can be good for you. Sunshine, as a rich source of vitamin D, is necessary for healthy development, and most people say they feel and look better with a suntan. But there's no doubt about it - the sun damages your skin.

We are living in a constantly evolving relationship with the sun, especially now that our own environmental foibles have thrown an age-old balancing act into question. The sun provides both the heat and light for life to survive, and the gravitational pull to hold the planet in place. Its warmth is one of our simplest and greatest pleasures. But its untrammelled power is equally life-threatening, as we are steadily learning.

Through the centuries, we have animated the sun, deified it, and dissected it scientifically in our efforts to explain and understand its power. Yet it remains an essential mystery. The Egyptians believed the sun was actually the eye of their sun god Ra. They, along with the Assyrians and Babylonians, and later the Greeks and Romans, acknowledged the sun's power to renew and restore. They were also probably the world's first sunbathers.

With the fall of the Roman Empire, and a shift in the seat of power from Mediterranean coastal countries to more northerly kingdoms, ideals of beauty changed, and a fascination for pale skin tones developed. Tanned skin soon denoted peasants and farmers, paler skin the non-labouring classes. This division of light and dark inspired generations of women to search for the perfect pale complexion with a variety of toxic skin tonics and powders that contained everything from mercury to white lead.

Although pale complexions were still in vogue in the 19th century, heliotherapy, the art of healing with sunlight, was also fashionable. It was championed by Niels R. Finsen, a Dane who founded the Light Institute for Tuberculosis patients and was awarded a Nobel prize in 1903. Suntanning as we understand the idea finally appeared in the 1920s when fashion arbiter Coco Chanel popularised the deliberate pursuit of a darker skin tone among cafe society's well-heeled leisure-seekers. In *Tender is the Night*, his depiction of the young swingers of his day, F. Scott Fitzgerald turned the tan into an identity badge for the in-crowd.

With that kind of social cachet to back it up, the suntan inevitably edged into the mainstream. In 1944 the first suntan lotion was marketed by a Miami pharmacist, and tanning became a sport of its own, its possible health benefits flung aside in the face of the search for the perfect tan.

One rather arcane anthropological interpretation suggests that tanning is the 20th century version of a sun

The more we know about the effects of the sun on our skin, the better we are able to protect ourselves. Practising safe sun won't curb enjoyment and can save your skin - and your life.

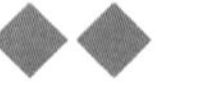

sacrifice in which we individually offer our bodies to the sun god. Dubious spiritual impulses aside, what is true is that tanning is unique in that it is the only semi-permanent body decoration that the Western world condones - most of our facial and body decorations are designed to wash off at the end of a day. If other cultures use permanent decoration such as tattooing and scarification as a form of communication, can the same be said of a tan? For the past 50 years, a good tan has signified attributes ranging from good health and good looks to wealth and a certain social status. Now that's subliminal communication of the best kind, and it's a difficult message to combat.

The Aztecs lived in constant fear that one day the sun would decide not to rise, and believed that humans had a responsibility to feed the sun to keep it alive. They routinely performed human sacrifice for its benefit, carving the heart out of a living being and offering it up (although anthropologists suggest this practice was also useful in scaring their enemies and keeping the Aztec population in check).

But combat it we must. The sun demands respect and a little healthy fear for more than its mystical and life-enhancing qualities. Look at the behaviour of the people who live in the sun. They stay out of it if they can. Many Mediterranean people prefer to stay sheltered while the sun is strongest, whilst North Africans generally cover the body to protect it further. The Cueva of Columbia alternate three or four hours' work with long cooling-off periods in the forest. And as long ago as the time of the Pharaohs, the oils, unguents and cosmetics used by the Ancient Egyptians to moisturise and decorate their skin probably acted as proto-sunscreens.

WHAT IS LIGHT?

The earth is constantly bombarded by electro-magnetic waves of varying lengths. From the longest to the shortest, the waves range from radio waves and infrared rays which heat, to visible light. (This includes all the light in the spectrum: red, orange, yellow, green, blue and violet.) The other waves are ultraviolet light, x-rays, gamma rays and, last of all, cosmic rays that never reach the earth.

Humans can see only the visible light rays, although the other waves can and do affect us. When we are in the sun, for example, the waves that harm normal skin are ultraviolet (UV) rays, not the visible light we can see with our eyes.

Fresh snow reflects 85 per cent of the sun's rays and dry sand 17 per cent. Some 30 to 50 per cent of UVA and UVB rays pass through cloud cover.

UVA, B AND C

Sunlight consists of different wavelengths of radiation: including ultraviolet A, ultraviolet B and ultraviolet C.

All three can damage your skin.

UVA rays gradually destroy the skin's elasticity and contribute to premature skin ageing and wrinkling. The longer wavelength and lower energy content of these rays generally means that they trigger melanin production without seriously burning the skin, but they also allow them to penetrate into the dermal layer, disturbing the body's collagen and elastin, and causing wrinkling and sagging. They can also trigger skin blisters, super fragile skin (called skin fragility syndrome), and sun allergies and photodermatoses. Evidence suggests UVA rays also contribute to the development of skin cancer. UVA rays are strong from dawn to dusk all year round - not just in summer or at noon.

UVB rays are responsible for tanning - but also for burning and the development of skin cancer. These rays are at their most intense at midday, in midsummer, in hot climates and at high altitudes. UVB rays usually attack the epidermis, the outermost layer of the skin.

UVC rays are the most damaging, but are filtered by the ozone layer and so don't reach the earth.

INFRARED

We feel infrared rays as heat. Present research indicates that in itself infrared is not harmful to the skin, but it may help increase the harmful effects of UV radiation. This is another reason to use good UVA and UVB protection.

RAY FACTS

According to one recent research paper, UVA rays are a thousand times less powerful than UVB rays, but still a threat. UVA coverage remains fairly constant throughout the seasons, throughout the day and even at varying altitudes. There are also about 20 times more UVA than UVB rays present at midday in midsummer, making them a potentially harmful force within the skin. And recent research suggests that UVA rays have a role in stimulating UVB rays into action.

Given the characteristics of these types of ultraviolet light, it seems at least one of these rays will be threatening your skin no matter where you go. No wonder the skin has had to arm itself accordingly.

THE OZONE FACTOR

Until recently, we were oblivious to the ozone layer. It simply did its job, filtering harmful UV rays from the earth's atmosphere. Then came the news that there was a hole in the ozone above the Antarctic and Chicken Little's prophecy about the sky falling down started to look like the stuff of nightmare. Thanks to a proliferation of manmade chemicals, primarily the now-banned chlorofluorocarbons (CFCs) and halons, which leak into the upper atmosphere and accumulate over time, the depletion in the ozone layer poses a whole new set of problems for mankind.

And the risks are just as great for animal, marine and plant life. Although we have yet to suffer the full effects of the depletion, reindeer in the Arctic Circle are already finding that their main food source, reindeer moss, has been affected, so they no longer have enough to eat. Friends of the Earth say plankton will be killed off by the increased levels of UVB which will pass the problem down through the marine food chain. And crop yields may also be affected.

BE SAFE UNDER THE SUN

The skin is the body's protective barrier. The largest organ in the body, it is designed to keep our insides in, and just about everything else out. The skin does have a defense system against the sun's harsh rays, but it was not designed for the extreme circumstances in which we have placed our bodies over the past 50 years.

So how does the body fend off ultraviolet radiation? About 60 per cent of the UVB rays and 20 per cent of the UVA rays the skin comes into contact with are absorbed by keratin, a fibrous protein contained in the skin's uppermost layer, the stratum corneum. Those that make it through this initial barrier help stimulate the production of a thicker epidermal layer, designed to provide a more substantial and fundamental physical barrier against the invisible rays.

The other protective barrier is a tan, long the symbol of good health and vigour, but in fact the indication of something rather more sinister.

WHAT IS A TAN?

A tan occurs when the skin tries to protect itself from the sun's harmful rays. Once the skin is exposed to the sun, melanocytes, specialised cells found in the basal layer of the epidermis, speed into action to produce melanin. Melanin is a protective darkening pigment that is designed to shield the skin from further intrusion.

SPF or Sun Protection Factors were first developed by Professor Rudolf Schulze in Germany in 1956.

In Caucasian skin, it takes two to four days for a tan to develop, the time it takes for the melanin to be produced and to rise to the upper layers of the epidermis. The amount of melanin the skin produces depends on our genes, not on any lotions or creams. Black and Asiatic people have a constant supply of melanin or pigment on hand at the surface ready to filter harsh rays. Olive-toned Mediterranean skins may tan with a fair amount of ease. However people with pale skin, blue eyes and red or fair hair, who tend to burn easily and tan with difficulty, produce less melanin which reacts much more slowly.

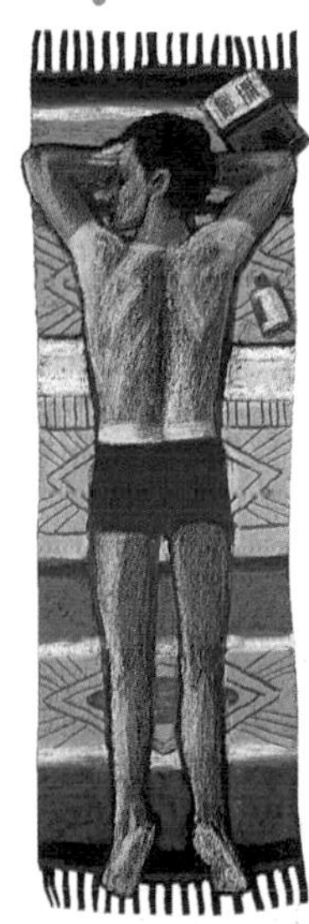

This group is at greatest risk from the sun. Such physical traits are usually characteristic of people from northerly countries, where cold weather and fairly regular cloud cover may have made it difficult for their ancestors to soak up enough vitamin D fortifying sunshine. In these conditions a low melanin content may have been a logical response to the weather systems. But modern man and woman has wrought havoc on the careful genetic alterations of generations by emigrating or holidaying in the sun.

American and European regulatory bodies use different standards to measure a sunscreen's protective capabilities, which means that different companies can offer different amounts of UVB protection while claiming as though they offer the same.

BLACK AND ASIAN SKINS

By the very nature of their skin, Afro-Caribbean and Asian people are better able to withstand the sun's damaging rays. Melanin, the pigment that gives their skin its darker colour, is also the substance the body uses to screen harmful UV rays. Because Asian and black skins contain a high percentage of melanin that is always in the surface layers of the skin, they have immediate protection from the sun.

Reduction in the ozone layer may lead to greater exposure to UV radiation. It is now predicted that a sustained 10 per cent decrease in ozone will be associated with a 26 per cent increase in non-melonoma skin cancer. All other things remaining constant, this would mean an increase in excess of 300,000 cases per year worldwide. (Statistics from Greenpeace.)

Black skins have a thicker epidermis to tackle harsh rays, and a more efficient vasodilatory system with which to handle excess heat. They also generally produce more sebum, which helps to filter UV light. But unfortunately, not all UV rays are screened by the extra protection, and some rays will penetrate to the dermal layer, initiating, albeit to a lesser degree, the same photo-ageing changes, such as elastosis, evident in Caucasian skins.

Black and Asian people do suffer from skin cancer, but it is an unusual occurrence. Recent research suggests that this might be a result of a genetic predisposition evident in people of all races, and not a direct result of over-exposure to UV radiation. Research into immunology at the University of Miami has shown that a particular gene called UVB-S, present in about 40 per cent of the population, makes the skin sensitive to UVB radiation. The immune systems of people with this gene shut down after UVB exposure. So, whether white, black or Asian, even heavily pigmented skins don't necessarily offer the immune system adequate protection from UVB rays.

HOW UV AFFECTS THE SKIN

UV radiation assaults the body on many levels and triggers a variety of reactions throughout it.

ON SUNBURNS AND SKIN CELLS

The common sunburn is often considered a precursor to a tan. Unfortunately, nothing could be further from the truth. Though they both tend to reflect a low melanin content in the skin, sunburns are triggered by a completely different set of circumstances than a tan.

Sunburns are generally thought to be caused by short UVB rays hitting the skin's surface and causing trauma to unsuspecting cells. The skin cells react as they would to any other kind of burn from hot water or heat - blood capillaries dilate in an attempt to rid the skin of excess heat, and the cells fill with liquid, slightly swelling the skin. Applying soothing anti-inflammatory and anti-bacterial products may ease the pain and decrease the risk of infection, but once the skin has been burned there is little that can be done to reverse the condition. The body has to go through its normal repair process, and the skin may blister and peel as this takes place. Severe erythema, as it is known medically, can be extremely painful, resulting in fevers, chills and nausea.

But that's not all the bad news. A more deadly aspect of sunburns is that they are a harbinger of skin cancer. Statistics show that even one sunburn in adolescence can double the chances of skin cancer later in life. This happens because the sunburned cells are replaced during the repair process with cells in which the DNA (the cell's genetic blueprint) has mutated due to UV damage. The skin has a memory for sunburn which can come back to haunt us.

Recent work has also revealed that sunburn, even of the mildest sort, can affect the immune system. Studies in America showed that, of a test group of subjects who suffered from sunburn, 95 per cent had a diminished ability to deal with a foreign intruder in the body, regardless of whether the intruder was placed near the sunburned site or not. In 30 per cent of the cases, the immune system was tricked into thinking the intruder was actually part of the body, so it did nothing at all. Further cause for alarm comes from experiments using mice which found that skin tumours a normal immune system could deal with actually increased in size when the mouse had a sunburn.

SUN AND AGEING

Sun is a major cause of ageing. Up to 90 per cent of the effects we formerly attributed to the inevitabilities of ageing - wrinkling, dryness, blotching, loss of skin tone, sallow skin - are in fact sun damage.

Check your own body. The skin on your face and hands receives the most exposure, so compare its condition to that of a part of the body which has never been exposed. The difference is glaring, especially on older people. But children who have been overexposed to the sun will already have started to reflect the damage to their skin by the time they reach their twenties, years before the natural ageing process would normally register its effects.

Damage seems to occur in areas where UVA rays are absorbed, reaching down into the dermal layer of the skin and altering the DNA, the genetic code that in normal circumstances ensures every cell is rebuilt to the

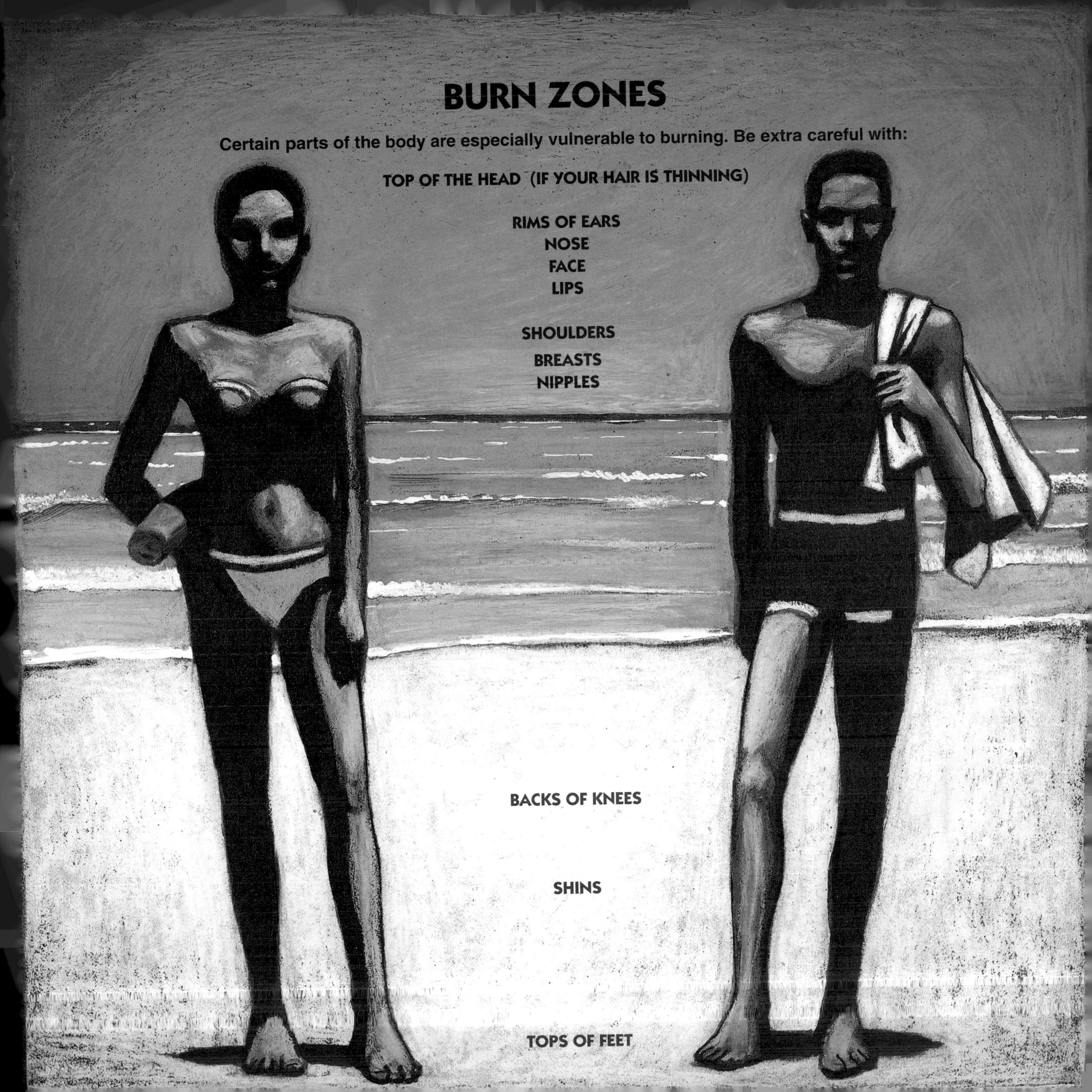
BURN ZONES
Certain parts of the body are especially vulnerable to burning. Be extra careful with:
TOP OF THE HEAD (IF YOUR HAIR IS THINNING)
RIMS OF EARS
NOSE
FACE
LIPS
SHOULDERS
BREASTS
NIPPLES
BACKS OF KNEES
SHINS
TOPS OF FEET

The threat to Australasians has been confirmed with findings that vets are treating hundreds of animals a year for skin cancer. The animals most at risk are light-furred creatures of European descent, such as white cats, white-faced Hereford cattle, English bull dogs and large white pigs. Accordingly, the Royal Society for the Prevention of Cruelty to Animals in Australia is recommending that pets be kept indoors between 11am and 3pm. Sun block and zinc creams can be applied to animals' noses and ears.

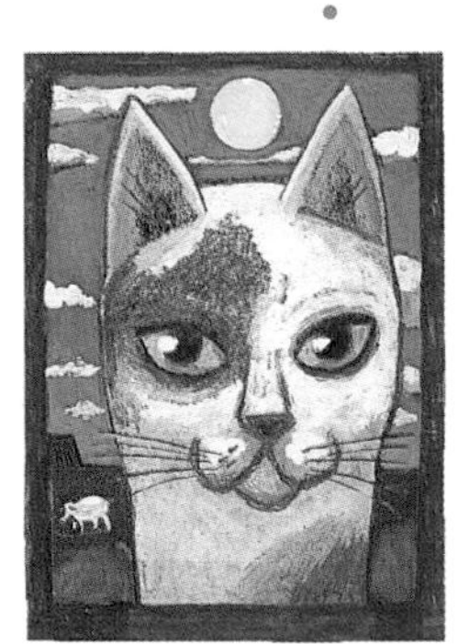

same design. The major villains in this process may be free radicals, rogue molecules of oxygen which oxidise or "rust" proteins and attack the DNA. They are caused in great numbers by UVA radiation. As well as contributing to elastosis, the breakdown of the supporting collagen and elastin fibres which give the skin its firm tone, free radicals can mutate genes so that they no longer replicate in the same manner. And UVB rays have their own part to play in the ageing process: they stimulate the production of the chemical interlukin 1 in the epidermal cells which sends a message to destroy elastin and collagen fibres.

If, at the end of this litany of sun-induced woe, it is becoming increasingly clear that excessive exposure to the sun speeds up the ageing process, perhaps some small encouragement can be derived from the deduction that early protection should help to avoid up to 70 per cent of skin damage caused by the sun.

SKIN CANCER

There can be no doubt about the correlation between UV exposure and skin cancer. The statistics are frightening. In the UK skin cancer is the second most common cancer - an estimated 30,000 new cases a year are diagnosed. In the USA the American Academy of Dermatology estimates that one in six Americans will contract the disease in his or her lifetime, and one in every three new cancers diagnosed is skin cancer. The figures are getting worse. In the USA and Scandinavia, skin cancer figures have doubled in the past ten years, and in Scotland, incidence of cutaneous melanoma, one specific type of skin cancer, is up by 80 per cent.

The reasons why skin cancer rates are rocketing are numerous, ranging from something as simple as the fact that we are living longer, and children are more exposed to UV radiation than they used to be, to the fact that more people can afford to take holidays in the sun. Any Caucasians who have overexposed themselves to the sun are possible victims. Those of Celtic origin, or those with particularly fair skins, red, blonde or light brown hair and blue eyes, have very little built-in protection and should be especially careful in the sun.

TYPES OF SKIN CANCER

BASAL CELL CARCINOMA

Accounts for 75 per cent of skin cancer cases in the UK. It develops in the hair follicles or basal layers of the epidermis, and is classified as a slow-growing cancer. Basal cell carcinoma usually shows up in people over 60, on the head, neck, arms and hands, the parts of the body regularly exposed to the sun. Because it is slow growing, it doesn't usually spread and has an excellent recovery rate. However if it is allowed to continue to grow, it can turn into an ulcer known as a rodent ulcer. There are several types of basal cell carcinomas, the most common of which is nodular basal cell carcinoma, which appears as pearly or waxy nodules 0.5 to 1cm in diameter on the skin.

SQUAMOUS CELL CARCINOMA

Develops in the epidermis or mature cells in the dermis and has a tendency to spread, making it more dangerous. If left untreated this cancer can be fatal; in the USA it is estimated to have caused 2,100 deaths in 1992. Squamous cell carcinomas are painless, crusty, red areas that show up in skin that has been exposed to the sun, especially the lower lip, ears and scalp on bald men. When treated immediately there is a high recovery rate.

MALIGNANT MELANOMA

The third and most deadly of the three types of skin cancer. According to the American Academy of Dermatology, incidences of malignant melanoma in the USA increased by 94 per cent while non-melanoma skin cancers increased by only 11 per cent between 1980 and 1989. Malignant melanoma is most often found on women's legs and men's trunks, although it can show up anywhere on the body, even the soles of the feet. If left untreated, it can spread to other organs in the body and can be fatal. In the UK, women are twice as likely as men to contract the disease.

SEVEN-POINT MALIGNANT MELANOMA CHECKLIST:

Although there are several types of melanoma, most of the warning signs are similar. Seven features are found more commonly in melanoma than in benign lesions. They are divided into three major features and four minor features. If you have one of the three major signs, you should see a dermatologist. If you have any concerns about moles on your body, seek medical advice as quickly as possible. The faster malignant melanoma is diagnosed, the more quickly it can be dealt with.

Major features of moles:

- Change in size
- Irregular shape
- Irregular colour

Minor features of moles:

- Largest diameter 7mm or greater
- Inflammation
- Oozing, crusting or bleeding
- Change in sensation (mild itch)

(With acknowledgement to Marie Curie Cancer Care and Professor Rona MacKie.)

WHO'S AT RISK?

Although UVB's burning rays are already acknowledged as an important factor in skin cancer, there is still some debate as to the role of UVA rays in the scheme of things. What is known is that different kinds of sun exposure do trigger different sorts of cancer. Basal and squamous cell carcinomas are, for example, most prevalent among people who have spent a significant amount of time in the sun over a period of years. Farmers, outdoor workers and sportspeople are much more likely to contract these two strains of the disease than other members of the public. Meanwhile, studies in Canada, Scandinavia, Scotland and Australia have discovered that office workers or urban dwellers who go on holiday and spend short periods of time in intense sun stand a much higher risk of developing malignant melanoma. The problem seems to be that Caucasian skin, exposed to intermittent bursts of hot sun, cannot acclimatise to harsh UV rays. This at least partly explains why the figures for malignant melanoma have risen so dramatically in recent years. Sunseekers may be getting a lot more than they bargained for on their package tour getaways.

The Body Shop's Watermelon Sun Care Range is formulated to be straightforward and easy to use. All the sunscreens offer both UVA and UVB protection.

A final statistic amid the growing number of cases of malignant melanoma may offer some hope for re-educating the public in future. Studies around the world confirm that sun exposure at a young age sets the stage for cancer later on in life. Conversely, one authoritative American study estimates that regular use of SPF 15 sunscreens during the first 18 years of life could reduce your "lifetime risk" of non-melanoma skin cancer by 78 per cent. Once again, the message is: take early protection.

SIMPLE STEPS TO SAFER SUN

PROTECT

Sun protection is a vital part of skin care and should be applied whenever you are outside - all year round.

Given the facts, it is plain old common sense to make proper sun coverage a health priority to protect the body not only from the ageing effects of the sun but its serious health risks too. By avoiding the hottest parts of the day when UV radiation is at its peak, and selecting the appropriate protection product, the risk of injury to the skin can be reduced.

If in doubt about the level of protection you need, choose a sunscreen with a high SPF - this leaves an extra margin of protection for uneven application and rubbing off. Don't make the mistake of thinking you won't get a tan with maximum protection creams. You'll simply tan more slowly and more safely.

CUTTING THROUGH THE CONFUSION

A sunscreen marked with a Sun Protection Factor (SPF) gives an indication of how long you can stay in the sun without burning when you use this product. The higher the SPF, the greater the protection. SPFs indicate protection against UVB rays only.

In theory, if your unprotected skin can take ten minutes of sun without burning, using an SPF 6 means you can stay in the sun approximately six times longer than if you were unprotected (6 x 10 = 60 minutes). In practice, things aren't so simple. Variables include the strength of the sun and the amount of sunscreen you apply and *reapply* after swimming, sweating and friction from clothes.

If it sounds confusing, it is. The vast array of products on offer with different SPF numbers (from 2 to 30 and beyond) and ways of measuring them, means it is difficult

ALOE VERA

Though it looks like a cactus, aloe vera is actually a member of the lily family. The plant generally grows to around two feet tall and has no stem. Instead, it is supported by a thick gel which fills the rubbery leaves. This particular species was named aloe vera (true aloe) in ancient times because it was thought to have the best medicinal properties.

Alexander the Great was persuaded by his tutor Aristotle to invade the island of Socotra off the coast of East Africa to guarantee a supply of aloe to heal the wounds of his soldiers.

Aloe vera is native to East and South Africa. Roman Catholic missionaries introduced it to the West Indies and Central and South America via Barbados in 1596. The Indians have since used it for centuries as a treatment for burns. They call it the wand of heaven.

Columbus took aloe with him for medicinal purposes on his voyages.

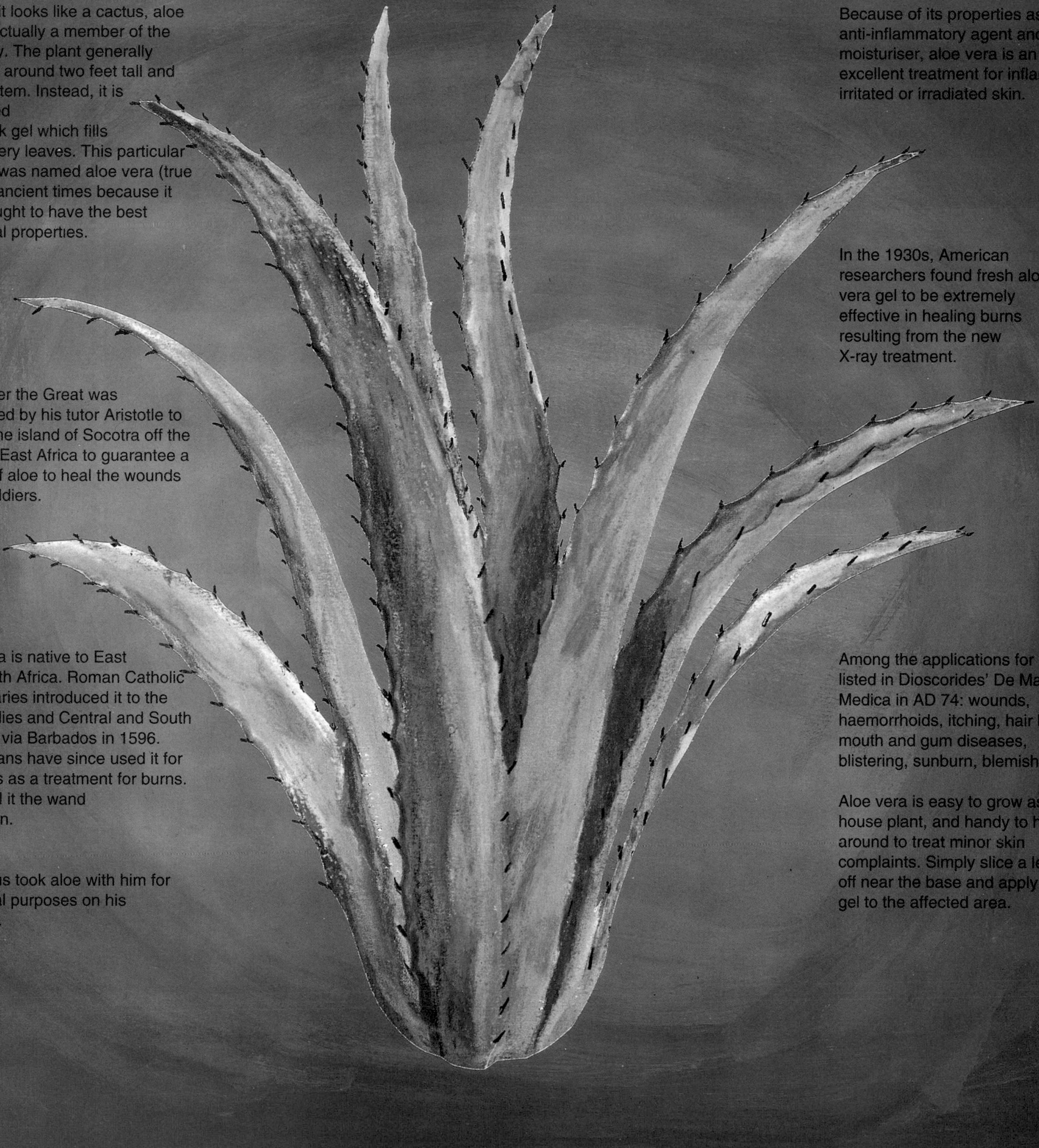

Because of its properties as an anti-inflammatory agent and moisturiser, aloe vera is an excellent treatment for inflamed, irritated or irradiated skin.

In the 1930s, American researchers found fresh aloe vera gel to be extremely effective in healing burns resulting from the new X-ray treatment.

Among the applications for aloe listed in Dioscorides' De Materia Medica in AD 74: wounds, haemorrhoids, itching, hair loss, mouth and gum diseases, blistering, sunburn, blemishes.

Aloe vera is easy to grow as a house plant, and handy to have around to treat minor skin complaints. Simply slice a leaf off near the base and apply the gel to the affected area.

to make informed choices. There is no international SPF system yet, so a product that is SPF 20 in America may be as protective as an SPF 10 in Europe. Add to that different systems of UVA ratings and it's hard to know what you are buying.

Regular use of a highly protective sunscreen for the first 18 years of life may reduce the risk of certain types of skin cancer by as much as 70 per cent.

SOOTHE

Skin which has been exposed to the sun will be especially dry, so it is vital to keep it well moisturised. The action of the sun's rays on your skin doesn't stop when you cover up, so an effective aftersun product can help minimise damage and prolong a tan.

Do follow an after-sun programme once out of the sun. Protection from sun damage needs diligence before and after exposure, as much as during. Any kind of sun exposure is traumatic to the skin, even when "armed" with a sun tan, and a thicker epidermis. The sun leaches precious moisture from the skin, which should be replaced as quickly as possible.

• If you have burnt your skin, try to drink as much cool water as possible. UV rays continue to do their worst once you are out of the sun, so take a cool bath or shower to lower the body's temperature slowly and hinder the process.

• Even if you're not burned, a cool bath or a soothing shower is a good idea to cleanse the body of excess dirt, sweat, salt or chemicals from swimming pools. Gently slough off any rough bits of skin.

• Apply after-sun moisturisers to help the skin in its process of repair. Aloe vera is one of nature's great post-sun soothers. And look for the anti-inflamatory ingredient alpha-bisabobol, a derivative of camomile, which will help bring down the swelling and redness in burned skin.

But remember, nothing can speed up the healing process.

PRETEND

It's easy to achieve a healthy looking glow without exposing your skin to the sun's harmful rays.

In the face of all the negative press about the harmful effects of the sun on the skin, a new generation of tanning products has taken the sun market by storm. Known as self-tanners, they were once the preserve of the deathly white melanin-deprived who were too shy to sit on the beach.

Ideally, everyone, regardless of colour, should feel comfortable with the shade of skin they were born with. But even if self-tanners don't redress our desire for a tan, they are proving effective as a halfway measure in weaning many off direct exposure to the sun.

Successful fake tanning is all about preparation.

• When applying a self-tanner, a good first step is exfoliation to rid the skin of dead skin cells and generally provide a smooth, even canvas. Then moisturise to make the skin supple and receptive.

• Take your time to apply these lotions. Use smooth, circular strokes and massage in well to avoid blotching and streaking. More effective than plastering it on is the application of several thin coats.

• Watch out for easy-to-miss spots like the backs of arms and knees, inner thighs and the side of the body.

• Wash your hands afterwards, and don't dress for at least half an hour as the lotion may stain clothes and leave the colour patchy.

• Several applications during the course of a day will help get the best coverage and colour.

• The colour fades as the skin naturally exfoliates. But regular exfoliation and bathing will help speed the fade.

Alternatively, faking it is easy with instant bronzing cosmetics which give a natural-looking glow to your face and body. Quick to apply and instantly removable, these cosmetics give you complete control over how tanned you become. Colourings, The Body Shop's make-up range, has products to suit all tastes and skin types.

CHILDREN AND THE SUN

If there is any hard and fast rule bred from our new consciousness of the sun's side effects, it is surely this: children should be protected at all times from excessive exposure to the sun. One severe sunburn before the age

The Body Shop's Self Tan Lotion contains dihydroxyacetone, a synthetic match to an ingredient found naturally in the body. It sits on the uppermost layer of the skin, the stratum corneum, and reacts with the amino acids in keratin and sweat to stain the skin a light brown. Walnut extract contains natural dyes that also stain the skin.

How to choose the right sunglasses. A good pair of sunglasses helps to protect eyes and stop you squinting, which causes crow's feet. Polarising lenses cut down on glare and are recommended if you're going to be near the water. Not all tinted lenses protect against UV rays - dark lenses can be misleading because the degree of tint is not an indication of UV absorbency. In fact, non-UV lenses can be dangerous. Low visible light causes the pupil to dilate, letting in more damaging UV light. To be sure, check with your optician.

of 20 can double a child's chance of skin cancer later in life.

An Australian study has suggested that a European child arriving in the country under the age of ten will be subject to the same rates of skin cancer as the regular population, but if that child arrives at the age of 15, his or her chances of contracting the disease are lower. Why? We absorb most of our UV radiation before the age of 20, turning our bodies into time bombs not only capable of ageing the skin, but causing cancer as we hit middle age.

Children spend much more time outdoors than adults, exposing themselves to three times more UV radiation than the average adult. To make matters worse, children have less natural protection against the sun. Their skin is thinner than adults', they have less melanin at hand to protect their skin; and the stratum corneum, the skin's outermost protective barrier, is not completely developed until the age of four.

HERE ARE A FEW POINTERS FOR EFFECTIVE SUN CARE FOR CHILDREN:

DON'T ever expose babies under six months of age to direct sunlight. Protect them with a hat, clothing and an unfragranced, uncoloured sun block.

DO keep children out of the sun during the middle of the day, when it is at its strongest.

DO protect children with a high SPF broad spectrum sunscreen. Cover all the body, especially sun-sensitive areas such as face, ears, neck, upper chest and arms with a high SPF. Try The Body Shop Sun Block SPF 20+. Apply generously before any outdoor activity - not just at the beach - and even on cloudy days. Reapply frequently. If children are going to be near water, a water-resistant sunscreen should be used.

DO make sure a hat or a cap with a visor is worn at all times in the sun. Long-sleeved T-shirts are a good idea if the sun is especially intense.

DON'T stop using sunscreens after a tan appears. Tanned skin is not sufficient protection against the sun's ultraviolet rays.

Finally, teach older children the importance of protective suncare. And set them a good example. Use an effective after-sun product. The Body Shop Aloe Gel is especially good for children.

EYE CARE - DO YOU?

Despite the fact that we worry incessantly about the impact of ultraviolet rays on our skin, we tend to forget about our eyes, often as not buying sunglasses for their fashion currency rather than their protective qualities. But ultraviolet light is as much of a threat to the eyes as it is to the rest of the body. Snow blindness, the inflammation of the cornea, is caused by excessive UV light, as are cataracts, which are actually the eye's efforts to protect itself with a yellow pigment that is its equivalent of melanin. As the pigment builds up slowly over the years, it creates a cloud-like substance floating over the iris.

For everyday wear, sunglasses should block 95 per cent of UVB rays and 60 per cent of UVA rays. For sports like skiing, glasses should block 99 per cent of UVB rays and 60 per cent of UVA rays. Leather side shields often featured on mountaineering glasses cut glare and prevent the eyes from drying out. However, according to experts, a baseball cap or any hat with a four inch brim will reduce the amount of sun getting to the eyes by up to 50 per cent.

Snow reflects 85 per cent of UV radiation right back in your face.

Intense exposure to infrared light can also burn the retina. Labourers in Victorian glass factories who worked in front of furnaces loaded with infrared light often lost their sight in middle age. Just as a sunscreen that can handle both UVB and UVA rays is essential, so are sunglasses that screen UVA, UVB and infrared rays.

LIP CARE

Lips are prime targets for sun damage. They are exposed all year round, have no melanin and are very thin-skinned. The lower lip is a common site for carcinomas and UVA rays hasten depletion of collagen, one of the reasons lines form and lips thin with age. When in the sun, make sure you treat your lips to constant applications of a lip balm with added sunscreen (try The Body Shop's Honey Stick, SPF 15). Opaque lipstick provides some physical sunblock, but products with an added sunscreen and moisturising properties are preferable.

SUN DOS AND DONTS

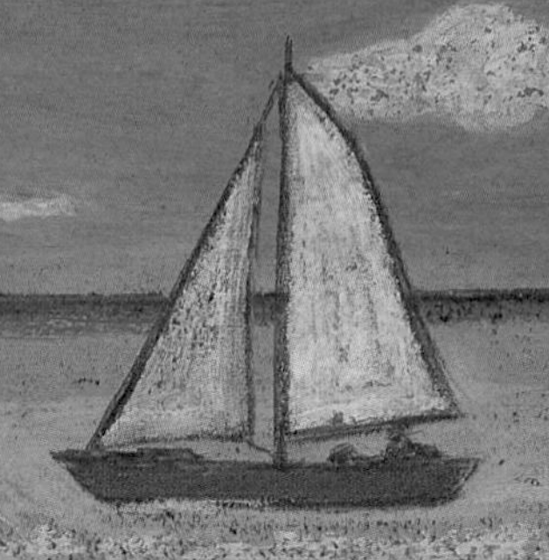

DO remember that UV rays are far more powerful closest to the equator where you'll require a higher level of protection.

DO choose a water-resistant formula if you are going to be near water, and reapply once you are out of the water.

DON'T forget that reflective surfaces like water and snow can increase the amount of UV rays penetrating the skin, and protect yourself accordingly.

DO avoid, whenever possible, going out in the sun between 11am and 3pm, especially during the summer months. This is when the the sun is directly overhead and UV rays have a direct path down to the earth.

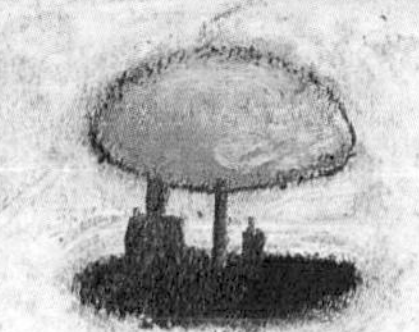

DO apply sun lotion generously at least half an hour before you go into the sun and, once in the sun, don't forget to reapply every few hours. Use twice as much sunscreen as you would a body lotion.

DO choose a sun product that contains both UVA and UVB sunscreens. At the moment, it is really up to the consumer to research the products he or she buys and ensure that adequate UVB and UVA or broad spectrum protection is offered. Because UVA sunscreens were not considered important until recently, no accurate system has been developed to assess UVA protection in sun products. So the Sun Protection Factor (SPF) refers to the amount of UVB protection a product offers the skin.

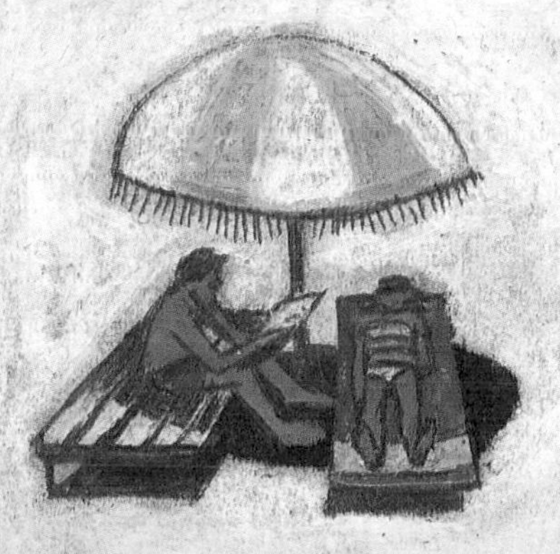

DO remember that the face always displays the first signs of ageing so give it extra protection. Use a higher SPF product than on the body. Wear a hat with a wide brim. If constant UVA exposure is an issue, consider wearing a light sunscreen year round to offer complete protection. Many basic cosmetic products now contain sunscreens.

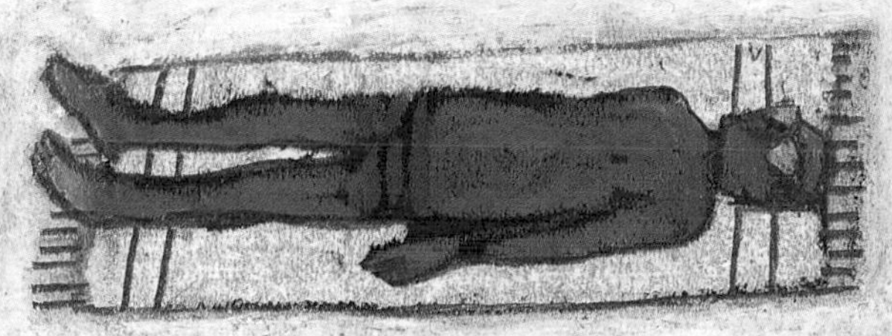

DO pay extra attention to vulnerable or exposed parts of the body, not just the ears and nose, but the collarbone, shoulderbone, tops of feet, breasts, nipples, shins and backs of knees.

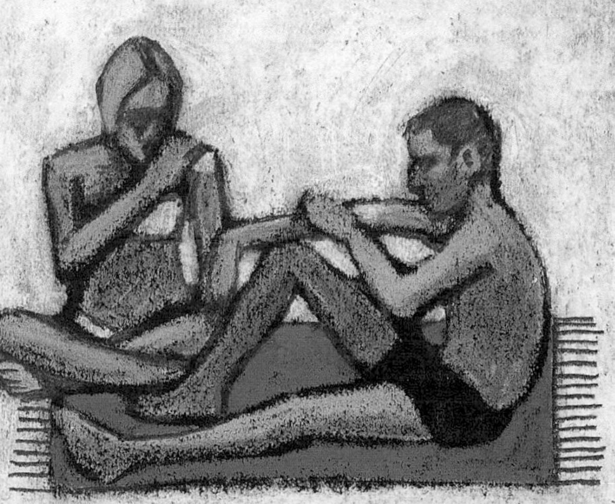

DON'T overdo it. Restricting yourself to 10-15 minutes of sun exposure on the first day of a holiday is a wise move. If you must tan, build up the skin's tolerance to the sun in steps.

Seasonal Affective Disorder (SAD) is a cause of depression and high suicide rates during the winter months. The problem lies with the pineal gland, which, if not regularly stimulated by the sun, is slow to produce melantonin, a hormone which affects our moods, sleep patterns, insulin production and general feeling of well being. The problem is easily solved - to restimulate the gland, you simply need to increase the amount of visible light encountered by the body. It is not, however, ultraviolet radiation, but full spectrum lighting that is required for the process. This type of light can be artificially produced and does not require extensive UV exposure.

HAIR CARE

The first flush of a sunburn makes the skin swell, smoothing out lines. You may think you look better but it's actually a sign of injury.

Although sunlight will not damage hair permanently, it can spoil its condition, colour and texture. Chlorinated water can cause damage to the hair, which may result in a colour change. Coloured or permed hair is particularly vulnerable.

Rinse hair after swimming to remove salt, sand and chlorine. Comb through a gel such as aloe for minimal protection. Alternately, twist hair into a chignon or wind into a top knot and cover with a bandana, scarf or hat for maximum protection. Gently shampoo in the evening after sun exposure and condition well. For best results, use specially formulated shampoos, conditioners and styling products.

(See Hair chapter for more information on hair care.)

SUNBEDS

Originally conceived as a foolproof way of getting a tan, sunbeds have proved to be increasingly dangerous. Alerted to the issue of UVB cancer-causing rays, most sunbed operators promote sunbeds with UVA rays, the rays that were considered "good" tanning rays until very recently. Unfortunately, as we have seen elsewhere in this chapter, this is far from the case.

Officials are striving to regulate the industry in the USA, where sunbeds were a billion-dollar business in the 1980s. As of 1992, only 24 states had any kind of regulations. Unfortunately, even in states with stringent rules, there are problems. One such state is North Carolina, where a survey of tanning salons found only one salon of the 32 surveyed to be within regulations. With the improved quality of self-tanning lotions on the market, it makes no sense to risk one's health on a tanning bed in pursuit of a darker skin tone.

MYTHS AND FACTS

Sitting in the shade is safe

WRONG Be extra careful near highly reflective surfaces such as sand, water or snow. Apply sunscreen even when you are underneath a beach umbrella - the rays can reflect off the sand. Sun protection is an absolute must when skiing. Because you're at a high altitude, your skin needs even greater protection. Additionally the cold saps the skin's protective moisture barrier.

Clothing will completely protect my skin from sunburn

WRONG Clothing will filter out some UV rays, and covering up is the best way to reduce sun on the skin - but choose the fabric carefully. If you can see through the cloth, the sun can get through. The more tightly woven the cloth, the better the protection.

A cloudy day means I won't get burnt

WRONG Sunlight can penetrate clouds. Daylight gets through and so do the ultraviolet rays. In fact, many people are badly burned on cloudy days because they think they are safe and do not use a sunscreen.

Water-resistant and waterproof sunscreens do not need to be reapplied after swimming

WRONG Products with these claims mean they will maintain their SPF for a set time in water - water-resistant ones for at least 40 minutes, waterproof for at least 80. (these definitions may change with new legislation). However, you must reapply your sunscreen whenever you come out of the water. Remember, towelling dry will often remove any sunscreen.

I have dark skin, so I don't need a sunscreen

WRONG Darker skins do contain more melanin which offers some natural protection against burning, but this does not mean that they are immune to the sun's harmful rays. Olive, brown and black skins can burn if unprotected. And all skin types are susceptible to the weathering and premature aging effects of UV rays.

I only need a sunscreen when I am on holiday

WRONG The sun affects your skin whenever you are outdoors. Sunscreens should always be part of your routine, not just while sunbathing on the beach. Protection is vital all year round.

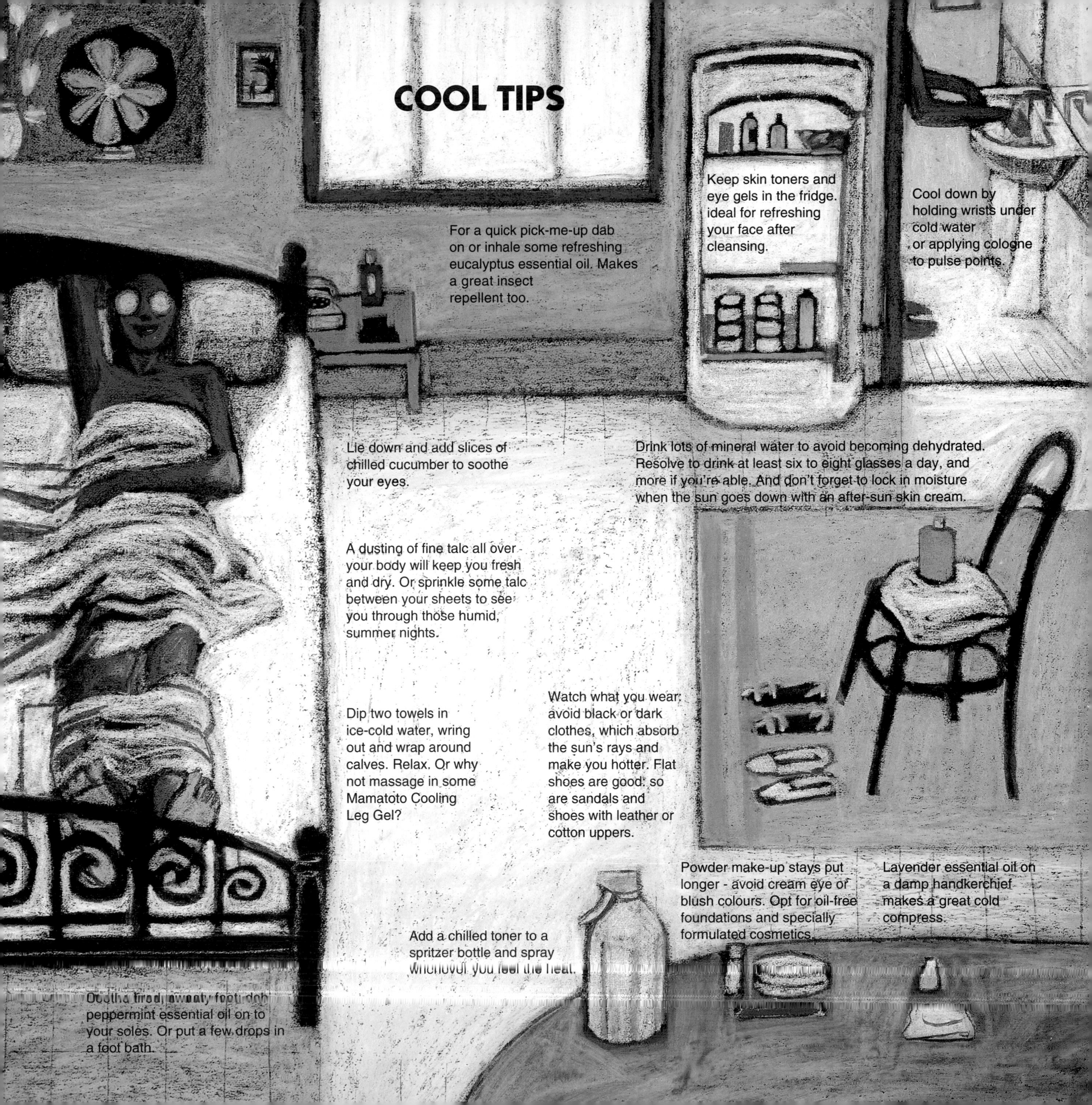

COOL TIPS

For a quick pick-me-up dab on or inhale some refreshing eucalyptus essential oil. Makes a great insect repellent too.

Keep skin toners and eye gels in the fridge. ideal for refreshing your face after cleansing.

Cool down by holding wrists under cold water or applying cologne to pulse points.

Lie down and add slices of chilled cucumber to soothe your eyes.

Drink lots of mineral water to avoid becoming dehydrated. Resolve to drink at least six to eight glasses a day, and more if you're able. And don't forget to lock in moisture when the sun goes down with an after-sun skin cream.

A dusting of fine talc all over your body will keep you fresh and dry. Or sprinkle some talc between your sheets to see you through those humid, summer nights.

Dip two towels in ice-cold water, wring out and wrap around calves. Relax. Or why not massage in some Mamatoto Cooling Leg Gel?

Watch what you wear: avoid black or dark clothes, which absorb the sun's rays and make you hotter. Flat shoes are good: so are sandals and shoes with leather or cotton uppers.

Powder make-up stays put longer - avoid cream eye or blush colours. Opt for oil-free foundations and specially formulated cosmetics.

Lavender essential oil on a damp handkerchief makes a great cold compress.

Add a chilled toner to a spritzer bottle and spray whenever you feel the heat.

Soothe tired, sweaty feet: dab peppermint essential oil on to your soles. Or put a few drops in a foot bath.

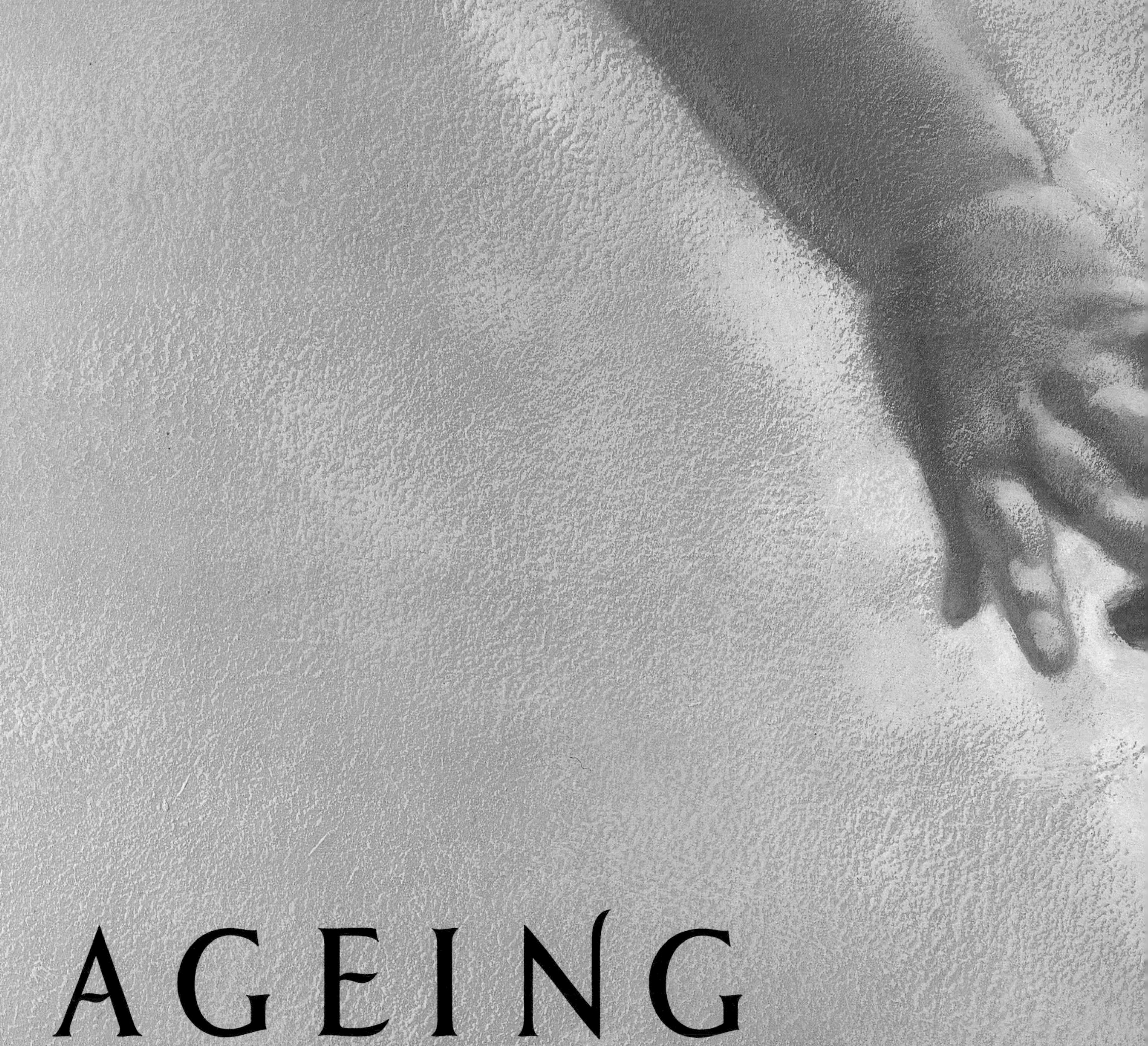

AGEING

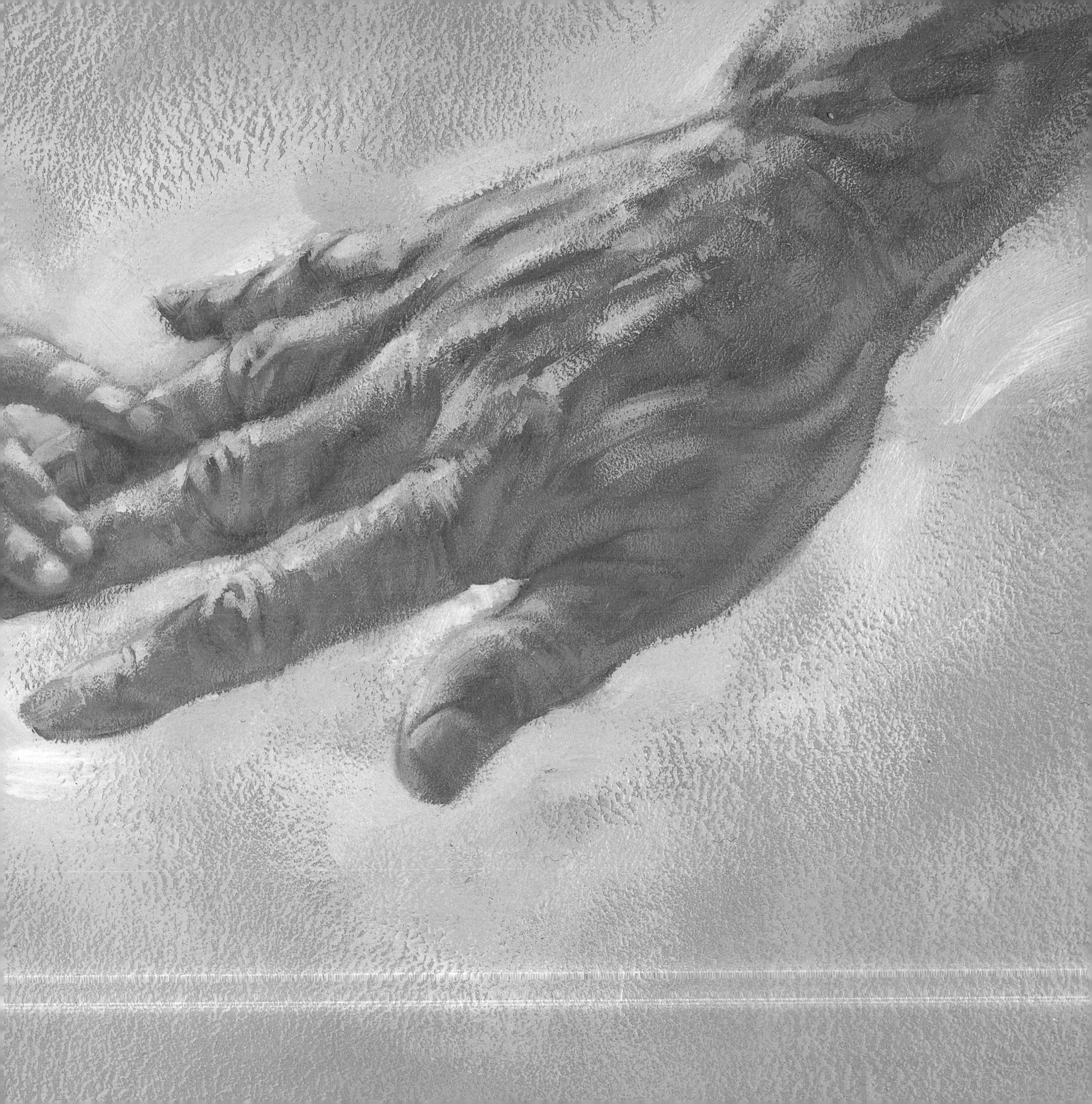

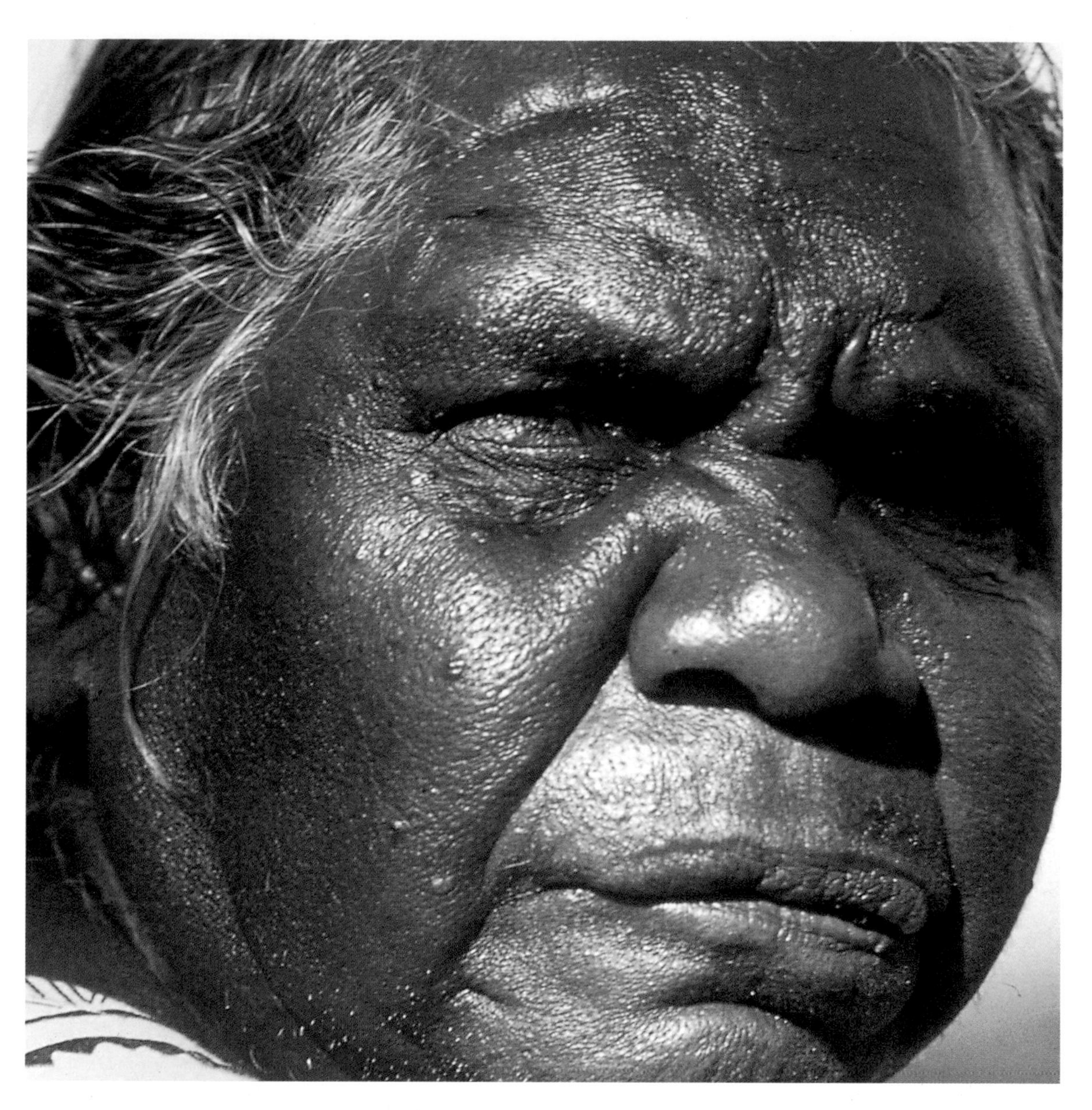

To a young Aborigine male in Australia, a seasoned old woman represents more than wisdom and experience - she is also an object of desire.

ageing

every culture has its own set of responses to ageing. In the West, we are slaves to chronology. We tend to base our assessment of the rights and abilities of others on their age. In fact, our culture's particular contribution to the list of isms that undermine humankind's finer instincts - racism, sexism and the whole motley crew - may well be ageism. And, equally, it may be the most pernicious, simply because it so blatantly ignores the facts of life in the late 20th century.

We're living longer and, on the whole, healthier lives than ever before. Neanderthal man lived 30 years on average. By the Renaissance, another eight had been added. In the 1880s, when German Chancellor Otto von Bismarck selected 65 as the age of retirement, average life expectancy was 45. The quantum leap came this century when at least 30 years were added to that figure. But private attitudes and public policy are still stuck in a time warp, maintaining the illusion that human capabilities seize up at an arbitrarily imposed date. And yet, by 2025, almost 20 per cent of the UK's population will be over 65, and China's elderly population will be as large as the entire population of the USA.

Design for the young and you exclude the old. Design for the old and you include the young.

Motto - Birmingham University's Centre for Applied Gerontology

In the sweep of history, this "life extension" has happened so quickly that it's no wonder we've scarcely acknowledged it, let alone come to grips with it. Given the statistics, the fear of ageing that is ingrained in our own culture starts to feel like an unrealistic kicking against the traces of time. But even societies that are more attuned to the need to keep their elderly as fully functioning members of the community must analyse their outlooks. At every level, from the upper echelons of government to the shopkeeper in the corner store, revisions of attitudes to ageing are essential for the future health and stability of humankind.

WHAT IS AGEING?

The human organism is undoubtedly a machine designed for living. Start with the rudiments. All mammals breathe once for every four heartbeats, so all mammals live for the same duration of relative biological time - except human beings. We live about three times longer than mammals of our body size should. In fact, we're the longest living mammal, ahead of the Indian elephant, the horse, the African elephant, hippopotamus, donkey, Indian rhinoceros and chimpanzee.

But are we made to age? Chronology and biology make their own set of distinctions. People who are low in DHEA, a hormone which regulates levels of cellular metabolism, immune functions and obesity, will typically be older biologically than they are chronologically. So in rare cases there is actually a physical basis for describing someone as "20 going on 70", even though when we make such a judgement, we are usually talking about a person's attitude. It's a way of acknowledging that ageing is a highly personal experience.

A Screen Actors' Guild study in the1970s found that positive portrayals of women on film begin to decrease when they hit 40. With men, they increase.

Logically, we should be reassured by the thought that the way we age is up to us, because such an idea lends us a degree of control over the uncontrollable. Instead, being human, our next step is illogical. We generalise wildly about ageing, sweeping vast numbers of people under one cheerless umbrella. The elderly especially are patronised. When we're not too scared to use the word "old", we chat patronisingly about "old folk" or "old boys and girls". When we are too scared, we talk euphemistically about "senior citizens" or "pensioners". Fear tends to spark that kind of over-reaction - we can thank our cultural conditioning for the tremors that the prospect of the passing of youth sets off in all too many hearts in the West. The only thing the Western world fears more than ageing is death: the next step. So our denial of the physical and emotional realities of ageing is really just the denial of death.

Given an ideal environment, the genetically planned cutoff point for homo sapiens is believed to be 115. But history records a range of variables. Legend has Karke, a Sumerian king, dying at 28,800. Biblical stalwarts Methuselah and Noah passed on at 969 and 950 respectively. More recently, Russian Shirali Mislimove died at an unsubstantiated 165, with his female counterpart Ashura Omarova claiming 195. In the United States, former slave Charlie Smith was allegedly 137 when he died in October 1979.

AGEISM - THE NEW BATTLEGROUND

MEN AND WOMEN AND AGEISM

Physically, a healthy 70-year-old male has more in common with a healthy 30-year-old than he does an ill man of his own age. His heart will pump blood as effectively under stress as that of the younger man. It is illness, not the wear and tear of ageing, that will stop a man reaching 70. In fact, if he makes it that far, the odds are on him reaching 80. And he'll look ten years younger than his female counterpart because a man's skin ages about ten years more slowly due to its greater thickness and oiliness.

But that's about the only edge nature gives the male of the species in the ageing game. The numbers suggest men in all cultures have a real problem coping with ageing. Males are susceptible to the myths about ageing - that it means an automatic decline in ability, agility, you name it. Self-esteem takes a real but rarely necessary whipping. Look at sex. How many men live in dread of a dying sex drive? The fact is that a man produces sperm well into his seventies, and there's no reason why his sex life shouldn't keep pace. But often men just aren't interested. One sad testament to this attitude is the suicide rate among men over 75: the highest in the general population. The rate among women of that age is less than half that of men.

Women simply seem to be better reconciled, physically and mentally, to the ageing process. Even with the greater risk of breast cancer they run in their fifties, women make up the majority of people over 65. Women of 65 and over are the fastest growing segment of the UK's population. But they have their own set of sad statistics. Many of them are alone, widowed on average at 56 and outliving their husbands by 18 years.

In the industrialised West, these women are a faceless majority, disenfranchised and stripped of their sex appeal by age and circumstances. "My pal [Robert] Redford gets furrows and character lines. I get wrinkles and crow's feet. It ain't fair!" wails Jane Fonda, an everywoman in the throes of middle age. What adds to a man's powers of attraction is deemed to subtract from a woman's allure, especially once menopause has put an end to her child-bearing years. The tangling of the isms means that, as the Western world's population grows older, ageism is supplanting sexism as the new social battleground.

TREATMENT OF THE AGED IN OTHER CULTURES

Contrary to lore, the elderly weren't universally venerated or respected or even looked after by their children in the pre-industrial West. Rather, it seems to have been a case of every man and woman for him- or herself. But even if they weren't living with their families, the elderly tended not to live alone. They would take in boarders for extra money. Bed and board - and the money it meant - was actually the contributing factor to a positive revamp in attitudes to the aged this century. During the Great Depression, the pensions paid to grandma or grandad were invaluable to families strapped for cash. The same situation still applies in Italy, where more than 70 per cent of people over 65 live in a family unit and contribute from their savings or social security

Basic to India's Brahmin philosophy is the belief that life is a learning curve: as you get older, you get better. Brahmins look to their artists for proof.

Life hasn't ever been any less complicated in other cultures. Although Western culture is wilfully inconsistent in its attitudes to ageing, we continue to insist that the true test of a society is how it cares for its aged. At the same time, we highlight our own shortfalls by pointing to the fairer deal that the ageing and elderly receive in other cultures. It's practically an anthropological truism to state that indigenous societies know how to treat their elderly properly because the wisdom and understanding of the oldest members of the tribe make them not only natural leaders but also the greatest cultural assets. The same line of reasoning is applied to our own pre-industrial past, where utopian visions of the closeknit family prevail.

SOBERING FACTS

In fact, the truth is rather less rosy. Up to one third of tribal societies kill their elderly, and 50 per cent practise some form of "death-hastening" behaviour. Yet these same societies also often claim respect for the elderly, based on a clear distinction between the useful elderly - teachers or religious leaders who are relied on to maintain the cultural and technical traditions that are critical to the community's survival - and the decrepit elderly who lose respect and become a burden when their contributions are no longer useful.

Societies most likely to kill their elders tend to be made up of non-hierarchical nomads living in harsh climates. The Inuit in the Arctic Circle are probably the best-known example. It is usually the Inuit elderly themselves who make the decision to "terminate without prejudice", often over their children's protests. But the Inuit have their own distinct concept of the relationship between parent and child. They believe a newborn is a full reincarnation of one of its grandparents so that the soul or "name" of someone about to die will shortly be returned to the community. Partings with the elderly are therefore less final and less difficult than in our society.

In societies where male status is based on hunting, the transition to old age is difficult because it involves loss of sense of self, whereas the expertise of women, whose status is not contingent on strenuous physical activity, often become more valued as they age. Once the taboos and restrictions that apply to the reproductive years are eased, the women of the tribe have more freedom to express themselves.

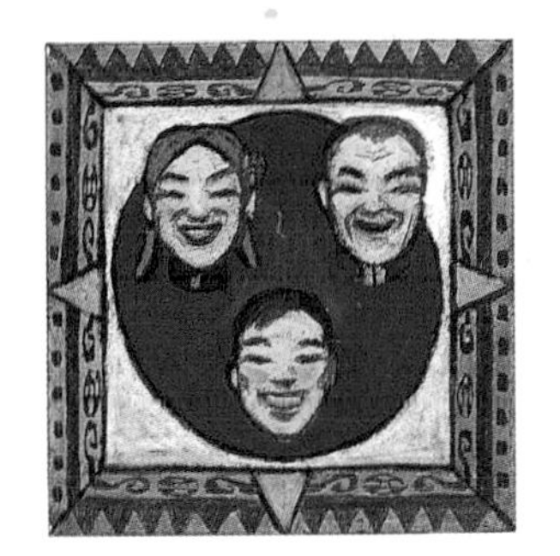

The Chipewyan Indians in Northern Saskatchewan are typical. For them, manhood is synonymous with the ability to hunt, which is a magical gift from a cosmic force. The magic remains as long as a man is strong enough to hunt. When he can no longer do this, it is believed the magic has left him and he is faced by the mortifying transition to a useless old age. On the other hand, the role of women in the tribe is not defined by a supernatural agent. As their skills - food preparation, raising the family, creating handicrafts - improve with age, they gain more respect and power within the community. In addition, the work of the women has a communal aspect so there is no shame in them seeking help from others, unlike the superannuated hunter who is used to relying only on himself.

On **is the Japanese concept of gratitude or debt one feels towards someone who has provided a service or favour, so *on* clearly promotes a strong connection between parent and child - 70 per cent of Japan's senior citizens live with one of their married children, usually the eldest son.**

ROLE REVERSAL

Perhaps the most extraordinary illustration of the power that accrues to women with time happens with the Gabra in East Africa. As with many other tribes around the world, a Gabra male's status in his community is determined less by his chronological age than by the "age set" he is currently in. Youth, bachelor, married man, elder - each of these grades carries with it a specific set of duties and responsibilities. A man can reach elder status at any time from his late thirties until well into his sixties.

But Gabra men don't stop at the oldest male age set. Once they have reached this milestone, the greatest honour they can achieve is to become honorary women, living out their last years with the rituals and roles of elderly women in their culture.

If this seems an unusually enlightened bridging of the biological and chronological gulfs that open up in the twilight years of our own lifespan, it pays to remember that the best antidote to ageism, sexism and racism is always enlightened awareness. The more we learn about the ageing process, the better equipped we are to face the realities of the future.

Breakthroughs in genetic research suggest that not only will scientists conquer our deadliest diseases but they will also be able to extend lifespan.

Already world leaders in life expectancy, the Japanese have initiated "The Golden Plan", a social/medical research programme aimed at making fundamental changes to society to ensure a longer, more enriching life for all.

WHAT HAPPENS?

In every body at any one time, a system of checks and balances governs the health of the organism. A delicate balance is struck between new cells and old cells, healthy cells and sick cells, cells that replace themselves, others that repair themselves. Among the latter are the cells of the vital organs - the heart, brain and kidneys, as well as the nerves and muscles. These regenerate, rather than replace. Among the cells that can replace themselves some, like those in the tendons, ligaments and cartilage of the joints, do so about 50 times in a lifetime. But others can go on replacing themselves more or less indefinitely, or at least for the conjectured lifespan of a healthy cell in ideal circumstances, which is mooted to be around 120 years.

CODE OF LIFE

At the heart of every cell is its genetic code, the DNA and RNA that pre-determine a cell's destiny. If DNA is the cellular architect and RNA the foreman, the cell's builders are the body's proteins, using amino acids as their raw material. This is the construction team which creates the body's connective tissue, the foundation of our skin, blood vessels, tendons, ligaments and cartilage.

Some protein molecules look like long spirals. From the time we're born, these spirals begin to bond together. At least some of such bonding, called cross-linking, is essential to the strength and elasticity of healthy tissue, and any excess cross-linking that occurs is controlled by the enzymes a young organism produces. But cross-linking eventually outstrips enzyme production and, as molecular strands continue to bond with age, they become tangled, rigid and inflexible. The construction team doesn't work so well together. It's members are slower, and they begin to receive garbled instructions from the architect. The edifice they've all been working to maintain begins to crumble. As cross-linking snarls the collagen and elastin proteins that are the major building blocks of the skin, wrinkles form. While the delicate webs of capillaries that nourish cells are slowly strangled, every part of the body is adversely affected. And by now, the process of ageing is in full cry.

FREE RADICALS AND AGEING

The worst of it is that the agent we blame for undermining the construction team's best efforts is the very same element we credit with life on earth - oxygen. The links that allow molecular spirals to tangle together and obstruct each other's work are forged by special molecules of oxygen, known as free radicals. These rogue toxins are actually a normal, even essential, part of all biological processes but as much as they encourage cellular life, they also seem bent on hastening its end. To name but two examples of their insidious effect: free radical damage to the nervous system has been implicated in Parkinson's Disease. And cholesterol, a steroid which is essential to the body's effective synthesising of vitamins and hormones, becomes dangerous once it is oxidised by free radicals. It attracts other cells to it, setting off a chain reaction that can result in the formation of artery-clogging plaque.

How variable is this process? Is the cross-linking that causes breakdowns in cell regeneration and replacement controllable? Increasingly, researchers believe it is. That's because cross-linking is a distinct physical phenomenon.

FIGHTING FREE RADICALS

Free radicals are not invincible. They can be headed off by anti-oxidants in the form of readily available vitamins and minerals. Among the most common of these free radical scavengers are vitamins A, B1, B5, B6 and C. A grapefruit won't turn brown (or oxidise) when it's cut because of its vitamin C content. Even better is vitamin E, which helps to protect cell membranes from oxidation. The minerals zinc and selenium promote the action of vitamins C and E.

> ***Bags under the eyes are usually inherited but regular physical exercise can help reduce them: it carries oxygen to skin cells and helps remove waste.***

Research into anti-oxidants is yielding some curious data. Manipulate your vitamins and minerals and you too can live a longer, healthier life. That seems to be the message.

A UCLA doctor claims that limiting calorie intake without decreasing vitamin or mineral intake could conceivably extend maximum human lifespan by 60 to 80 per cent. And life extension may be as close as a glass of house red. Because blood levels of one potent anti-oxidant, Super Oxide Dismutase (SOD), increase according to copper intake, the copper content in red wine has been singled out as one possible reason for the longer lives led by the French.

AFFECTING THE SENSES

We might live longer in relative terms than any other creature, but the steady decay of our senses suggests we're as primed as the rest of the animal kingdom for the survival of the fittest, the strongest and especially the youngest. Our main lines of defence - our immune system - start packing up at 30, but by then our main faculties have already begun to decline.

SIGHT

Our eyesight is at its best at the age of 17. It is then that the pupil is largest, catching most light, and the eye muscles are at their most flexible, able to focus and refocus rapidly.

By our early forties, the lens of the eye has thickened to the point where it begins to cause problems. A thicker lens scatters light on the retina, making glare a bigger problem (meaning more squinting and therefore more wrinkles). The hardening lens is too big for the eye muscles to focus properly on close objects. But paradoxically, those with near sight may find their vision actually improves as their lenses harden.

The amount of light reaching the retina declines with age. Our night vision is reduced and we need more light to read. The cornea, lens and fluid in the eye yellow with age, absorbing the shorter wavelengths of visible light and making blue and green harder to distinguish. Colour awareness generally is reduced. The violet spectrum is harder to detect.

Live long enough to pursue this process to its logical conclusion and you're likely to end up blind.

SOUND

A dog hears sound - a whistle for instance - at 40,000 hertz, or vibrations, per second. A child can also hear that well. In fact, human hearing peaks by the age of seven. By 16, that capability is halved, as cells begin their breakdown deep within the ear. A cricket chirps at 15,000 hertz - the average 30-year-old would have trouble hearing anything above that. By the age of 70, the upper limits of hearing have dropped to 6,000 hertz, or the high notes on a pipe organ, though normal human speech is fortunately still audible - it's pitched below 4,000 hertz.

But hearing has deteriorated precipitously since the rock music era dawned and especially since the launching of the personal stereo made it possible to pump noise at high volume directly onto the eardrum. Baby boomers will be lucky to have the hearing their parents enjoyed at the same age.

TASTE

We're born with tastebuds on the roofs of our mouths, on the walls of our throats and all over our tongues. So any taste in our mouths is a flavour explosion when we're infants, which helps explain why small children feel

Even though hearing deteriorates at a steady rate, we never lose the ability to hear a cry for help. In technical terms, a distress scream lies between F-sharp and G in the fourth octave above middle C. These frequencies alert the nerves of the human ear like no other sound, no matter how feeble the hearing. And, to ensure that a human distress call will always register as such, we broadcast no other sounds in this segment of the vocal spectrum. It is strictly for "emergency broadcasts".

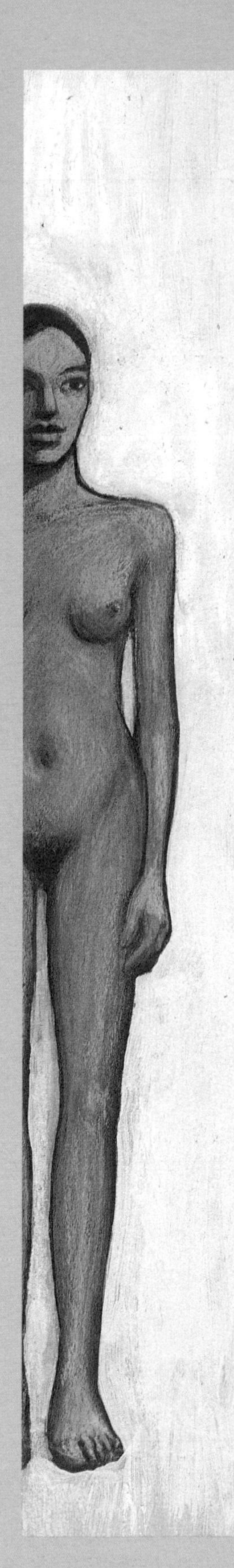

HOW THE BODY AGES

WOMEN:

Brain: At 60, the brain has four times as much information as at 21.

Memory: At 70, reaction time slows by 15 per cent.

Eyes: Lenses steadily thicken and harden throughout life. Amount of light reaching retina declines. Bags under the eyes are hereditary.

Sleep: A two-week old sleeps 20 hours a day. A 65-year-old sleeps five hours or less.

Ears: At seven, you can hear sounds at frequencies up to 20,000 hertz. At 70, you can't hear above 6,000 hertz (everyday human speech is below 4,000 hertz).

Tastebuds: Papillae on the tongue have 245 tastebuds at 30, but only 88 tastebuds at 80.

Skull: Thickens with age (about a quarter of an inch per decade).

Bone: Bone mass peaks at 35. It then decreases at an average rate of 0.5 per cent per year, increasing to anywhere between 1 and 5 per cent in the first five years after menopause. Women are eight times likelier to develop osteoporosis than men.

Breasts: Tissue changes, becoming more lumpy.

Nails: Growth rate - 0.94mm a week at 20 and 0.60mm a week at 70.

Muscles: 3 to 5 per cent loss of lean muscle tissue every decade after 30.

Heart: Women are at low risk of heart disease until after the menopause - perhaps oestrogen offers natural protection, which may be why women on Hormone Replacement Therapy have low rates of stroke and heart disease.

Lungs: Capacity reduced between 30 to 50 per cent by the age of 80.

Weight: By 50, around 44 per cent of women are overweight. Women gain, on average, almost 10lb between 35 and 45 and two more between 45 and 55. But after 65, bodyweight diminishes and muscles weaken.

Sexual Organs: Small decrease in size after the menopause.

Back: By mid-seventies, spinal discs have lost 30 per cent of their water.The space between them narrows, resulting in a one-and-a-half inch loss in height. By 75, a woman may have lost 30 to 40 per cent of the bone mass in her spine.

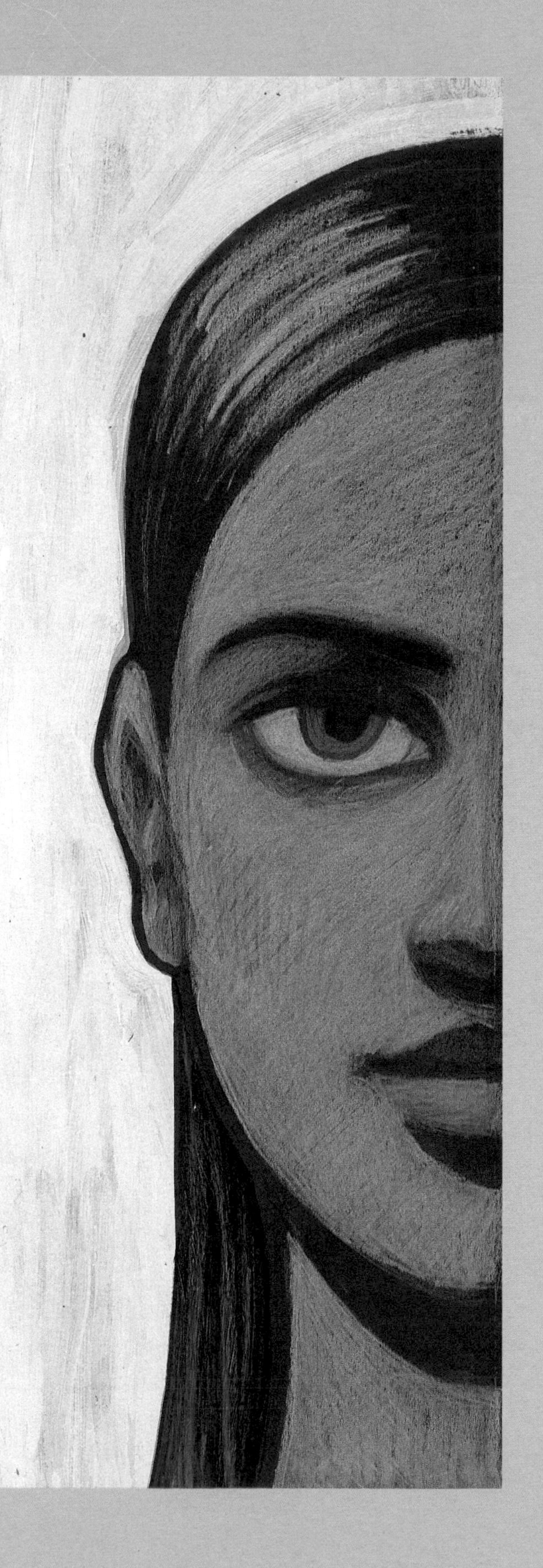

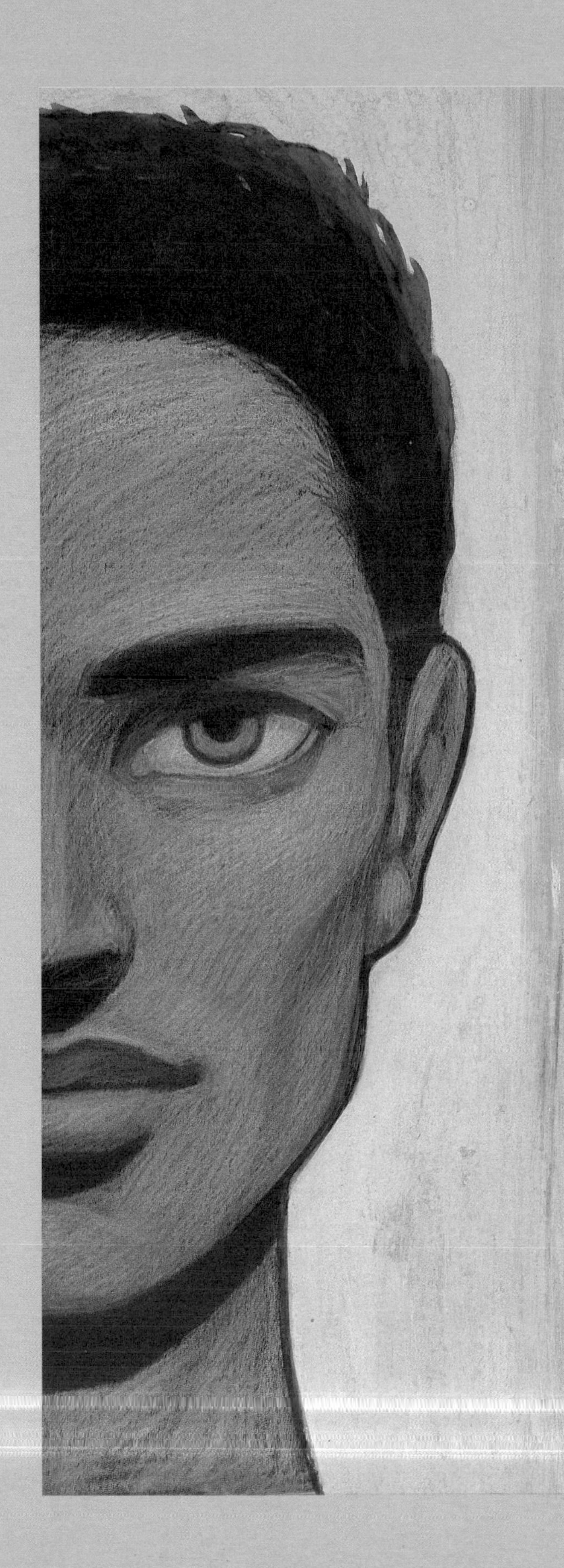

MEN:

Brain: At 60, the brain has four times as much information as at 21.

Memory: At 70, reaction time slows by 15 per cent.

Hair: Thins, grows finer (at 70, hair is as fine as a baby's).

Skull: Thickens with age (about a quarter of an inch per decade).

Eyes: Lenses steadily thicken and harden throughout life. Amount of light reaching retina declines. Bags under the eyes are hereditary.

Sleep: A two-week old sleeps 20 hours a day. A 65-year-old sleeps five hours or less.

Ears: At seven, you can hear sounds at frequencies up to 20,000 hertz. At 70, you can't hear above 6,000 hertz (everyday human speech is below 4,000 hertz).

Voice: After 50, a man's speaking voice rises from a C to an E flat because vocal chords stiffen and vibrate at higher frequency with age.

Tastebuds: Papillae on the tongue have 245 tastebuds at 30, but only 88 tastebuds at 80.

Nails: Growth rate - 0.94mm a week at 20 and 0.60mm a week at 70.

Muscles: 3 to 5 per cent loss of lean muscle tissue every decade after 30.

Bone: Bone mass loss occurs after 45.

Heart: If *you* stay healthy, *it* will stay healthy - a normal 80-year-old heart is as effective as a normal 30-year-old heart.

Lungs: Capacity reduced between 30 to 50 per cent by the age of 80.

Weight: Metabolism begins to slow at 25. You need 2 per cent fewer calories per decade to maintain weight. The body's ability to store fat is unharmed by age.

Sex: Frequency of orgasm: 104 per year at 20, 22 per year at 70. Men produce sperm into their seventies.

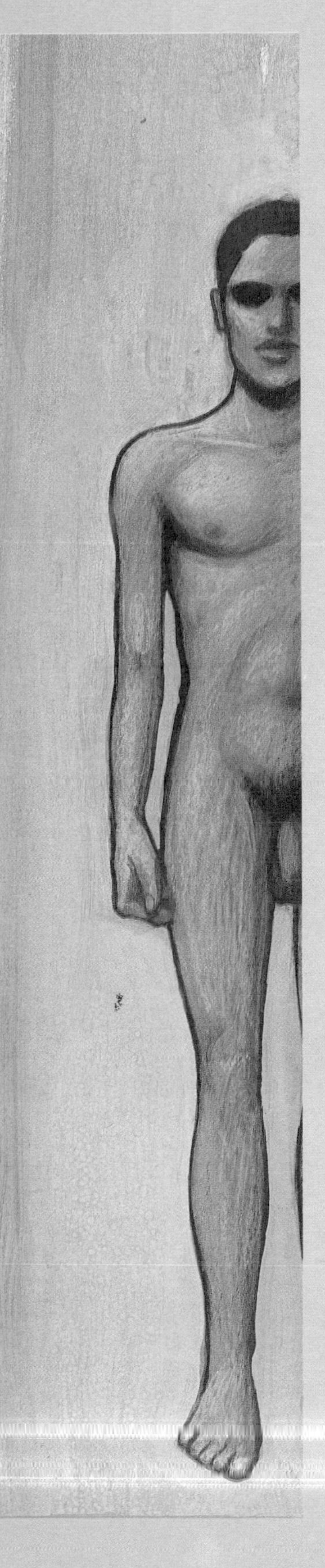

In an 18th century treatise, Hermippus Redivivus claimed men aged because they lost vital "particles" every time they breathed out. His suggested particle replacement therapy was to breathe in the exhalations of young women.

compelled to sample the detritus of the great outdoors. But by the time we're ten, tens of thousands of tastebuds are already lost and those that are left are concentrated on the tip, at the back and round the rim of the tongue on tiny ridges called papillae. The average 30-year-old has about 245 tastebuds on each papilla.

Tastebuds are assisted in their work by secretions from the mucous membranes, which help pulp chewed food. But, as the tastebuds degenerate, so these secretions dry up. To the average 80-year-old, with a mere 88 tastebuds remaining on each papilla, food will be relatively flavourless. Here is biological backup - as if it were needed - for Oscar Wilde's conviction that youth is wasted on the young.

TOUCH

What little research there is into tactility unsurprisingly suggests age diminishes our sense of touch, at least as touch is measured in terms of response to pain. That is logical enough. Age, after all, brings with it an assortment of aches and pains. Our genetic programming is doing us a favour if it can dull our responses to such unwanted newcomers.

But response to pain is at least as psychological as it is sensory. In this area, male reactions are the same, whether young or old. Men won't readily admit to feeling pain because of their need to be seen as strong. Women, on the other hand, have no problems admitting they feel pain in behavioural studies but, in real-life situations, they are as stoical as men.

SMELL

Smell, the oldest sense and humankind's most reliable helpmate in the evolutionary fight for survival, is appropriately the faculty that suffers least from the ageing process, perhaps because it is connected most directly to the brain. It is only after the age of 65 or so that our ability to distinguish variations in concentrations of smell begins to wane. However, smokers can expect their sense of smell to give up the ghost much earlier, which is just one of the pernicious effects that cigarettes have on the ageing body. Others include nutrient depletion, calcium imbalance and accelerated cross-linking.

PHYSICAL CHARACTERISTICS

WEIGHT

Basal metabolism (the rate at which a resting body converts food to energy) begins to slow at 25, and then continues to slow by about three per cent every decade. What this really means is that you'll require two per cent fewer calories per decade to maintain your ideal weight. Without that adjustment, middle age spread will get all the help it needs. Chronic dieters are further challenged by a metabolic rate reduction of up to 14 per cent!

Here's a further caveat about dieting. Women tend to gain nearly 10lb in the decade between 35 and 45, then another 2lb in the following decade. But current research suggests at least some of this fat may have a critical physical function. After menopause, body fat is one of the three sources of oestrogen. So statistics that state that around 45 per cent of women are overweight by the age of 50 (as opposed to 21 per cent of 20 to 24-year-olds) may have to be revised. If, as has been suggested, "ideal" body weights have been set too low, then many middle-aged women may be dieting themselves into hormone deficiencies.

HEIGHT

Adults can expect to shrink an inch in the course of a day between leaving bed in the morning and returning to it at night. This is because our intervertebral discs contract while we're upright.

STRENGTH

Muscles make up our lean body mass. Everyone starts to lose about three to five per cent of this mass for each decade after 30. If you don't exercise, you'll tend to lose even more. And the less muscle mass you have, the harder it is to burn calories, which basically means less muscle, more fat. Here's an additional fattening factor: though the body doesn't absorb as much protein as it ages, and therefore needs a higher proportion of protein in its diet, it can't store excess protein or carbohydrate without first converting it to fat.

In addition to muscle mass, women will also lose 30 per cent of their bone mass between 35 and 65, increasing the risk of osteoporosis in later life.

HONEY

Honey is one of the earliest known humectants, a substance which holds moisture.

In Valencia, Spain, cave drawings dating from 7,000 BC show a man harvesting honey from hives. Because they did not know exactly how it was produced, the ancients worshipped honey as a gift from the gods and credited it with mystical powers.

In Ancient Egypt, honey was mixed with acacia gum and crocodile dung to form a preventive barrier used as a contraceptive. The Egyptians also made a disinfectant with frankincense, myrrh, cinnamon bark and honey, boiled together, formed into pellets and used to fumigate houses, scent clothes and keep breath fresh.

Honey is much more than a sweetener - its exceptionally high potassium content makes it an excellent antibacterial agent, which is why both the Egyptians and Romans used it to preserve corpses.

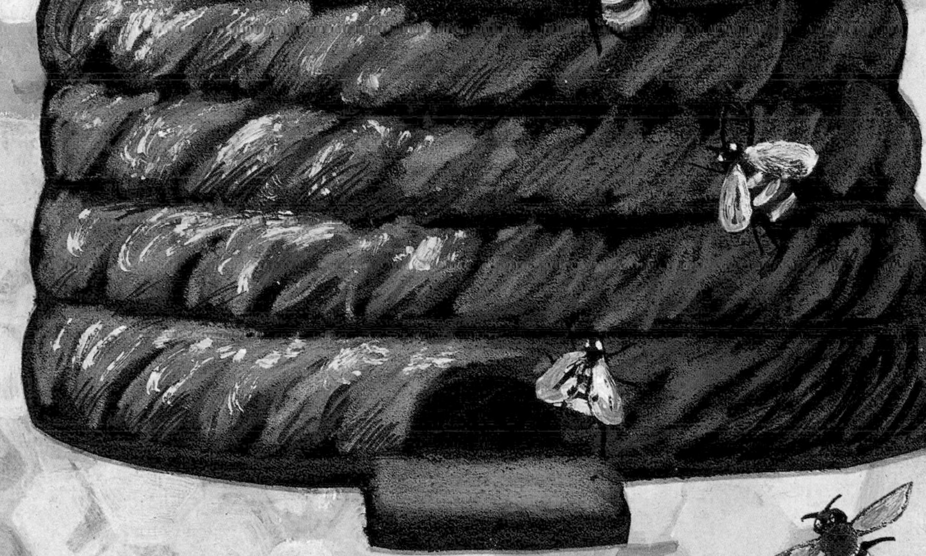

The concept of the "honeymoon" derives in part from the medieval Northern European custom in which newlyweds would drink a cup of mead every day for the first month of their married life.

A good hive can produce about 20 lb of honey a day - amazing when you consider that each pound of nectar necessitates 60,000 to 80,000 trips by individual bees between the flower fields and the hive.

From Ancient Rome to present-day India, honey crops up as a key ingredient in face masks worldwide. Here's an Indian recipe:
Combine 1 oz honey, 3 oz ground barley and the white of an egg. Leave on your face overnight, then rinse off with tepid water in the morning.

Cleopatra used a mixture of lapis lazuli, malachite, ochre and honey to paint her eyelids.

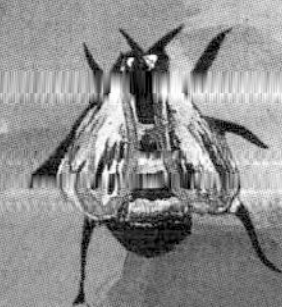

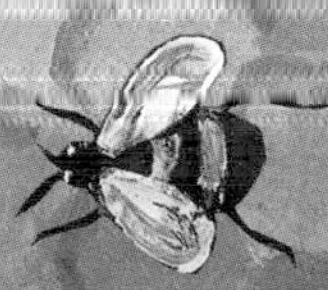

MEMORY

At last, some cheer. The brain uses 25 per cent of the body's basal metabolism. Even though ageing may entail a 15 per cent slowing down in reaction time or memory time by the age of 70, slowdown is not the same thing as loss. The brain's ability to store words and facts is perfectly adequate for the informational intake that adult experience demands. A 45-year-old knows three times as many words as a 20-year-old, and a 60-year-old's brain contains four times as much information. Still, the brain needs a regular workout to keep it in shape.

According to a recent UK survey, 40 per cent of men and 55 per cent of women would like to continue working after retirement age.

NOW THE GOOD NEWS

Regular exercise acts as an antidote to many of the ravages of time. Exercise can increase physical function in a young person by 10 per cent, but in an old person it can make as much as 50 per cent of a difference. Regular exercise fulfils five anti-ageing functions:

- bone strengthening
- heart strengthening
- weight regulation
- flexibility
- joint mobility

In addition, exercise lowers blood pressure; reduces the risk of heart attack, stroke, arthritis and emphysema; relieves depression; aids sleep and helps keep chests clear during colds, thus reducing the risk of pneumonia and bronchial complaints that can be deadly in the aged.

One reason why Italians have the healthiest diet in the world: the average Italian eats 264 lb of fruit a year. His counterpart in the UK eats just 59 lb.

Exercise also promotes blood circulation, which helps the look and feel of the body's largest organ, the skin. Energetic activity brings extra nutrients to the skin's surface, warming it and actually increasing its collagen content so it thickens and becomes more flexible.

Regular exercise is particularly important for ageing women because it helps the body to absorb calcium, thus reducing the risk of osteoporosis. Exercise becomes even more important if, for some reason, an elderly woman finds she is not getting outside as much. One of the good effects of daily exposure to the sun is to stimulate production of vitamin D, which also promotes the absorption of calcium. So calcium levels which may be threatened by less time outdoors can be maintained with a little more exercise.

AGEING AND THE COSMETICS INDUSTRY

MIND AND BODY

The attitude you adopt to your own ageing will have a huge effect on the way you age. You'll look as good as you feel - and if you look good, you'll feel better. That is one of the basic principles of psychoneuroimmunology (PNI), a relatively new field of research which seeks to clarify this obvious link by analysing the primal connections between mind and body.

No matter how superficial, even deceptive, the whole idea of the painted, preserved face may seem, it's attitude that counts. PNI would have been old news to the ancients. From the moment human beings began mulling over their appearance they sought to assist nature, with a special emphasis on preserving for as long as possible the appearance of youthfulness. The Fountain of Youth has always been a kind of massmarket philosopher's stone, turning ageing flesh to gilded youth. And the appeal it exerts hasn't faded with time. Cosmeticians have been able to trade off it for thousands of years, all because of that underlying truth. It has allowed four millennia worth of charlatans to manipulate the innermost hopes, dreams and fears of millions of women - and men.

ANTI-AGEING - TRUTH OR ILLUSION?

In the past decade, the cosmetics industry's response to the greying of the West has been to wage an anti-ageing campaign with such vigour that a casual observer might have thought the Fountain of Youth was shifting position on a daily basis. In the USA, federal intervention was eventually required to tone down some of the more outrageous claims of the cosmetics giants and to restore a sense of balance.

The bald fact is, of course, that no cosmetic product can make a jot of difference to the ageing process. Several major cosmetics companies are currently working on a new breed of products that will inevitably carry claims they can reverse signs of ageing. Should any product be able to penetrate the dermis to the point where it *can* stimulate such a process, it most definitely isn't a cosmetic. It's either a drug or a new species of genetic engineer and therefore subject to a whole different set of regulations. One of these will doubtless be a stipulation for the use of animal testing, which will kick that particular issue back into the forefront of debate in the cosmetics industry.

How susceptible is the average human being to the notion that a cosmetics product can restore the illusion of youth? There will always be those who hope against hope and who believe the hype. Others may know that nothing can stop skins getting older, but in the act of trying to look their best, they're acknowledging the fact that they still care enough about themselves to make an effort. It's not hard to calculate the psychological benefits - increased confidence and boosted self-esteem among them - especially for any man or woman who is passing into middle age or beyond. It has nothing to do with culturally imposed ideas about chronology and appearance, or anything that demands surgical intervention. For a happy, healthy exterior, look good, feel better, look best.

MEETING THE NEEDS OF AGEING SKIN

MOISTURE

The criteria for a healthy appearance remain the same as skin ages. It is the skin's moisture content that is responsible for its healthy glow, but levels of sebum, the skin's essential fluid, diminish from adolescence onwards. Moisture supplements become more important for ageing male and female skin, with special attention

ANTI-AGEING THROUGH THE AGES

- In Greek myth, Medea's recipe for reviving her husband Jason's father Aeson was: "pebbles from the farthest Orient; hoarfrost gathered from under the moon; wings and flesh of the infamous horned owl; entrails of a werewolf; the skin of the Cynyphian water snake; the liver of a long-lived stag; the head of a crow nine centuries old; and a thousand other things..."

- The Syriac Book of Medicine suggests: "Lay the lung of a camel on the face of the patient, for a complexion like wax."

- Ancient Egyptian additives to anti-ageing formulas included: writing fluid, hippopotamus fat, gazelle dung, and ground donkey teeth mixed with honey.

- An anti-wrinkle cream in Ancient Rome consisted of honey, wine lees and finely ground narcissus bulbs.

- The anti-ageing secret of a 14th century Bavarian queen was a combination of boars' brains, crocodile glands and wolf's blood.

- Henri III, a 16th century king of France, slept in a night mask of flour and egg whites, sponged off in the morning with chervil water.

- In the 17th century, women slept in "face gloves": masks of silk, linen or leather stretched over cream-covered faces to "iron out" the lines.

- Anti-wrinkle treatments in the18th century included: snails, sheep's trotters and wax injected under the skin (one disadvantage was that it melted when it got hot).

- Here's an 1825 recipe for a night cream: heat 2 oz each of onion juice, white lily and honey and 1 oz white wax in a new earthen pipkin until the wax has melted. Stir with a wooden spatula until cold, apply at night and don't wipe off till morning

NUTRITION FOR LIFE

The role of diet in health for life cannot be over-estimated. Dietary factors are implicated in as many as 35 per cent of all deaths from cancer.

Clearly, there are some foods that simply don't do us any good. Equally, there are others that help boost our immune systems and combat the natural wear and tear of ageing, especially the oxidising process that is increasingly targeted as a major cause of ageing. And the amount we eat is significant: eating more than the body needs contributes to "oxystress" in the system. One sensible guideline recommends people in mid-life (30 to 50) to obtain only 10 to 15 per cent of their calories from fat (as opposed to the current 40 per cent), 20 to 25 per cent of their calories in the form of protein.

The following table is intended simply to indicate the part each vitamin or mineral plays in long-term health maintenance. We haven't gone into supplements or recommended dietary allowances because they are subject to a huge range of variables dependent on everything from individual need and ethnic differences to the amount of processing the food in your regular diet may have undergone. On the outer reaches of anti-ageing research, the supplementary dosage levels bandied around by researchers - for vitamins C and E for example - can be quite dizzying. At the same time, an excess of some minerals, such as iron , can be as potentially damaging as a deficiency. However, if you feel you may be lacking in particular vitamins or minerals, a straightforward blood test from your doctor will help define deficiencies.

Vitamin A	**Vitamin B1 (Thiamine)**	**Vitamin B2 (Riboflavin)**	**Niacin**
Fat-soluble vitamin - necessary for good night vision; keeps skin and body's linings healthy; helps body resist infection, promotes growth, maintains teeth, hair, bones and glands in good condition	Water-soluble vitamin - helps the body use carbohydrates as energy; maintains normal appetite and healthy digestion; contributes to functioning of heart and nervous system	Water-soluble vitamin - converts protein, fat and carbohydrate into energy; helps produce antibodies to defend against infection; helps form red blood cells	Water-soluble vitamin - helps keep nervous system and digestive tract healthy; helps body extract energy from carbohydrates, protein and fat
Sources: liver, kidneys, eggs, milk, yellow and green fruit and vegetables (e.g. carrots, spinach, apricots, peaches, broccoli, asparagus)	**Sources:** whole-grain and enriched cereals, pork, beef, lamb, nuts and legumes	**Sources:** green vegetables, blackstrap molasses, brewer's yeast, liver, nuts, whole grains	**Sources:** liver, meat, fish, poultry, peanuts and enriched cereals

Vitamin B6 (Pyridoxine)	**Vitamin B12 (Cyanocobalamin)**	**Folic Acid (Folacin)**	**Vitamin C (Ascorbic Acid)**
Water-soluble vitamin - metabolises protein and helps normal functioning of nervous system; essential for proper maintenance of immune function; protects against atherosclerosis and heart disease	Water-soluble vitamin - aids synthesis of haemoglobin and helps maintain healthy red blood cells	Water-soluble vitamin - important in the manufacture of compounds used to make genes; keeps red blood cells healthy	Water-soluble vitamin - excellent anti-oxidant; helps to fight cancer by preventing formation of carcinogens in body; vital in manufacture of collagen; helps absorb iron; maintains healthy teeth, gums and bones
Sources: liver, beef, lamb, pork, salmon, whole-grain cereals, lima beans, carrots, tomatoes, potatoes, green leafy vegetables, bananas, avocados	**Sources:** liver, kidneys, fish, eggs, milk, milk products	**Sources:** dark green leafy vegetables, liver, kidneys, milk and milk products, salmon, tuna, dates, whole grains	**Sources:** citrus fruits, broccoli, cabbage, brussel sprouts, cauliflower, spinach, peppers, cantaloupe, strawberries, papaya

Vitamin D	Vitamin E	Calcium	Phosphorus	Iron	Sodium	Potassium
Fat-soluble vitamin - aids absorption of calcium and phosphorus, thus helping bone formation; maintains normal action of heart and nervous system	Fat-soluble vitamin - excellent anti-oxidant, particularly good for preventing the oxidisation of vitamins A and C; maintains cell membranes and general health of the blood	Macronutrient mineral - crucial for the development and maintenance of strong teeth and bones; necessary for digestion; aids in blood clotting	Macronutrient mineral - as phosphate, it's necessary for the formation of teeth and bones; helps body make genes; ensures calcium absorption	Micronutrient or trace mineral - necessary for production of haemoglobin which carries oxygen through the body	Macronutrient mineral - maintains body's acid/alkali balance; sends nerve impulses; aids muscle contraction; helps maintain balance of fluids inside and outside body's cells	Macronutrient mineral - works with sodium to maintain body's balance of fluids and acid/alkali balance; sends nerve impulses
Sources: egg yolk, liver, certain fish such as salmon. Interaction of skin and sun	**Sources:** polyunsaturated oils and margarines, green vegetables, almonds, sunflower seeds, whole grains, eggs, liver, oatmeal	**Sources:** milk, sardines and salmon (canned with their bones)	**Sources:** dairy products, meat, fish, eggs, peanuts	**Sources:** spinach, brussels sprouts, broccoli, strawberries, eggs, liver, fish, chicken, cereals	**Sources:** milk, cheese	**Sources:** bananas, oranges, dried fruit, kiwi fruit, tomatoes, potatoes

Chloride	Fluoride	Magnesium	Manganese	Iodine	Selenium	Zinc
Macronutrient mineral - maintains body's acid/alkali balance; major component of hydrochloric acid in stomach, needed for good digestion	Trace mineral - helps build strong bones and teeth (a deficiency can contribute to osteoporosis)	Macronutrient mineral - aids release of energy from carbohydrates and synthesis of protein; stimulates nerve and muscle action; helps retain tooth enamel	Trace mineral - needed for normal bone development; functions as an anti-oxidant	Trace mineral - vital component of the hormone thyroxin, which regulates the thyroid gland that controls the body's basal metabolic rate	Trace mineral - an anti-oxidant, working much like vitamin E; protects against carcinogens; prevents release of free radicals	Trace mineral - helps body metabolise protein and carbohydrate and produce insulin; promotes T-cell immunity as a vital guard against infection (unless such infection is bacterial)
Sources: table salt, meat, milk, eggs	**Sources:** Sardines with their bones, fluoridated water	**Sources:** whole-grain breads and cereals, nuts, beans, milk, fish, green leafy vegetables	**Sources:** nuts, whole-grain cereals, bananas, green leafy vegetables, liver, pineapples	**Sources:** saltwater fish, shellfish, iodised salt	**Sources:** butter, cereals, fish, cider vinegar, garlic, asparagus	**Sources:** spinach, liver, shellfish, whole grains, brewer's yeast, mushrooms

A severe housing shortage in China means families are often forced to stay together out of necessity. But pensioners receive a state pension which approximates to the wages earned by their working children so, rather than become a financial burden, elderly people can contribute their full share to household expenses.

needing to be paid to delicate areas where skin is naturally thinner, such as on the neck and under the eyes. But you want moisture without over-oiliness. Products containing vitamin E fit the bill, and a rich night cream will work with the body to promote healthy-looking skin.

The numbers of people over 100 are increasing. In 1977 there were 300 centenarians in the UK. A decade later, that number had increased tenfold.

TEXTURE

Young skin is made up of an evenly criss-crossing web of fibres cemented together by the proteins collagen and elastin. The even texture means that the skin reflects light uniformly, which accounts for healthy skin tone. And the regular renewal of skin cells about once every 25 to 28 days helps the process. As skin ages, this rate of renewal slows. At the same time, free radical oxygen molecules "cross-link" with collagen and elastin, which lose their pliability, and the crisscross begins to tangle and become irregular. Light is no longer reflected uniformly, which lends skin the dull tone we associate with age.

Although loss of some skin tone is inevitable, there are ways to postpone it for as long as possible. Start young with the daily use of a sunscreen and you won't be giving free radicals any help. Regular facial massages will stimulate blood circulation and the production of collagen in the dermis. And regular facial scrubs will remove dead skin cells and stimulate cell renewal.

FIRMNESS

Sebum, collagen and elastin all help to support the network of fibres that makes up the epidermis and keeps young skin plump and firm. As the support system is slowly eroded by free radicals and the network begins to crumble, skin thins, loosens, and eventually wrinkles form. Among the bad habits that speed up such degenerative processes are overexposure to the sun, cigarette smoking and excessive dieting, which can stretch and damage the skin so that it loses its flexibility. Restrict smoking and dieting and use a sunscreen to protect the skin from ultraviolet damage.

SMOOTHNESS

Skin texture depends on an uninterrupted process of cell renewal. Once this becomes irregular as the cycle slows, the surface of the skin itself becomes irregular. The same process that undermines firmness works against smoothness. Some of the tiny lines that crisscross the skin's surface fade, others deepen to become wrinkles.

Regular exfoliation is the best way to remove dead skin cells and stimulate production of new ones, but ageing skin needs facial scrubs and masks with gentle action.

AND DON'T FORGET....

The skin of the body needs as much attention as that of the face. Body scrubs, body creams and rich body butters will maintain the tone and texture of the largest organ in the body. Bath oils and moisturising shower gels ensure that bathing doesn't strip away the skin's vital oils.

One ageing giveaway is the skin on hands. Over exposure to sun is the villain behind age spots. Daily use of a moisturising sunscreen is one solution. Feet also demand proper care, because foot irritants such as bunions and corns become more of a problem with age. Regular pumicing to exfoliate dead and hardened skin from the heel and soles of the feet will help. Then apply Peppermint Foot Lotion to moisturise.

And for allover well-being, remember the virtues of aromatherapy oils in massage or as a bath additive. A little assistance to a positive attitude goes a long way.

AGEING AND THE FUTURE

The greying of the population will change the face of Western society like no other social force. The most negative predictions describe a social security disaster, with a shrinking work force facing the impossible task of subsidising a growing army of retirees. Take the USA as an example. It currently costs $90 billion a year to care for those suffering from Alzheimer's Disease. That

MATURE SKIN CARE

FACE	NORMAL TO DRY	NORMAL TO OILY
Cleanser	Honeyed Beeswax & Almond Oil Cleanser Orchid Oil Cleansing Milk Glycerine & Oat Facial Lather	Glycerine & Oat Facial Lather Passion Fruit Cleansing Gel
Face Mask	Peanut & Rosehip Face Mask	Parsley & Mint Face Mask
Freshener	Honey Water	Cucumber Water
Moisturiser	Vitamin E Cream Jojoba Moisture Cream Aloe Vera Moisture Cream Neck Gel	Carrot Moisture Cream Vitamin E Cream Neck Gel
Eyes and Lips	Elderflower Eye Gel Under Eye Cream Lip Balms Honey Stick	Elderflower Eye Gel Lip Balms Honey Stick
BODY	**NORMAL TO DRY**	**EXTRA TREATMENT FOR VERY DRY SKIN**
Moisturiser	Cocoa Butter Hand & Body Lotion Mango Body Butter Avocado Body Butter Cocoa Butter Stick	Mango Body Butter Cocoa Butter Stick
Hands and Nails	Hawthorn Hand Cream Sweet Almond Oil	Cocoa Butter Hand & Body Lotion
Feet	Peppermint Foot Lotion Pumice Foot Scrub Cooling Leg Gel	Peppermint Foot Lotion
Bath and Personal Hygiene	Bath Oil Orange Cream Bath Oil Aromatherapy Relaxing Bath Oil Aromatherapy Reviving Shower Oil Roll on Deodorant	Pre-shower treatment - Mango Body Butter
Aromatherapy	Warming Cream Relaxing Moisture Cream Aromatherapy Relaxing Bath Oil Aromatherapy Reviving Shower Oil Lavender Essential Oil Rose Essential Oil Neroli Essential Oil Ylang-Ylang Essential Oil	Relaxing Moisture Cream

RECIPE FOR LONGEVITY

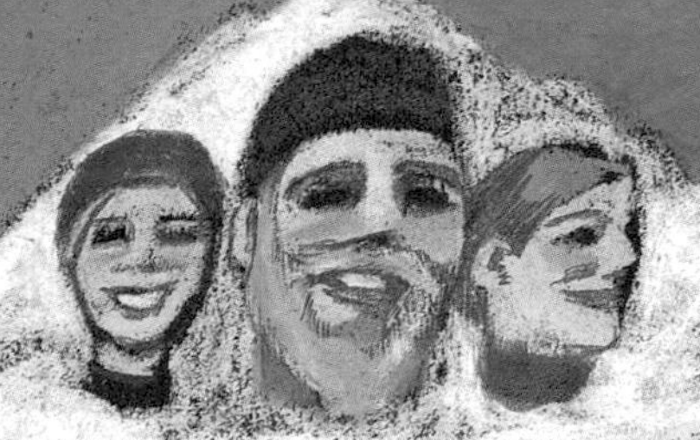

The longest-lived peoples in the world are the Georgians of the Caucasus Mountains in Southern Russia the Vilcabamba Indians of the Ecuadorean Andes and the people of the Hunza Valley in Kashmir. All three...

live at high altitudes with little air pollution

exercise regularly and consistently

live in extended families, which offer cradle-to-grave security

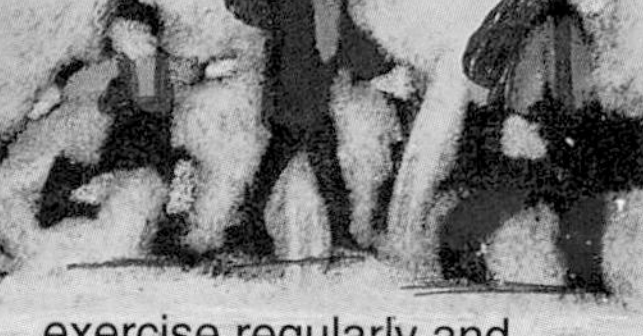

don't use preservatives or artificial colourants

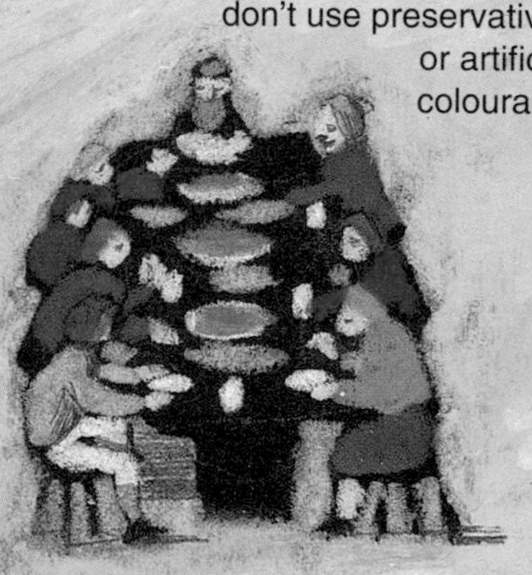

eat a frugal diet, high in fibre, low in salt, fat and refined sugar and rarely fry in oil

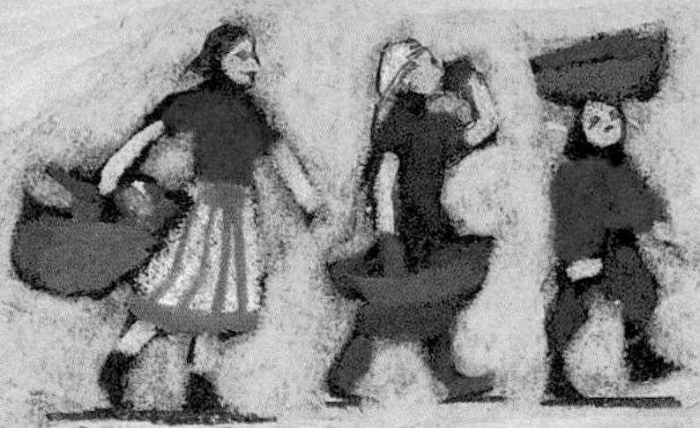

consume plenty of fresh fruit and vegetables

practise holistic medicine, using traditional herbs and medicines to prevent and cure disease

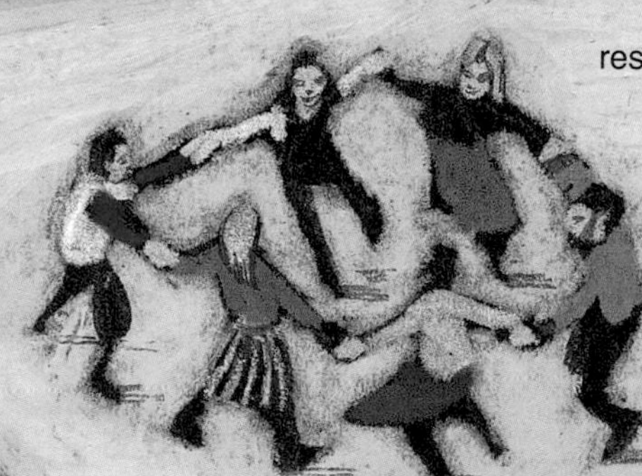

respect their elders, who lead busy active lives into their 100s

emphasise relationships and harmony over the pursuit of wealth or success

never experience loneliness

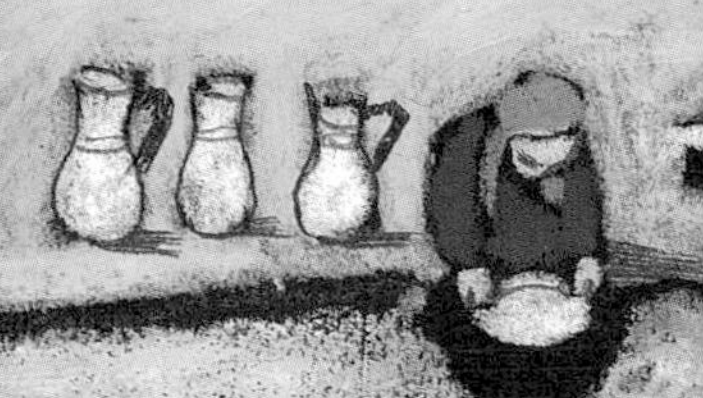

drink water with a high mineral content from fresh mountain streams

seldom drink or smoke

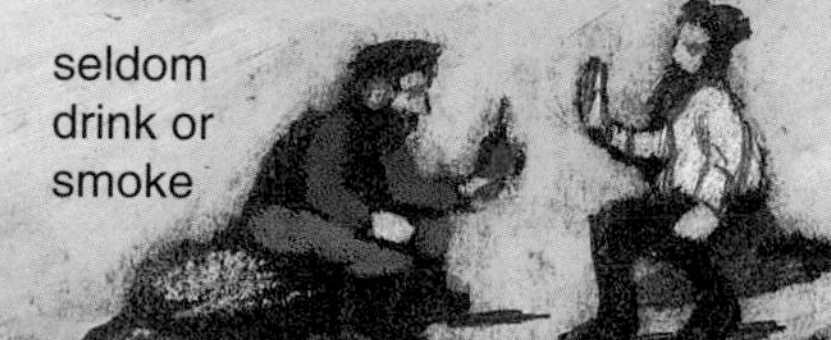

enjoy regular sex, even up to the age of 100

amount is expected to increase eightfold as baby boomers enter the Alzheimer's curve, and the disease is just one of the syndromes that is becoming more prevalent with our longer lifespans. Without a change in the current system, pension and healthcare costs will be gobbling up more than 60 per cent of the US federal budget by the year 2040.

So it's clearly a change that is called for. But the change will have to be at least as much about popular attitude as it is about public policy. Consider the results of this May 1991 poll on Attitudes to Ageing conducted by National Opinion Polls on behalf of British Gas:

Good things about getting older in the UK today (asked of a cross-section of people over 55):

More free time / not working	36 per cent
Hobbies / pastimes / leisure	17 per cent
Nothing	29 per cent

Bad things about getting older in the UK today:

Financial difficulties	45 per cent
Declining health / mobility	36 per cent
Loneliness / isolation / no family	20 per cent

It is obvious we must shape a more positive scenario for the future. We need to blur the arbitrary distinctions we make between young, middle-aged and old, and value each stage in our lives, or at least accept them as a natural progression. The Hindus offer us a role model. They see life as a cycle in four stages: student, householder, ascetic and mendicant. The householder phase ends somewhere between 45 and 55, when grown children can supply the material needs of the household. The older Hindu is then expected to turn away from worldly affairs and devote his remaining years to wisdom and moksha, or liberation from the universe's endless cycle of birth, death and reincarnation. At this point, his status in the community is at a peak.

A DIFFERENT WORLD

Why should 60 be an age at which everything stops? Imagine a world in which workers have multistage careers, based on constant retraining - reaching 60 would simply mean a switch to another kind of work.

Here are some other changes we may expect to see in the first decades of the new century, according to experts in the UK and the USA:

- Technology that is currently geared towards the young will have to change, focusing on function rather than gimmicks.
- The home will become a centre of convenience for work, play, and education: mail order will boom.
- The rapid shift from scene to scene in television and films will have to slow down because it takes longer for ageing eyes to focus. This means that the "MTV attention span" may be extended.
- Packaging will improve, with bigger type sizes, clearer colours and more convenient wrapping.
- There will be a greater demand for value and quality. Consumer bodies will be more vocal.

In other words, it almost looks like society has to become more attuned to people's needs, which makes sense given those who will be initiating the changes. People now in their forties and fifties grew up in a world that wasn't dominated by video. The written word still had some currency. There was a stronger sense of personal and social morality.

THINGS TO COME?

The shifts that accompany progress can go in two directions, either rendering old ways obsolete or turning the elders' knowledge of tradition into an anchor for young people cast adrift by rapid change. At the moment, it would seem that the denigration of old ways has alienated young people all over the world from traditional values. Imagine, again, an alternative, where the 50-year-olds of today become the wise old men and women of the future, a generational bridge between the pre-nuclear and post-nuclear ages, a bloodline back to an age of optimism.

It's clear what we need: tolerance, respect, generosity and a healthy dollop of optimism. We have to believe positive change will come. There is a beauty in all of that. And even as we endeavour to redefine it, we come back to words written by John Keats nearly 200 years ago:

"Beauty is truth, truth beauty, - that is all
Ye know on earth, and all ye need to know."

GLOSSARY OF COSMETIC TERMS

The Body Shop makes no unrealistic claims or promises about its products. They simply cleanse, polish and protect the skin and hair. So the language we use to talk about them is equally straightforward. We want to be honest with our customers. But this glossary also includes terms used by other cosmetics companies. You'll see how creative cosmetic English can be.

ACID - any solution on the pH scale with a value between nought and seven. Skin and hair are slightly acid.

ACNE - a chronic skin disorder, common in adolescence and characterised by overactive sebaceous glands and tender red swellings or bumps just beneath the skin.

ACNEGENIC - a product may be labelled acnegenic which means it will not cause or exacerbate acne. It is however extremely unlikely that a single product would be the sole reason for acne - diet and hereditary factors are sure to have some effect.

ADHESION AID - a substance which helps a product stay on the skin. Often required in colour cosmetics.

ALKALI - a substance which has a pH greater than seven when dissolved in water. Soaps and many detergents are alkaline.

ALLERGEN - a chemical substance that can cause an allergy. Fragrances are considered to be the most common group of allergens in cosmetic ingredients. This is because fragrances contain a large number of materials and the more materials there are the greater the chance someone will be allergic to it.

ALLERGY - a condition of abnormal sensitivity to a substance in which delayed swelling, itching and inflammation can occur when even a small amount of the substance touches the skin.

ALLERGY-TESTED - all The Body Shop's cosmetic products are thoroughly tested to ensure they are safe for normal use. So-called allergy-tested products are supposed to be less likely to cause an allergic reaction because they omit a common allergen - usually the perfume. However this term is misleading since it is not possible to make completely "allergy-free" cosmetics as there is always someone who is allergic to something.

ALPHA-HYDROXY ACIDS (AHAs) - see FRUIT ACIDS

AMINO ACIDS - molecules containing amines and organic acid groups. They can link together in long chain polymers to form proteins, the basic constituents of skin and hair.

ANHYDROUS - a substance that contains no water.

ANTI-AGEING - a cosmetic product labelled anti-ageing is either misleading or it is a drug, not a cosmetic. What this term generally seeks to imply is that the product will erase wrinkles. There is no moisturiser on the market today that can stop the normal ageing process or permanently reverse the signs of ageing. An oil and water emulsion can only rehydrate the skin, temporarily plumping out fine lines and smoothing the skin. Retin-A is said to be the "anti-ageing miracle" cream but its primary function is the treatment of chronic acne and it is only available on prescription. Materials such as vitamin E can remove free radicals formed by exposure to the sun, air and pollutants which accelerate skin ageing.

ANTIHYDROTIC - a substance that reduces the amount of sweat secreted from the sweat glands. Antiperspirants contain antihydrotic ingredients.

ANTIMICROBIAL - an ingredient sometimes included in cosmetic formulations as an antiseptic or a preservative to prevent microbial growth which would spoil the product.

ANTIOXIDANT - an agent such as vitamin E that prevents oils and fats deteriorating and becoming rancid due to the effect of oxygen.

ANTIPERSPIRANT - applied to the underarms it reduces the level of perspiration and eliminates odour by counteracting the bacteria that thrive on warm, moist areas of skin. Antiperspirants are generally based on aluminium compounds, usually aluminium chlorohydrate which has an astringent effect, contracting the pores and checking the secretion of perspiration.

ANTISEPTIC - a substance which prevents the growth of bacteria either by killing the organisms or by preventing their growth.

ASTRINGENT - a skin tonic which tightens the pores and gives a refreshed feeling to the skin. Some astringent products contain volatile alcohols which evaporate rapidly and exert a cooling effect on the skin.

BACTERIA - micro organisms which often cause disease.

BACTERICIDE - a substance able to destroy or prevent the growth of bacteria.

BASAL CELLS - cells in the germinative layer of the epidermis. It is from here that new epidermal cells are constantly being generated.

BIODEGRADABLE - describes any material which can be broken down and digested by micro-organisms or by the effects of sunlight or oxygen.

BLACKHEAD see COMEDONE

BOTANICALS - plant extracts.

BUFFER - a material or materials added to keep the pH of a product constant. The buffer system will prevent the pH drifting in some products, which can cause instability.

BUTTER - fatty substance that is solid at room temperature and melts on the skin.

CARCINOGENIC - describes a substance that can cause cancer, a disease caused by rapid undifferentiated cell growth that blocks the functioning of normal healthy cells.

CARRIER OIL - an inert oil (usually vegetable or mineral) which is used to hold or dilute less stable substances such as fragrant essential oils. A carrier oil does not alter the properties of the other substance, it simply reduces its concentration.

CELL - the smallest living unit of which all organisms are composed.

CELLULITE - the name given to subcutaneous fat alleged to resist dieting. Also called orange peel skin as it resembles the "pitted" appearance of an orange. Said to consist of fat cells containing a higher concentration of toxins than ordinary fat cells.

CLEANSER - a substance, usually a detergent, which removes dirt and grease from the surface of the skin or hair.

COLLAGEN - a fibrous substance found in the dermis consisting of long-chain molecules which intertwine giving the skin support, strength, elasticity and suppleness. Collagen is sometimes incorporated in cosmetic products - it is mainly extracted from cattle hides and is a by-product of the meat industry.

COLOURANTS - colouring materials used in cosmetics and toiletries. There are three types of colourants: lakes which consist of an insoluble metallic coloured salt deposited on an inert substrate such as talc; pigments which are insoluble and frequently occur in nature among rocks and sand and soluble dyes which are used primarily to colour the cosmetic rather than the skin.

COMEDONE - commonly known as a blackhead, an "open" comedone is a pore blocked with sebum. There is some dispute over whether the black part is oxidised sebum blocking the opening of the pore or whether it is melanin from the surrounding skin. A "closed" comedone is a waxy looking white lump composed of blocked sebum but covered by a thin layer of epidermis. It is typically referred to as a whitehead.

CONDITIONER - a substance which aims to restore the healthy, oily coating of the hair that may have been stripped by colouring, perming, rough drying, excess heat or washing with a harsh shampoo. It smooths and flattens the cuticle giving the hair a soft, shiny appearance

CORTEX - the central section of hair containing the colour pigment.

CUTICLE - the hard outer layer of the hair shaft consisting of scales which should normally lay flat - if the hair is damaged, the cuticle is rough.

DANDRUFF - technically called pityriasis capitis. Dead skin flakes build up on the scalp and fall away in grey-white clumps, which usually makes the head itchy. It is generally recognised that dandruff is exacerbated by the presence of certain micro-organisms.

DENATURE - to change the nature of a substance by physical or chemical means such as the action of heat or acid. For instance ethyl alcohol can be denatured and rendered unfit for human consumption by adding a bitter nauseous substance.

DEODORANT - a substance used to mask the smell of the body's natural secretions. It may contain an antiseptic or bactericide to destroy or prevent the growth of bacteria which cause body odour. Deodorants do not reduce the level of perspiration.

DEPILATION - any method of hair removal which allows regrowth, for instance plucking, shaving or dissolving the hairs away.

DERMIS - the tough elastic layer of skin below the epidermis. Consisting of collagen and elastin, it is tough to protect the body from bumps and knocks and elastic so the skin always "fits" the body. The dermis contains sebaceous glands, sweat glands, hair follicles, the blood supply and the nerve endings which perform the skin's sensory function.

DESQUAMATION - the natural shedding of dead skin cells from the stratum corneum, the top layer of skin.

DETERGENT - usually a synthetic, organic, water-soluble cleansing agent. It has wetting and emulsifying properties enabling oil and water to mix and wash off dirt.

DISPERSANT - a liquid or gas used to disperse small particles or droplets, as in an aerosol.

DISTILLATION - the purification of liquids through evaporation followed by condensation.

ECZEMA - a chronic skin disorder characterised by red patches of itchy, flaking or blistering skin.

ELASTIN - the fibres that constitute most of the elastic tissue in the body, such as the walls of arteries and the dermis.

EMOLLIENT - a lubricating substance that softens and smooths the skin. Most emollients are oils or oil-derived compounds which can help reduce moisture loss when applied to the surface of the skin.

EMULSIFIER - an agent used to emulsify or mix oils, fats or waxes with water to give a stable dispersion. Common emulsifiers are soaps and detergents.

EMULSION - a stable mix of two liquids which are immiscible (do not usually mix) such as oil and water. One liquid is made to disperse in another by means of an emulsifying agent. Energy in the form of stirring or heating is usually required. An oil-in-water (o/w) emulsion means fine droplets of oil are suspended in a larger amount of water. Water-in-oil (w/o) emulsion is fine droplets of water dispersed in oil.

ENZYME - any of a unique class of proteins which act as catalysts in biochemical reactions. Enzymes are formed in living cells. Each enzyme initiates its own particular chemical process.

EPIDERMIS - the outer layer of skin which protects the living tissue from the ravages of the environment, e.g. sun damage, dryness, bacteria and chemicals. The outermost, "cornified" layer of the epidermis consists of dead (keratinised) skin cells which fla ke away. The underlying layers aid the replacement of the outer layers which counter wear and tear.

ESSENTIAL OIL - the volatile, odorous constituent of a plant that holds the fragrance of leaf or flower in concentrated form. Essential oils are usually obtained by steam distillation. They are used in aromatherapy.

EXFOLIANT - a grainy scrub agent designed to help clear the skin of its residual dead skin cells.

EXFOLIATION - the deliberate removal of dead skin cells from the surface of the skin.

FILLER - an inert material used to dilute active powders to the required level, e.g. pigments in colour cosmetics.

FIXATIVE - the agent that prevents the volatile ingredients in perfumes from evaporating too quickly.

FOAM BOOSTER - a material added to shampoos, shower gels and foam baths to improve and stabilise the foam

FOLLICLE - a tiny pore in the dermis of the skin from which hair grows.

FRAGRANCE - usually a mixture of natural or synthetic odorous materials formulated by a perfumer to create a desired perfume.

FRAGRANCE FREE - a cosmetic product containing no added fragrance or fragrant materials.

FRAGRANCE WARDROBE - a cosmetics industry marketing ploy which suggests that, rather than adopting the traditional approach to scent (find the one that's you and stick to it), you use a selection of fragrances to match your various moods.

FREE RADICALS - in cosmetics, these are often activated oxygen molecules which are suspected of encouraging the ageing process. When a molecule breaks up, often in response to environmental stresses, particularly overexposure to the sun, it releases highly reactive particles which appear to cause knock-on damage to healthy skin, though the process is not yet fully understood.

FRUIT ACIDS (alpha-hydroxy acids) - these are naturally occurring chemicals, derived from fruit or milk, that help peel dead skin cells from the skin's surface, thus promoting smoother, healthier skin. AHA is a buzzword at the moment in the cosmetics industry, but they are difficult to formulate effectively.

FUNGICIDE - a substance which kills, inhibits or prevents fungal growth.

GELLING AGENT - a material that can trap large amounts of water or oil in its structure and make a gel.

GERM - a micro-organism such as a bacterium or virus which causes infection and diseases.

GERMICIDE - a substance which will kill bacteria

HOLISTIC - refers to a philosophy, attitude or treatment that deals with the whole person because of the belief that it is more beneficial to take an all-encompassing overview and consider the effect of actions on an integrated system - the whole - rather than focusing on one specific area.

HUMECTANT - a substance able to attract and hold moisture. Used in cosmetic creams to prevent the cream from drying out when exposed to air. Humectants such as glycerin are used to help maintain the moisture balance in the skin and hair.

HYDROGENATION - the chemical process of adding hydrogen gas under high pressure to liquid oil. It is used to convert liquid oils to semi-solid fats at room temperature.

HYPO-ALLERGENIC - describes products that are supposed to be less likely to cause an allergic reaction because they omit known allergens - such as perfume. However this term is misleading because it is not possible to make completely "allergy-free" cosmetics - there is always someone who is allergic to something.

IRRITANT - a chemical that causes a skin reaction at the site of contact.

KERATIN - an insoluble protein contained in skin, hair and nails.

LIPIDS - substances composed of fats, waxes and oils and found in the skin.

LIPOSOME - a particle consisting of a double layer lipid membrane enclosing an aqueous compartment. Liposomes are said to be small enough to penetrate the epidermis, thus carrying moisture below the surface of the skin, but their supposed properties are surrounded by a great deal of controversy.

LUBRICANT - acts like an emollient, but usually forms more of a water-tight barrier. In cosmetics it can help reduce moisture loss from the surface of the skin.

MATT - dull, not shiny.

MEDULLA - the core running through the middle of the hair shaft.

MELANIN - colour pigment in the form of granules produced by cells called melanocytes and found in the hair and skin. Dark skins have a high concentration of strongly coloured melanin and very active melanocytes. Fair skin has only partially coloured melanin granules which become more strongly coloured when exposed to the sun.

MICRONISED - ground up into very small particles.

MICROSOME - a name given to a very small form of liposome.

MOISTURISER - a substance which reduces moisture loss from the skin, usually by forming a water-impenetrable barrier on the surface of the skin.

NON-COMEDOGENIC - describes a product that is supposed to be less likely to cause or promote the formation of open or closed comedones. However, a product is unlikely to be the sole cause of comedones.

OPACIFIER - a material added to a product to prevent light passing through it. It usually makes a product appear white.

ORGANIC - relating to, derived from or characteristic of living plants and animals.

PABA - a chemical sunscreen included in suntan lotions to protect the skin from the burning rays of the sun.

PEARLISER - an opacifier that has a pearly sheen.

pH - a scale determining whether a substance is acid or alkaline. The pH scale ranges from 0 to 14. 0 to 7 values are acid, 7 is neutral and and 7 to 14 values are alkaline. Materials at either end of the scale, i.e. about 1 to 3 and 11 to 14, will cause damage to the skin.

pH-ADJUSTER - many products are pH-adjusted by the addition of small amounts of weak acids or bases in order to balance with and be effective on the skin and hair. A toiletry product carrying the words pH-adjusted implies that others are not - this is a completely misleading term and relatively meaningless.

PHOTO-AGEING - the effect on skin cells of the ultraviolet rays of the sun. It results in fine lines, wrinkles and premature ageing.

PHOTO-SENSITIVITY - a skin condition whereby the application of certain chemicals causes an allergic reaction when the skin is exposed to sunlight.

PITYRIASIS - the medical term to describe dandruff.

PORES - the openings to the sweat gland tubes on the surface of the skin. Sweat glands secrete continuously and act as an excretory organ, excreting water, salt and other materials. They also regulate body temperature.

POROSITY - the degree to which a single hair will absorb chemical or organic applications.

PRESERVATIVE - a chemical ingredient included in cosmetic formulations of creams, lotions, etc., which prevents the growth of bacteria, yeasts and fungi in the substance.

PROTEINS - large molecules made up of amino acids which form the basis of human skin and hair.

RETIN-A - retinoic acid, a derivative of retinol (vitamin A). Developed as a treatment for acne, but said to be effective in diminishing wrinkles.

SCRUB - a formulation containing small granules in a cleansing base which is massaged onto the skin to remove, or exfoliate, the surface layer of dead skin cells.

SEBORRHOEA - a disorder of the sebaceous glands which causes an excessive secretion of sebum.

SEBUM - the waxy, oily secretion from the sebaceous glands which acts as a lubricant, giving gloss and shine to the hair and softness to the skin. It also provides some protection against bacteria.

SELF-TANNING LOTION - a product containing dihydroxyaceton (DHA) which reacts with amino acids in the uppermost layers of the skin to form a substance that is, in its chemical make up and colour, very similar to melanin, the substance that gives us a tan in the sun. This process is best compared to an apple turning brown after it has been cut in half.

SHINE - a glossy effect produced by reflected light.

SLIP AID - a material used in powder or pigment-based products to make them easier to apply to the skin.

SOLUBILISER - a material which is mixed with oils and perfumes to make them soluble in water.

SOLVENT - a liquid which is used to dissolve the active ingredients in a product. Water is a solvent.

STRATUM CORNEUM - the horny layer of dead skin cells which forms the outermost layer of the epidermis, the top layer of skin.

SUN PROTECTION FACTOR/SPF - a guide to the effectiveness of a sunscreen product. If you can stay in the sun for one hour with no sunscreen without burning, an SPF 4 sunscreen theoretically allows you to stay out four times longer, i.e. four hours. This is a very general measure and has not been regulated across the cosmetics industry. Nor does it allow for skin type or the varying intensity of the sun according to place, time of year and time of day.

SUPERFATTING - an agent added to to cleansing products such as shampoos or soaps to replace some of the natural oils lost from the skin or hair when cleansed.

SURFACTANT - a surface acting agent which lowers the surface tension between oil and water and enables them to mix. Surfactants can also act as emulsifying agents, detergents and solubilisers. A primary surfactant is the main detergent used in a product for its cleansing and foaming properties. A secondary surfactant is a detergent which is added to improve some of the properties of the primary detergent, such as mildness or foam.

TONER - a skin toner or tonic is not strictly a cleansing product but has a cooling and refreshing action on the skin. It will temporarily tighten the pores thereby reducing the secretion of perspiration and sebum.

TOP NOTE - the first impression a fragrance makes upon the sense of smell. The most volatile part of the perfume, it is one of the most important factors in the success of a perfume but it does not last beyond the first sniff.

TREATMENT - the application of a specific product to treat a specific condition.

ULTRAVIOLET - the ultra violet rays of the sun are made up of a wide ranging band of radiation consisting of UVA, UVB and UVC. Short wavelength, high energy UVC rays are filtered out mainly by the ozone layer in the atmosphere. They pose the greatest threat to plant and animal life. UVB rays cause the skin to burn, promote the production of melanin and stimulate epidermal growth which thickens the stratum corneum. Sunscreens once just filtered out UVB allowing UVA rays through to promote a tan. Now it is known that all UV light is harmful and a contributing factor to skin cancer and skin ageing.

UVA SUNSCREEN - protects the skin from the tanning and ageing rays of the sun.

UVB SUNSCREEN - protects the skin from the rays of the sun that cause sunburn.

VITAMINS - vitamins are essential, in small quantities, for the normal functioning of the body's metabolism. They cannot usually be synthesised in the body, but occur naturally in certain foods. An insufficient supply of any particular vitamin results in a deficiency disease.

INDEX

Page numbers in *italic* refer to the illustrations

We thrive on communication with our customers.
Ideally, this book will be the starting point of a whole new set of conversations.
That is why we want to hear from you with your own product tips, family remedies or anecdotes.
Look at it this way - whatever you send us may become the seed for
the *next* book The Body Shop does!

HERE ARE SOME ADDRESSES YOU MIGHT FIND USEFUL:

INTERNATIONAL HEADQUARTERS
The Body Shop
Watersmead
Littlehampton
West Sussex BN17 6LS
United Kingdom

THE BODY SHOP ANTIGUA
PO Box 1449
Heritage Quay
Antigua

THE BODY SHOP AUSTRIA
Schlossgasse 14
A-1050 Vienna
Austria

THE BODY SHOP AUSTRALIA & NEW ZEALAND
1 Jacksons Road
Mulgrave
Victoria 3170
Australia

THE BODY SHOP BAHAMAS
PO Box 4882
Nassau
Bahamas

THE BODY SHOP BAHRAIN
PO Box 32165
Bahrain

THE BODY SHOP BERMUDA
22 Reid Street
PO Box HM 2463
Hamilton HM JX
Bermuda

THE BODY SHOP BRUNEI
Lot G6A
Wisma Jaya, Jalan
Permancha
Bandar
Seri Begawan
Brunei

THE BODY SHOP CANADA
33 Kern Road
Don Mills
Ontario M3B 159
Canada

THE BODY SHOP CYPRUS
199 Ledra Street
Nicosia
Cyprus

THE BODY SHOP DENMARK
Biblioteksvej 68
DK 2650 Hvidovre
Denmark

THE BODY SHOP EAST MALAYSIA
Sabah:
Shop Lot 32, 1st Floor
Towering Industrial Centre
Mile 5
Jalan Penampang, Panampang
Koto Kinabalu
Sabah
East Malaysia

Sarawak:
The Motorship Co. Building
Lot F.1
MPL Saguking Warehouse
Jalan Patau-Patau
87000 Labuan
East Malaysia

THE BODY SHOP FINLAND
Vuorikatu 22 A 15
00150 Helsinki
Finland

THE BODY SHOP FRANCE
12 rue de Castiglione
75001 Paris
France

THE BODY SHOP GERMANY
Graf Landsberg - Str 1 H-K
41460 Neuss
Germany

THE BODY SHOP GIBRALTAR
164 Main Street
Gibraltar

THE BODY SHOP GRAND CAYMEN
PO Box 30197
Grand Caymen
British West Indies

THE BODY SHOP GREECE
Empedokleous St.57-59
Pagrati 116 33
Athens
Greece

THE BODY SHOP HOLLAND, BELGIUM & LUXEMBOURG
P O Box 483
1400 AL Bussum
Holland

THE BODY SHOP HONG KONG
21/F Shun Ho Tower
24 Ice House Street
Hong Kong

THE BODY SHOP ICELAND
Box 1742
Laugavegur 51
121 Reykjavik
Iceland

THE BODY SHOP INDONESIA
JJ Punai 111 Blok T7-9
Bintaro Village, Sektor II
Bintaro Jaya, Jakarta 15412
Indonesia

THE BODY SHOP IRELAND
82 Grafton Street
Dublin 2
Eire

THE BODY SHOP ITALY & MALTA
43 G.Borg Olivier Street
St. Julians
Malta

THE BODY SHOP JAPAN
Hongo Takeshita Building 2F, 25-14
5-Chome, Hongo, Bunkyo-ku
Tokyo 113
Japan

THE BODY SHOP KUWAIT
PO Box 181
Saafat 13002
Kuwait

THE BODY SHOP MEXICO
Domingo Diez 1589-9
Cuernavaca, Mor. CP. 622
Mexico

THE BODY SHOP NORWAY
c/o International Headquarters
The Body Shop
Watersmead, Littlehampton
West Sussex BN17 6LS
United Kingdom

NEW ZEALAND - SEE AUSTRALIA

THE BODY SHOP OMAN
PO Box 4475
Ruwi
Oman

THE BODY SHOP PORTUGAL
Rua da Reboleira 5
4000 Porto
Portugal

THE BODY SHOP QATAR
The Centre
PO Box 5316
Doha
Qatar

THE BODY SHOP SAUDI ARABIA EAST AND CENTRAL PROVINCE
PO Box16296
Riyadh 11464
Saudi Arabia

THE BODY SHOP SAUDI ARABIA WESTERN PROVINCE
PO Box 41168
Eshrawaat Street
Baghdadia
Jeddah 21521
Saudi Arabia

THE BODY SHOP SINGAPORE
391A Orchard Road
12-01 Ngee Ann City
Tower A
Singapore 0923

THE BODY SHOP SPAIN
Calle Padilla 17
6th Derch
28006 Madrid
Spain

THE BODY SHOP SWEDEN
Box 17532
11891 Stockholm
Sweden

THE BODY SHOP SWITZERLAND
Postfach 3330
8031 Zurich
Switzerland

THE BODY SHOP TAIWAN
5F-3, 150 Section 5
Min Sheng E Road
Tapei, Taiwan
R.O.C.

THE BODY SHOP THAILAND
10/F Grand Amarin Tower
1550 New Petchburi Road
Makasan,Rachtavee,
Bangkok 10310
Thailand

THE BODY SHOP UAE
PO Box 12386
Dubai
UAE

THE BODY SHOP U.S.A.
P.O. Box 1409
Wake Forest
North Carolina 27588-1409
USA

THE BODY SHOP WEST MALAYSIA
No.7, 3rd Floor
Jalan Semangat
46100 Petaling Jaya
Selangor
Malaysia

HEAD-SPINNING ❦ TAIL-WAGGING ❦ HE

CATCHING ❦ EAR-SPLITTING ❦ MO

TEETH-GRITTING ❦ NAIL-BITING ❦

BUTTOCK-CLENCHING ❦ STOMACH-CH

RAISING ❦ CHIN-WAGGING ❦ NOSE-DIV

TOE-TAPPING ❦ HAND-PICKING ❦